# Visual Attention and Cortical Circuits

# Visual Attention and Cortical Circuits

edited by Jochen Braun, Christof Koch, and Joel L. Davis

A Bradford Book
The MIT Press
Cambridge, Massachusetts
London, England

This book was set in Times Roman by Achorn Graphic Services, Inc., on the Miles 33 System.

Printed and bound in the United States of America.

Library of Congress Cataloging-in-Publication Data

Visual attention and cortical circuits / edited by Jochen Braun, Christof Koch, and Joel L. Davis.
     p. ; cm.
   ''A Bradford book.''
   Includes bibliographical references and index.
   ISBN 0-262-02493-4 (hc : alk. paper)
   1. Visual cortex. 2. Attention.   I. Braun, Jochen.   II. Koch, Christof.   III. Davis, Joel L.,
1942–
   [DNLM: 1. Visual Cortex—physiology. 2. Visual Perception—physiology. WL 307
V834 2000]
QP383.V58 2000
152.14—dc21

                                                                    00-039447

Dedicated to the memory of Helen T. Davis

# Contents

# Preface

This volume presents the results of a small workshop, "Visual Attention and Cortical Circuits," held in early 1999 at Two Harbors, Catalina Island, some twenty miles offshore from Los Angeles. The aim of the workshop was to enlarge the common ground between the psychology, neurobiology, and theory of selective visual attention in the mammalian visual system, and to place key findings into a shared framework. The cover picture of this volume (*Red Bridges,* by Aristarch Lentulov) was chosen because it expresses the optimism and hope associated with sturdy bridges (e.g., between disciplines). We felt that this aim could be best achieved by a small and intensive workshop, in parallel with the publication of a book. Although the participants did not represent a full cross section of current attention research, they did share an affinity for interdisciplinary approaches to attention. Piecing together the contributions of psychophysics, biology, and computational theory on the subject of attention remains, at least for now, an untidy affair with much room for argument.

The book focuses mainly but not exclusively on the effects of visual attention in the ventral and dorsal streams of visual cortex in humans and monkeys, and the associated changes in visual performance. As a result, there is a fair amount of overlap between chapters. Naturally, each chapter exemplifies the approach of one particular group, but the book as a whole also makes several larger points. A brief overview chapter summarizes the main findings of the fourteen substantive chapters, and also attempts to formulate some of the larger points that emerge.

The book is aimed at researchers and advanced students from a variety of fields, including but not limited to neurology, neurobiology, psychology, cognitive science, and computer vision. The presentation is as simple and clear as possible, and the contributors have made a significant effort to make the material accessible and to provide illustrations of the highest quality. Our aim as editors was to ensure that all chapters presuppose a similar degree of expertise, so that they can be readily compared. In view of the range of disciplines represented, and the different conventions observed by each, this was not always easy.

The workshop was funded by the Office of Naval Research and by the National Science Foundation-supported Center for Neuromorphic Systems Engineering at the California Institute of Technology. We are extremely grateful for their support. We also thank Geraint Rees for his most helpful comments on the overview chapter. Special thanks are due to Jacklin Ferris of Banning House Lodge, who made us want to stay much longer. Finally, we appreciated the friendly welcome by the people of Two Harbors, and the spooky persistence of the resident pair of ravens (*Corvus corax*) trying to join our morning sessions.

Jochen Braun and Christof Koch
California Institute of Technology

Joel Davis
Office of Naval Research

# Overview

**Jochen Braun and Christof Koch**

In everyday language, "attention" describes our willful ability to be aware of one thing at one moment, and another thing at the next. Introspectively, attention contributes to our mental dynamic and explains, for example, why the contents of our consciousness shift even when the world stays the same. Psychological research has refined these introspective notions about attention and has created sophisticated conceptual tools for building a comprehensive theory of attention. In neurobiology, attention is recognized as one of the factors that contribute to neural responses and that relate to the task rather than to the stimulus (extraretinal factor). In a typical experiment, the retinal stimulus is held constant while attention is directed to one stimulus or the other by cueing or by changing the task that has to be performed. If the neural response changes as a result of such manipulations, attention is presumed to be involved.

It seems evident to us that the psychology and neurobiology of attention have much to learn from one another. To help along the convergence of the two fields, the present volume tries to enlarge the mutual vocabulary, to highlight work drawing on both sides, and to juxtapose corresponding results from each side. The strength of psychology lies in the immense breadth of its empirical base, and its consequent ability to reach valid generalizations about attention. Neurobiology contributes additional information about neural architecture and function, which is not available through psychological means. In our eyes, the goal must be a comprehensive theory that accounts simultaneously for psychological and neurobiological results on attention.

The goal of linking neural activity to psychophysical performance and, eventually, to phenomenal experience is, of course, not limited to the attention field, but is shared by vision research in general. On the road to this goal, attention offers a means for controlling neural activity and phenomenal experience that is orthogonal to manipulations of the stimulus. This evidently constitutes a splendid opportunity for trying to relate the two domains. Thus, although the study of attention is clearly worthy in and of itself, it also enlarges our arsenal of tools for linking perception to the neural substrate. Many contributions to the present volume place particular emphasis on this potential for linkage.

The following remarks emphasize what we take to be the highlights of the book and are meant to make the contents more accessible. We organize our remarks around the several larger points that emerge from the book as a whole, and describe how various chapters add to each point. Most chapters contribute to more than one such point.

## "Attention" May Involve More Than One Neural System

To carry out its overall function of adapting perception to changing behavioral goals, it is likely that attention will have to integrate several subfunctions. One subfunction may be to assemble advance information about which parts or aspects of the sensory environment are likely to become relevant in the near future (guidance). Another subfunction may be to modulate sensory processing accordingly, that is, to selectively enhance the currently relevant information (execution). Yet another subfunction of attention may be to trigger a particular behavioral response as soon as a relevant stimulus appears (decision). The extent to which different subfunctions involve distinct neural systems remains one of the major open issues. Several chapters consider attention at this global level and discuss possible neural correlates of attentional guidance, execution, and decision.

Chapter 1 (Corbetta and Shulman) draws a distinction between *expectation signals* (advance information about future visual events) and *attentional modulations* (altered responses to current visual events). To isolate expectation signals, the authors rely on the differential time course of expectation signals as revealed by event-related fMRI. The results show expectation signals in *intraparietal* areas, *inferior temporal* areas, and motion-sensitive *occipital* areas, but not in prefrontal areas. Chapter 4 (Duncan) considers the role of *prefrontal* areas in attentional planning and control. The author synthesizes the results of several neuroimaging studies and concludes that prefrontal regions contribute not only to attentional control but also to a wide range of other cognitive problems and demands. In other words, the prefrontal regions in question seem to serve more general functions, which at times may include attentional control. Chapter 8 (Thompson, Bichot, and Schall) reports further fascinating information about the *frontal eye fields* of monkeys. Once a monkey has learned the relevance of particular stimulus attributes, some frontal eye field neurons respond more strongly to stimuli with these attributes but not others, suggesting that frontal eye field responses may code directly for task relevance. In addition, when perceptual information is marginal or ambiguous, some frontal eye field responses seem to reflect the behavioral report of the monkey rather than the physical stimulus. This raises the possibility that frontal eye fields contribute to both guidance and decision functions of attention. Chapter 12 (Shimojo, Watanabe, and Scheier) focuses on an ambiguous visual percept that is disambiguated by auditory stimuli. This rare instance of auditory dominance over vision turns out to hinge on a modulation of cross-modal attention. The effect is sufficiently dramatic to be used in studying the development of attentional function in human infants.

## Attention Modulates Early, Intermediate, and Late Stages of Visual Processing

It seems likely that attention will ultimately turn out to involve many parts of the brain, from the lateral geniculate nucleus to visual cortex and temporal, parietal, and frontal cortices, as well as their associated thalamic nuclei. In particular, attention modulates most, and perhaps all, visually responsive areas of cortex, including area V1. Chapter 1

(Corbetta and Shulman) includes an overview of functional imaging studies demonstrating the effect of attention on early stages (area V1), intermediate stages (areas V2, V4, MT), and late stages (inferotemporal and parietal areas) of visual processing. Chapter 2 (Heeger, Gandhi, Huk, and Boynton) uses fMRI to demonstrate attentional modulations in area V1. Moving stimuli are presented in both visual hemifields, and observers are asked to discriminate the speed in either one or the other. As attention shifts back and forth between the two hemifields, the fMRI signal changes substantially (20 to 30%). In the macaque monkey, chapter 5 (Ito, Westheimer, and Gilbert) reports large attentional effects on the response of individual neurons in area V1. Chapters 6 (Maunsell and McAdams) and 7 (Reynolds and Desimone) provide representative examples for the effect of attention on neurons in areas V2 and V4, and chapter 8 (Thompson, Bichot, and Schall) demonstrates attention effects in area FEF.

For the most part, psychological approaches to attention have not had enough time to accommodate these findings. However, the fact that attention acts at multiple levels will lead to behavioral implications. Chapter 11 (Braun, Koch, Lee, and Itti) reports that attention alters visual perception in several different ways, and proposes that this multiplicity may reflect attentional effects at different cortical levels.

## Attention Is Constrained by Cortical Interactions

Attention appears to modulate visual cortical responses by modulating local cortical interactions (i.e., interactions within a given area). This explains why attention tends to have its largest effects when the stimulus configuration gives rise to strong interactions between stimulus components. Furthermore, cortical interactions seem to severely constrain the effect attention can have. Once attention is focused on a given location in the visual field, its effect on neural responses (increase, decrease, or neither) seems to be determined largely by the stimulus (i.e., bottom-up) rather than by the behavioral task (i.e., top-down). The reasons for this surprising restriction are unclear; perhaps it is a safeguard to prevent top-down signals (''imagination'') from overwhelming sensory information and giving rise to hallucinations.

Chapter 5 (Ito, Westheimer, and Gilbert) investigates the facilitatory effects of stimuli well outside the receptive field on neurons in primary visual cortex (contextual facilitation). As it turns out, attention seems to modulate this contextual facilitation, producing substantial increases or decreases in the response. However, the effect of attention is observed only in the presence of contextual stimuli. This may explain why numerous earlier studies failed to find large attention effects in area V1. Chapter 7 (Reynolds and Desimone) takes a slightly different tack and considers the response of neurons in areas V2 and V4 to *two* stimuli in the receptive field. When one stimulus is attended and the other ignored, the effect of attention may be excitatory, inhibitory, or neutral, depending on the stimuli in question. In general, attention shifts the response toward the level obtained with the attended stimulus alone, thus eliminating the influence of the ignored stimulus. Chapter 6 (Maunsell and McAdams) agrees that attention effects are larger with multiple stimuli in the receptive field, but proposes that attention alters neural responses directly (multiplicative scaling) rather than indirectly by modulating interactions. In spite of this fundamental difference, the models offered by chapters 6 and 7 are remarkably similar.

The notion that attention modulates, and is constrained by, bottom-up processing is also consistent with certain perceptual effects of attention. Chapter 11 (Braun, Koch, Lee, and Itti) probes bottom-up interactions (divisive inhibition) by measuring psychophysical thresholds for simple patterns. The results suggest that attention intensifies the competitive interactions in question. Surprisingly, there is no evidence for task dependence in the effect of attention, even though the measurements include five different visual tasks that could certainly have benefited from task-specific modulations.

## A "Saliency Map" Remains Central to Thinking About Attention

The notion of a saliency map dates back to the late 1970s and early 1980s, and was intended to synthesize psychophysical results of Bela Julesz and Ann Treisman (e.g., Julesz, 1990; Treisman, 1993) with newly gained insights into the functional anatomy of visual cortex (e.g., Felleman and Van Essen, 1991). As formalized by Koch and Ullman (1985), a saliency map is a topographic representation of visual space which combines and summarizes information from the several distinct cortical areas that process elementary visual features such as shape, color, and motion (feature maps). Its activity distribution is thought to guide both overt and covert orienting responses (i.e., both eye movements and shifts of attention). One of the many attractions of the saliency map architecture is that it accommodates both bottom-up and top-down flows of information (e.g., Itti and Koch, 2000).

Chapter 8 (Thompson, Bichot, and Schall) demonstrates several of the presumed functionalities of a saliency map in the *frontal eye fields*. Visually responsive neurons in the frontal eye fields index the global salience of a stimulus in a given context (i.e., whether it is the only one of its kind or whether there are other stimuli like it elsewhere). After a period of training on a visual task, such neurons also signal the relevance of a given stimulus in the context of the current task. Thus, it appears that both bottom-up and top-down salience are reflected in the frontal eye fields. Chapter 10 (Sperling, Reeves, Blaser, Lu, and Weichselgartner) elaborates the saliency map idea into a model that accounts quantitatively for a wealth of psychophysical data. In many of these data, apparent motion is used as a sensitive assay for attentional input to figure-ground segmentation. Saliency is viewed as a real-valued variable determining ''figureness'' and controlling access to recognition processes. Interestingly, attention is found to change saliency/figureness without altering the phenomenal appearance of stimuli, suggesting that there may be separate pathways for saliency and feature information.

Chapter 14 (Tsotsos, Culhane, and Cutzu) presents a computational model of visual cortex in which the saliency map and feature maps form part of a single hierarchical architecture. Saliency and feature information are represented by separate units, and each level of the hierarchy determines saliency through a winner-take-all process. Consistent with chapters 8 and 10, saliency can be influenced both bottom-up and top-down (i.e., both by the stimulus and by the task). A strong prediction of the model in chapter 14 is that attentional latencies should *decrease* from lower to higher visual areas, in sharp contrast to stimulus latencies, which *increase* in this order. Perhaps the most appealing aspect of this model is the economical way in which it combines the functions of guiding attention and modulating sensory information.

## Comparing the Results of Different Methods Can Be Tricky

Ideally, the results of behavioral measurements, functional imaging, and single-unit recording would paint a coherent picture of attentional function. One obstacle to attaining this happy state of affairs is the near impossibility of measuring the same variable with different methods. Chapter 1 (Corbetta and Shulman) discusses some of the discrepancies one encounters while assessing neural populations of different size (i.e., by single-unit recording, measuring evoked potentials on the scalp, or functional brain imaging based on hemodynamics). Chapter 13 (Pouget, Deneve, and Latham) highlights some of the difficulties of relating brain activity to behavioral performance. Behavioral performance is limited by the *total information* contained in the response of a neural population, which in turn depends on both the size of the responses and the degree to which they are correlated. Any method that considers only response size, without taking into account response correlations among neighboring neurons, cannot provide a definitive measurement of information content. Indeed, it has been shown (Steinmetz et al., 2000) that attention acts not only on the former but also on the latter; that is, attention changes, and usually increases, the nature of the correlation among neurons, thereby changing the stimulus information available to postsynaptic structures (Niebur and Koch, 1994).

Luckily, matters are not hopeless. Chapter 2 (Heeger, Gandhi, Huk, and Boynton) quantitatively relates functional imaging data to behavioral performance. To obtain this match, it is necessary to make certain assumptions about neural response properties, including absence of response correlations. Similarly, chapter 3 (Lavie) establishes at least a qualitative correspondence between functional imaging and behavioral measurements. Chapter

5 (Ito, Westheimer, and Gilbert) compares psychophysical measurements and single-unit recordings from the same animals. The contextual facilitation observed psychophysically is strengthened by attention in one animal and weakened in another animal (presumably due to different training regimes). Gratifyingly, single-unit recordings in area V1 produce consistent results (i.e., stronger facilitation in the first animal and weaker facilitation in the second). Such a remarkable agreement between different methods remains all too rare. Chapter 9 (Motter and Holsapple) introduces a highly efficient technique for measuring the spatial distribution of attention in a situation that is potentially suited for single-unit recordings. The technique infers the probability of target detection as a function of distance from the current focus of attention, on the basis of eye movement recordings during a visual search task. These data may be the most detailed measurement of attention in monkeys to date, and promise significant new insights once they are correlated with simultaneous single-unit recordings.

## The Processing of Unattended Stimuli Remains a Contentious Issue

One of the longest-running debates about attention concerns the processing of unattended stimuli. According to proponents of late selection, even unattended stimuli are subject to perceptual processing, because attention affects primarily postperceptual processes such as memory and responses. The early selection view is, however, that attention also affects perceptual processes, implying that the perceptual processing of unattended stimuli can be prevented.

Chapter 3 (Lavie) proposes to resolve this debate with the help of a *perceptual load* model. According to the model, unattended stimuli are processed only to the extent that there is spare attentional capacity, in other words, only to the extent that attention is not already fully engaged. Thus, if the demands on attention are slight, one may obtain results consistent with late selection (i.e., processing of unattended stimuli), whereas if demands on attention are heavy, one obtains the outcome predicted by early selection (i.e., no processing of unattended stimuli). Chapter 11 (Braun, Koch, Lee, and Itti) also reports both types of results, consistent with either early or late selection. However, here a distinction is made between different types of perceptual processing. Although much processing seems to depend on attention (early selection), simple attributes of salient stimuli seem to be processed independently of attention (late selection). Interestingly, the extent to which unattended stimuli are processed seems closely related to the computation of saliency. Namely, the processing of unattended stimuli seems to encompass only salient stimuli, and only features that enter into the computation of saliency. Chapter 14 (Tsotsos, Culhane, and Cutzu) makes detailed predictions about the processing of unattended stimuli, and also marshals some psychophysical evidence in support. The prediction is that the processing of unattended stimuli depends on their distance to the focus of attention: processing is suppressed in the immediate vicinity of, but permitted at greater remove from, the attentional focus.

## Theories of Attention Are at Last Becoming Neurally Plausible

As attention becomes the subject of more and more neurobiological studies, the theorizing about attention will inevitably break away from established psychological molds. In particular, the need to accommodate neurobiological data will probably erode the usefulness of abstractions such as ''early/late selection,'' ''capacity allocation,'' and ''processing bottleneck.'' These notions are clearly too coarse to account for detailed observations such as, for example, those in chapter 5 (Ito, Westheimer, and Gilbert). On the other hand, the pendulum should not swing too far. At the moment, only psychological theories exhibit the requisite universality, and rather than dismissing psychological concepts as outmoded, it will be necessary to ground them in the neural substrate.

An example illustrates the envisaged shift in theoretical thinking. A recent book (Pashler, 1998) concludes that visual attention may be conceptualized either as an ''exclusionary process'' or as an ''allocation of resources.'' In both cases, attention limits the number of stimuli that can be processed in parallel to N. The difference is that an exclusionary process would ensure that N stimuli (i.e., the maximal number) are processed at all times, whereas a resource allocation would allow fewer than N stimuli to be processed, as long as this is consistent with task demands. When translated into a neural context, ways of reconciling the two notions become apparent. Assume that a hierarchical winner-take-all operation computes saliency, thereby determining which stimuli are ''figure'' and gain access to recognition processes (chapters 10 and 14). Since the number of salient stimuli depends on the stimulus configuration, rather than on task demands, this qualifies as an exclusionary process. Assume further that attention biases the saliency computation in favor of certain stimuli or locations (chapters 6, 7, 10, and 14). Since attention is free to select any set of locations, this is a resource allocation, even though not every selection will be equally effective (i.e., some will alter the saliency computation and others will not). Thus, the neural implementation of attention may involve both exclusionary processes and resource allocations, and it may be pointless to try to decide between the two.

Various chapters in the present volume offer theories or models of attention. There are cognitive theories with qualitative predictions (chapter 3) and computational theories that account quantitatively for particular observations (chapters 6, 7, first theory in chapter 10). Both types mirror the structure of the data they are meant to explain. Another type of theory seeks to build upon a general knowledge of visual function and cortical circuits, which a priori has nothing to do with attention (second theory in chapter 10, chapters 11 and 13). In its most developed form, such a structural theory makes predictions at multiple levels, many of them unforeseen and counterintuitive (chapter 14). Although all types of theories have their place, we feel that today the most promising approaches are those which combine the comprehensiveness of psychological theories with a general understanding of neural architecture and cortical circuits.

In conclusion, a comprehensive understanding of attention must take account of both psychological and neurobiological observations. Some correspondences between the two fields may be obvious, others less so. For example, the limited capacity of attention may be intimately related to the competition for saliency in visual cortex. In fact, it seems quite possible that saliency *is* the limited capacity, in the sense that competitive interactions in cortex constrain the number of stimuli that can be salient, and thus be processed, in parallel. Thus, the effort of translating and correlating the respective vocabularies of different disciplines seems well worthwhile. We hope that this volume will improve the mutual comprehension of all those working on attention.

## References

Felleman, D. J., and Van Essen, D. C. (1991). Distributed hierarchical processing in the cerebral cortex. *Cereb. Cortex* 1: 1–47.

Itti, L., and Koch, C. (2000). A saliency-based search mechanism for overt and covert shifts of attention. *Vis. Res.* 40: 1489–1506.

Julesz, B. (1990). Early vision and focal attention. *Rev. Mod. Phys.* 63: 735–772.

Koch, C., and Ullman, S. (1985). Shifts in selective visual attention: Towards the underlying neural circuitry. *Hum. Neurobiol.* 4: 219–227.

Niebur, E., and Koch, C. (1994). A model for the neuronal implementation of selective visual attention based on temporal correlation among neurons. *J. Comp. Neurosci.* 1: 141–158.

Pashler, H. (1998). *The Psychology of Attention.* Cambridge: MIT Press.

Steinmetz, P. N., Roy, A., Fitzgerald, P. J., Hsiao, S. S., Johnson, K. O., and Niebur, E. (2000). Attention modulates synchronized neuronal firing in primate somatosensory cortex. *Nature* 404: 187–190.

Treisman, A. (1993). The perception of features and objects. In A. Baddeley and L. Weiskrantz (eds.), *Attention: Selection, awareness, and control* (pp. 1–35). Oxford: Oxford University Press/Clarendon Press.

# Visual Attention and Cortical Circuits

# 1 Imaging Expectations and Attentional Modulations in the Human Brain

**Maurizio Corbetta and Gordon L. Shulman**

## 1.1 Introduction

Neurobiological research since 1980 has clearly established that visual perception does not depend solely on the neural activity evoked by individual objects, but is also powerfully influenced by contextual sensory information and the behavioral states of the observer. For example, the activity of individual neurons in visual cortex (including area V1) does not depend only on the attributes of the object in the classical receptive field (luminance, contrast, color, orientation, and so on). Rather, the context created by other objects inside or outside the neurons' receptive field (Knierim and Van Essen, 1992; Gilbert, 1996; Ito et al., 1998; Ito et al., this volume; Reynolds and Desimone, this volume) and the level of arousal and interest of the observer are important as well (Wurtz et al., 1980; Motter, 1993). Some of the sensory interactions mediating this context dependence become ingrained during the development of visual cortex, hardwired by the selective pressure of the visual environment over years. Other interactions reflect the ability of visual cortex to learn new visual patterns and configurations over a time scale of minutes or hours (perceptual learning; e.g., Karni et al., 1995; Ito et al., chapter 5 in this volume). In contrast, changes in the behavioral state of the observer can alter the response of visual neurons on the more rapid time scale of milliseconds to seconds. For instance, variations in the level of vigilance occur throughout the day and produce tonic and rather nonselective changes in the level of visual activity (Wurtz et al., 1980; Mountcastle et al., 1987). Cognitive signals such as behavioral goals, expectations, memories, or thoughts, however, produce briefer and more selective modulations of visual activity (for reviews, see Desimone and Duncan, 1995; Maunsell, 1995). This ongoing modulation of visual perception is necessarily selective because at any one time many visual objects compete for awareness, and because multiple cognitive signals can potentially bias perception.

This review focuses on the psychological and neural mechanisms underlying the use of advance visual information, such as knowledge about the color, motion, or location of a target object, for its detection or discrimination in a visual scene. This is a common situation, as when we search for a face or a colored hat in a crowd of people, or when we guess the trajectory of a tennis ball coming our way. In the laboratory this behavior is studied by providing the observer (human or animal) with a cue that carries advance information about some task-relevant target object, and by testing the accuracy or speed of target detection/discrimination in a subsequently presented test display. It is well established that the cue helps the detection/discrimination of relevant objects, and impairs the detection/discrimination of irrelevant objects (Eriksen and Hoffman, 1972; Posner, 1980; Hawkins et al., 1990; Sperling et al., chapter 10 in this volume). Little is known about how the brain organizes this complex behavior. Where in the brain are cognitive expectations or goals about visual objects or features coded? What is the format of these signals, and how/where in the visual system do they interact with incoming sensory information? What is the effect of such interaction on visual processing, and hence on visual perception?

In the first part of this chapter, we discuss some of the advantages and disadvantages of functional neuroimaging as compared with other neurophysiological methods for measuring neuronal activity during visual tasks. Second, we review some psychological theories as to how cued information influences visual processing. Then, we discuss experiments that demonstrate the effects of focused attention on visual processing. Finally, we present a new functional imaging experiment employing event-related fMRI to dissociate the encoding and maintenance of cue information from its subsequent effect on visual analysis (processing?). Whenever possible, the imaging results will be discussed in relationship to current psychological and neurophysiological findings/ideas on visual selection.

## 1.2   Tracking Neural Activity during Visual Attention

Tremendous progress has been made in our ability to monitor brain activity at different spatial and temporal resolutions (for reviews, see Wurtz et al., 1984; Hillyard and Picton, 1987; Raichle, 1994). Single-unit recordings in awake, behaving primates, scalp recordings of evoked electrical activity, and imaging of local changes in brain hemodynamics (blood flow or deoxygenation) in human subjects are the main methods used to record activity of the brain during cognitive tasks. Each method provides a view of the brain in action that is biased toward a particular spatiotemporal resolution. Single-unit recordings offer excellent spatial (microns) and temporal (milliseconds) resolution within a cortical region in the monkey, but typically sample only a small fraction of the neurons (cortical areas) involved in a task. Evoked potentials have an excellent temporal resolution, but are biased toward neural activity coming from the surface and have a poor spatial resolution (several centimeters). Finally, functional imaging surveys the whole brain (both cortical and subcortical regions) simultaneously with a spatial resolution of a few millimeters, but with a temporal resolution that is coarser (several seconds) than real-time neural activity. An additional problem with imaging is that the local hemodynamic signals which are recorded represent only an indirect measure of neural activity, and the details of the coupling between blood vessels and neurons are presently unknown. There is good evidence, however, that hemodynamic signals precisely colocalize (within hundreds of microns) with neuronal activity recorded by single units in monkey's visual cortex (Ts'o et al., 1990). Furthermore, hemodynamic signals vary linearly within certain parameter ranges with several psychophysical visual functions (e.g., contrast sensitivity; Boynton,

1996) and cognitive variables (e.g., load during working memory tasks; Nystrom et al., 1998).

More direct information about the coupling of neuronal activity and hemodynamics will become available once fMRI for monkeys is more fully developed (Stefanacci et al., 1998; Logothetis et al., 1999). An important recent development in human fMRI is the capability to record focal changes in blood oxygenation caused by single sensory, cognitive, or motor events (event-related fMRI; Zarahn et al., 1997; Dale and Buckner, 1997; Friston et al., 1998; Rosen et al., 1998). This constitutes a significant improvement over earlier PET or fMRI designs in which activity had to be recorded, averaged, and displayed over many trials (blocked design). Event-related fMRI allows the randomized presentation and analysis of separate trial types. Recently, our laboratory has further extended this approach to the analysis of different events within a trial (Ollinger et al., 1998). For example, regions of activation related to the presentation of a cue can be now differentiated from regions related to the presentation of a test stimulus or a motor response (Shulman et al., 1999). This method is very helpful for tracking the slow temporal evolution of the hemodynamic signals.

## 1.3 Psychological Theories about the Selection of Simple Visual Features

Psychological studies have characterized the experimental conditions under which advance information about simple visual attributes facilitates the perception of relevant stimuli, and impairs the perception of irrelevant stimuli (Pashler, 1998). Highly discriminable cues such as location, color, and size are very effective in facilitating perception of subsequently presented stimuli. The facilitation is greatest when the discrimination is difficult or in the presence of irrelevant stimuli. Under optimal selection conditions there is little evidence of processing of irrelevant stimuli (but see Braun et al., chapter 11 in this volume). These findings are consistent with the notion that cue information interacts with processes involved in the sensory and/or decisional analysis of both relevant and irrelevant stimuli, and that this interaction relatively facilitates the processing of relevant stimuli. It is currently debated whether an object can be selected directly on the basis of information about its intrinsic features such as color, size, or direction of motion, independently of its location, or whether location analysis is indispensable for object selection (Moore and Egeth, 1998; Shih and Sperling, 1996).

Pashler (1998) reviews two general accounts of the effects of cues on the analysis of incoming sensory information. On one account, advance information enhances the sensory processing of the signal (signal enhancement mechanism). On the other account, advance information allows observers to disregard channels containing noise, that is, information that could degrade a perceptual decision if allowed to influence the decision. The ability to disregard information from irrelevant channels can improve perception for merely statistical reasons by minimizing the chance of a false alarm, that is, erroneous detection based on noise information. Noise suppression might be implemented through a variety of mechanisms: raising the threshold for decision and/or suppressing sensory information in the irrelevant channel. A related issue, which has driven much of the psychological research on attention since 1960, is at what level of processing selection mechanisms operate (Deutsch and Deutsch, 1963; Duncan, 1980; Broadbent, 1982; Treisman, 1969). Selection mechanisms (both signal enhancement and noise suppression) might work at early (anatomically and temporally) or late stages of visual processing, that is, respectively influence sensory and/or decisional stages of analysis.

Can we use these ideas to generate predictions about patterns of neural activation related to the encoding, maintenance, and use of visual expectations, and their influence on sensory/decisional visual processes? In terms of imaging research, a straightforward prediction about putative mechanisms of visual selection is that the site of neural modulation should differ, depending on the underlying mechanism. In particular, a mechanism that enhances signal should involve predominantly task-relevant pathways, whereas a mechanism that suppresses noise should at least partly involve irrelevant pathways. For example, if a subject is required to attend to discriminate a feature of a stimulus (e.g., its speed) while ignoring other features (e.g., its color or shape), most of the signal should be present in motion-sensitive regions, whereas most of the noise should come from color- and shape-sensitive regions. Modulations in motion-sensitive areas would support signal enhancement accounts; modulations in color- and shape-sensitive areas would favor noise suppression accounts (figure 1.1). Similarly, if a subject is required to attend to a location in the visual field and to discriminate the orientation of stimuli presented at attended or unattended locations, modulations at either attended or unattended parts of retinotopically organized cortical areas would support, respectively, signal enhancement or noise suppression accounts. Finally, modulations that occur early in the visual system (e.g., area V1) are unlikely to alter decisional stages of analysis. In this case it is important to show that modulations occurring anatomically early in the visual system do not reflect temporally late feedback signals from postperceptual levels.

An important caveat in considering a neural implementation of psychological mechanisms is that the visual system comprises more than thirty visual cortical areas that are hierarchically organized and reciprocally linked by several hundred connections (for a review, see Van Essen and DeYoe, 1995). Hence, psychological distinctions (and models) about information-processing stages—such as input, sensory analysis, stimulus identification, and decision—must take into account the great complexity of the underlying neural implementation. In the brain, different stages of processing are likely to overlap across multiple areas; decisions may be generated at different levels, depending on task demands;

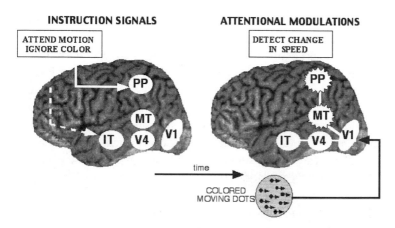

**Figure 1.1**
Expectation signals and attentional modulations. Expectation signals are neural signals that encode/maintain visual expectations about a visual attribute (perceptual set) (*left*). PP, posterior parietal cortex; MT, middle temporal cortex; V4, area V4; IT, inferior temporal cortex; V1, area V1. The preactivation by expectations of relevant pathways (solid line to PP) is consistent with capacity allocation (signal enhancement) mechanisms; the preactivation of irrelevant pathways (broken line to *IT*) is consistent with noise suppression mechanisms. Expectation signals interact with incoming visual information and produce attentional modulations. The neuroimaging evidence during attention to stimulus features suggests modulation of task-relevant pathways (e.g., MT and PP).

and the flow of information is likely to be bidirectional from lower to higher levels, and vice versa. Moreover, attentional effects on perception and behavior may well reflect modulations at multiple cortical levels from sensory to motor centers.

## 1.4   Expectation Signals and Attentional Modulations

Focusing attention on simple visual features not only facilitates the perception of relevant stimuli in a visual scene, but also powerfully modulates the neural activity in visual cortex evoked by those stimuli. Logically, it seems important to separate processes (or neural signals) relating to the establishment and maintenance of visual expectations established by a cue (which we call *expectation signals;* ''template signals'' in Desimone and Duncan, 1995), on the one hand, from processes/signals reflecting selective modulation of sensory activity evoked by a test stimulus (which we call *attentional modulations*), on the other hand. These two kinds of signals presumably have different time courses, since expectation signals must precede attentional modulations. They may also have different spatial distributions within the brain. For example, whereas attentional modulations may emphasize visual areas involved in the analysis of the test stimulus, expectation signals may involve both nonvisual areas, necessary for their encoding and maintenance in time, and visual areas, which receive (and possibly maintain) them (figure 1.1).

Finally, a crucial aspect of human cognition is that similar behavioral goals and expectations can be generated from information that occurs in widely different formats. For instance, the search for a red car in a parking lot might be initiated verbally (e.g., a friend's comment, ''My car is the red one''), by information stored in long-term memory (e.g., I know that my car is red), or by recently presented sensory information (e.g., ''Where is the red car we saw enter the parking lot?''). In all these cases, an expectation is established that guides the search for the red car. Hence, similar expectation signals may be expected for cues presented in different sensory modalities (e.g., vision, audition) or formats (e.g., iconic, symbolic, linguistic).

Although many studies have demonstrated the existence of attentional modulations in both monkey and human visual cortex (for reviews of primate studies, see Desimone and Duncan, 1995; Maunsell, 1995; and Motter, 1993, 1994a, 1994b; for human studies, see Hillyard and Picton, 1987; Corbetta et al., 1991; Dupont et al., 1993; Haxby et al., 1994; Mangun et al., 1993; Beauchamp et al., 1997; Buckner et al., 1997; Tootell et al., 1998; Wojciulik et al., 1998; Martinez et al., 1999; Shulman et al., 1999; Gandhi et al., 1999), little is known about how cognitive expectations and goals are encoded and maintained in the brain. Below, we first review what has been learned through neuroimaging about attentional modulations in the visual system, and then consider a new experiment aimed at isolating expectation signals.

### 1.4.1   Attentional Modulations

Imaging studies since 1990 have clearly demonstrated several general rules about attentional modulations in the visual system.

First, directing attention to simple visual features such as color, motion, shape, and location, or more complex objects such as faces, words, or buildings, modulates activity in task-relevant pathways, that is, in visual areas specialized for processing the selected visual attribute or object. For example, in our original positron emission tomography (PET) study (Corbetta et al., 1990, 1991) subjects performed a match-to-sample task on a random display of colored moving bars. In different scans, subjects either attended to/discriminated a particular kind of change of the stimuli (selective attention to either color, motion, or shape), or attended to/discriminated any kind of change (divided attention between color, motion, and shape), or simply detected stimulus onset (passive viewing). Discrimination thresholds were lower with selective than with divided attention, confirming that selective attention enhances perception. PET measurements demonstrated higher activity in the visual system during selective attention as compared with passive viewing or divided attention. In other words, activity was higher when attentional resources were concentrated on one particular pathway than when they were presumably spread across multiple pathways. For example, during motion discrimination, activity was enhanced in extrastriate visual areas known to be sensitive to visual motion (namely, in a collection of areas called MT+ that includes area MT/V5).

The selective modulation of task-relevant pathways while focusing attention on a particular stimulus feature has been confirmed by other studies. O'Craven et al. (1995) found a 27% increase in blood oxygenation level-dependent (BOLD) signal in area MT+ when subjects attended in the same display to moving versus static random dots. Beauchamp and colleagues (1997) found that the BOLD signal dropped by 56% in MT+ and the intraparietal region (another motion-sensitive region) when subjects diverted attention from stimulus speed to stimulus color in a colored random dot display. The signal fell by 150% when subjects diverted attention from the random dot display to a small central fixation point in order to detect changes in its luminance. This study therefore indicates that activity in the same visual area can be modulated by attending to the task-relevant feature and/or location, and that the two effects may be additive.

In addition, many other studies have found an effect of cueing location alone (Corbetta et al., 1993; Vandenberghe et al., 1996, 1997; Woldorff et al., 1997; Tootell et al., 1998; Brefczynski and DeYoe 1999). Directing attention to the location of flashed stimuli to be detected/discriminated modulates activity in visual areas that code for stimuli at the attended location. Finally, other studies have found modulations in task-relevant pathways by directing attention to more complex stimuli such as faces or buildings (Haxby et al., 1994; Wojciulik et al., 1998). For example, Haxby and colleagues, using PET, observed more ventral occipital activity during face processing and more dorsal parietal activity during location discrimination on the same set of visual stimuli. Wojciulik and colleagues found that activity in a ventral region specialized for face perception was 145% stronger when subjects processed faces than when they processed objects on the same set of stimuli.

It is less clear if the described attentional modulations reflect a relative increase of activity in task-relevant pathways or a relative suppression in task-irrelevant pathways. This is important in deciding between signal enhancement vs. noise suppression accounts. Direct comparisons between attended versus unattended conditions are not helpful because the corresponding modulation may reflect either a relative increase or a relative decrease in activity. Instead, it is necessary to gauge the sign of the modulation with an independent control condition. The approach used in many experiments has been to introduce a passive viewing condition, in which subjects are presented with the same set of stimuli and have to respond with a key-press to the onset of each display. The word ''passive'' is unfortunate because it may suggest large differences in the level of vigilance from the ''active'' tasks. Instead, a passive viewing control may be quite effortful, because subjects have to maintain accurate eye fixation, detect the onset of temporally asynchronous visual stimuli, and prepare/execute an appropriate detection response. A more appropriate term may be "detection" task. The logic behind a passive viewing task is to provide an independent sensory-motor baseline in which selective attention is not explicitly and endogenously directed toward certain stimuli or features. Admittedly, the control is problematic because attention is unchecked. On the other hand, it is not unreasonable to think that in this task attention is mostly drawn by the physical properties of the display, and thus evenly distributed across stimuli or stimulus features.

In our original experiment (Corbetta et al., 1990, 1991), we found no modulation in regions coding for the irrelevant feature as compared with a passive viewing control or a selective attention condition. In other experiments, which involve focusing attention toward one visual field location and bilateral presentation of target or distractor stimuli, attentional modulations have been found contralateral to the attended side (the side representing the attended location). In contrast, little or no modulation has been observed ipsilateral to the attended side, contrary to what one would expect if the role of spatial attention was to filter out irrelevant information from unattended locations (e.g., Vandenberghe et al., 1996, 1997; Woldorff et al., 1997). These effects have been correlated with improved psychophysical performance and early temporal modulations on scalp electrical potentials (for a review, see Hillyard et al., 1998). Recent elegant experiments by Tootell and colleagues (1998) and Brefczynski and DeYoe (1999) found that directing attention toward multiple locations in the visual field enhances cortical activity at the corresponding locations of retinotopically organized visual areas, including area V1 (see also Gandhi et al., 1999; Martinez et al., 1999; Somers et al., 1999).

These findings show directly that attending to a particular visual location enhances visual performance at that location by modulating activity at the corresponding points of retinotopically organized visual cortex. Tootell and colleagues (1998) also reported that the allocation of attention to peripheral field locations produced a suppression of activity in adjacent cortical regions representing the fovea, which was unattended during the experiment. Interestingly, the region of cortical suppression did not extend to other cortical locations that were coding for distractor (irrelevant) stimuli presented in other visual quadrants, either in the same or in the opposite hemisphere. Hence, the suppressive modulation is spatially incongruent with the source of noise, and it is unclear whether this reflects the neural correlate of a noise suppression mechanism.

Another common finding is that attentional modulations involve multiple visual areas within a task-relevant pathway, including at times primary visual cortex (area V1). In our original experiment, we found modulations at early (near calcarine sulcus, primary visual cortex), intermediate (MT+), and late (parietal) stages of the visual hierarchy. Similarly, Buchel and colleagues (1998) found modulations in areas V1/V2, V3, V5, and parietal cortex during attention to motion as compared with passive viewing. Haxby and colleagues (1994) showed that attention to faces modulated a large swath of tissue in ventral occipital cortex, overlapping with the multiple foci identified by Corbetta and colleagues (1991) for shape discrimination. These are likely to correspond to intermediate and higher levels of the ventral stream of processing (areas V4, TE, TEO). Recently, there have been elegant demonstrations that attention to specific visual field locations enhances activity in corresponding retinotopic locations of multiple early-intermediate visual regions (Kastner et al., 1998; Tootell et al., 1998; Brefczynski and DeYoe 1999), including area V1 (Tootell et al., 1998; Somers et al., 1999; Heeger et al., chapter 2 in this volume).

These imaging findings indicate that attentional modulations occur within a sensory pathway at early, intermediate, and late stages of processing. It is therefore likely that both perceptual and decisional processes are modulated. The predominance of modulation in task-relevant pathways suggests that attention may influence the signal more than suppressing the noise from irrelevant channels. The modulations might reflect top-down expectation signals that act directly at multiple levels of a sensory pathway (Olshausen et al., 1993). Alternatively, the occurrence of modulations at different levels may reflect a cascade effect due to existing connectivity caused by a top-down signal that primarily acts at a single level in the hierarchy of visual areas (Tsotsos et al., chapter 14 in this volume).

Open questions for future research include the quantification of these attentional modulations (in terms of both volume and magnitude) across multiple visual areas, their relationship to individual psychophysical performance, and how they relate to the attentional modulations recorded with other methods. For example, Treue and Maunsell (1996) reported a neuronal enhancement for attended stimuli of 86% and 113% in areas MT and MST, respectively, during a speed discrimination task in which attended and unattended targets were placed within the same receptive field. The size of this modulation is comparable with the one obtained in imaging experiments on attention to motion (e.g., 56–150% in Beauchamp et al., 1997).

However, there are also some discrepancies between methods. Heeger and colleagues (this volume) report strong attentional modulation in area V1 with fMRI during spatial attention. For many years, modulations of area V1 have been difficult to demonstrate by single-unit recordings in monkey. Similar attentional modulations in area V1 have been reported in fMRI studies from other laboratories (Martinez et al., 1999; Somers et al., 1999), and represent a robust and easily replicable finding. Martinez and colleagues compared attentional modulations in area V1 observed with different methods (fMRI and ERP), and suggested that the hemodynamic modulations may reflect temporally late feedback signals into area V1 from higher visual areas. They reached this conclusion because no attentional modulation was evident on the earliest visually evoked electrical potentials.

It is possible, therefore, that single-unit recording and functional imaging may sample neuronal signals in area V1 on different temporal scales.

Another puzzle is that attentional modulations in single-unit experiments are much stronger when target and distractors are placed within the same receptive field. For example, the neuronal enhancement reported by Treue and Maunsell (1996) fell from 86% to 19% in area MT, and from 113% to 40% in MST, when the distractor stimulus was placed in the opposite visual hemifield rather than next to the target stimulus in the receptive field of the recorded neuron (Maunsell and McAdams, this volume). The weakness of attentional modulations when stimuli are not positioned within the same receptive field is also a common finding in the ventral system (including area IT, where receptive fields are large and span both visual hemifields) (Moran and Desimone, 1985). In contrast, very strong attentional modulations can be obtained with both evoked potential and imaging methods by placing target and distractor items in opposite hemifields. The argument usually put forward in the single-unit literature is that modulations at the single-neuron level are best observed when there is competition between stimuli in the same receptive field (e.g., Desimone and Duncan, 1995).

This raises the paradox that correlates of neural competition between stimuli far apart on opposite sides of the vertical meridian would be observed only in areas with bilateral receptive fields. It is unclear whether the brain has such neurons, but there is strong psychophysical, imaging, and evoked potential evidence indicating that spatial competition between stimuli is resolved rather early in the visual system (possibly as early as area V1 under certain conditions). Therefore significant differences must exist between modulations observed at the population (e.g., imaging and evoked potential) and the single-unit level. Although there are many potential explanations for this discrepancy, one possibility is that the extracellular recording of the spiking activity of single neurons in visual cortex does not capture some critical neural codes reflecting the allocation of attention to spatial locations. For example, typical single-unit recordings would not detect systematic temporal correlations in the firing of neuronal populations within an area, which might underlie important behavioral, surface electrical, or hemodynamic modulations related to attention (Engel et al., 1991). It will be critical in the near future to develop more quantitative models of the relationship between vascular and neuronal signals. This will require comparing in the same animal, and under the same task conditions, hemodynamic signals, single-unit firing rates, and other measurements characterizing larger neuronal populations (e.g., multiunit recording, cross-correlation analysis).

## 1.4.2   Expectation Signals

An important ambiguity in all imaging experiments reviewed so far is their failure to distinguish between visual expectation and the effect of that expectation on visual processing. Expectations (e.g., what type of stimuli are task-relevant) are typically induced by top-down signals that are triggered by an appropriate cue, and that encode and maintain the relevant perceptual set. These neural signals must be separate from the modulations they induce on the sensory activity evoked by a subsequent stimulus (attentional modulations). Blocked PET and fMRI designs average activity over many trials, and therefore blur differences between processes that are active at different times within a trial. The ability to distinguish between earlier expectation signals and later attentional modulations is critical for the question of how visual expectations are implemented in the brain, and whether they resemble previously described mechanisms of signal enhancement or noise suppression. Signal enhancement models would predict expectation signals to be present predominantly on task-relevant pathways, whereas noise suppression models would predict expectation signals to be localized predominantly on task-irrelevant pathways. The reviewed imaging evidence, which finds predominant modulations in task-relevant pathways, is ambiguous in this respect because expectation signals, visual responses, and related attentional modulations were temporally confounded.

At present, little is known about the neural basis of visual expectations (or expectation signals) even from a single-unit perspective. Several neuronal correlates of expectation signals have been described. Many authors have reported an increase in the baseline firing rates of neurons in several brain regions when the monkey can anticipate the location of an upcoming target stimulus (Bruce and Goldberg, 1985; Colby et al., 1996; Luck et al., 1997). The effect is endogenous and spatially selective, that is, the attended location coincides precisely with the neuron's receptive field. Luck and colleagues (Luck et al., 1997; Reynolds and Desimone, chapter 7 in this volume) have distinguished the tonic modulation of the baseline response from a time-locked neuronal enhancement of the visual response triggered by the presentation of a target stimulus. They have argued that the tonic baseline increase reflects a selective biasing signal for location (expectation signal), whereas the enhancement is the result of a change in the gain of the sensory response caused by the biasing signal (the attentional modulation of the test stimulus).

Other studies have recorded cue-specific neural activity from several extrastriate and prefrontal areas during the cue period of delayed match-to-sample tasks. Typically, the animal is shown a sample object (or cue, which generates the expectation signal) and has to determine whether it matches subsequent objects (Fuster, 1973; Chelazzi et al., 1993; Miller et al., 1996). Interestingly, cue-related activity can be recorded in visual cortex (e.g., in area V4) even when the cue information is delivered in a tactile format (Haenny et al., 1988). Such delay activity therefore represents a neuronal correlate of visual expectations about upcoming stimuli. However, in the presence of intervening distractor stimuli (i.e., stimuli that do not match the cue), cue-specific delay activity is disrupted in extrastriate visual cortex but is maintained in prefrontal areas (Funahashi et al., 1993; Miller et al., 1996). Desimone and Duncan (1995) have therefore proposed that these prefrontal areas are the source of expectation signals that produce attentional modulations in posterior visual areas.

Overall, these studies clearly demonstrate that expectation signals generated by the presentation of visual cues are present in visual cortex prior to the presentation of a test stimulus, which is consistent with psychological theories in which cue information preactivates sensory channels. However, these signals have been recorded from one visual cortical region at a time (but see Miller et al., 1996), so that expectation signals and attentional modulations have not been characterized simultaneously over the entire brain on the same task. Furthermore, one cannot rule out the possibility that expectation signals generated through iconic cues (as in most match-to-sample paradigms) might be partially confounded with visual activity. Finally, we can generate expectations about visual attributes or scene in a variety of ways: through vision, audition, or touch of a sample attribute/object, verbal information derived either from outside cues (e.g., visual or auditory words) or internal processing, verbal or visual memory, imagery, and so on. How are all these different sources of expectation/bias organized and funneled in the visual system, in formats that are compatible with those of cortical visual areas? Is a common set of brain systems (e.g., working memory systems) involved in maintaining on-line different expectations?

### 1.4.3 Dissociating Expectation Signals and Attentional Modulations with Event-Related fMRI

The main purpose of this experiment (fully reported in Shulman et al., 1999) was to develop a method to separate BOLD signals related to the encoding/maintenance of expectation signals, from their effect (attentional modulation) on a subsequent visual response evoked by a test stimulus. Therefore, we used psychophysical tasks in which expectation signals could be generated in one condition, but not in a control condition, while matching basic sensory-motor variables. To avoid concerns about sensory activations produced by iconic cues, we elected to instruct subjects through symbolic cues, which require active transformation and do not contain motion energy. The task is a cued motion coherence detection task, modified after Ball and Sekuler (1981) and Newsome and colleagues (Britten et al., 1993). Ball and Sekuler have previously shown that stationary direction cues improve motion detection. Newsome and colleagues have extensively used a motion detection coherence task to understand the contribution of area MT in monkey to motion processing. The motion system is the best understood sensory system in both monkeys and humans. Several motion-selective regions have been recently described in the human brain (for review, see Tootell et al., 1996). This information allows us to label more precisely areas in which attentional modulations are found, and thus better define the putative stage of attentional selection.

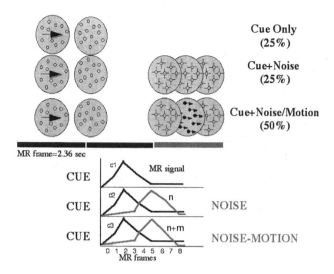

**Figure 1.2**

(*Top*) Stimulus sequence of a cue trial, a cue + noise trial, and a cue + noise/motion trial. The circular aperture was centered on the fovea and was 3.25° in diameter. In the actual display, no solid line defined the outer limit of the aperture. The cue was presented for 1600 ms. Dot density (n = 50) and size were the same for the cue and test periods. Dynamic noise is indicated by the starred dots, and coherent motion is indicated by the arrowed dots (speed 4.3° per second). The motion could be in any of eight directions (given by 45° increments from upward motion). 50% of the trials during the MR session were cue + noise/motion trials, 25% were cue + noise trials, and 25% were cue trials, with the three trial types randomly mixed. The temporal relationship of each trial event to the corresponding MR frame (scan) is indicated. The MR frame (2.36 s) is the time necessary to take a snapshot of the whole brain. (*Bottom*) Linear decomposition of the hemodynamic response function. The MR signal during a cue + noise/motion trial is modeled as composed of two functions, one for the cue period ($c^3$) and one for the noise plus motion (n + m) period. Direct parameter estimation is performed with a linear model for these two functions at each MR frame. Cue trials provide a direct estimation of the MR signal during the cue period in isolation ($c^1$). Cue + noise trials provide a direct estimation of the MR signal during the cue ($c^2$) and noise (n) periods in isolation. This information is used to estimate components during the cue period across all trial types ($c^{123}$), the noise (n), and the noise plus motion (n + m) periods.

In the fMRI experiments we ran three types of scans: *directional cue, passive cue,* and *motion localizer.* During *directional cue* scans three types of trials were randomly intermixed (figure 1.2). All trials began with a stationary arrow cue, presented at fixation on a random field of static dots for 1600 ms. The arrow cued one of eight possible directions of subsequent motion. Following the extinction of the cue, subjects held fixation on a small cross at the center of the random field of static dots for 3120 ms, for a total cue period of 4720 ms. Therefore, most of the cue period was spent encoding and holding in mind the direction of the arrow. The first type of trial ended following the completion of the cue period (*cue trials,* 25% of total). These were necessary to isolate expectation signals during the cue period. In the second and third types of trials, the static dots were randomly replotted following the cue period (once each display frame), producing dynamic random noise during the test period. In *cue + noise/motion trials* (50% of total), a percentage of the dots moved coherently (in the direction of the earlier arrow cue) during a brief interval (300 ms) at some randomly chosen time within the test period. Subjects detected the motion by pressing an MR compatible key-press with their right hand. The percentage of coherent motion was adjusted in each subject to yield just above threshold performance (d′ approximately 2.0). In *cue + noise trials* (25% of total) only dynamic noise was presented (i.e., dots never moved coherently), and subjects had to withhold a response. Each trial lasted on average 4720 ms, and the intertrial interval was randomly varied between 4720 ms, 7080 ms, and 9440 ms.

During *passive cue* scans, subjects passively viewed trial sequences that were identical except that the cue was a filled square (rather than an arrow) and that subjects did not make a response. *Passive cue* scans served as a control condition in which the cue generated no expectation about direction of motion. These scans also provided a control for the sensory activity evoked by the onset of the cue and the test stimulus. Differences in magnitude of the response to the test stimulus during directional and passive cue trials provided a measure of (attentional) modulations produced by a motion set generated through directional arrow cues during the detection of coherent motion.

Finally, to determine which areas were activated by sensory motion, subjects received *motion localizer* scans in which periods of continuous radial dot motion were alternated with control periods in which the dots were stationary. Subjects looked at the display and maintained fixation on a central crosshair. Areas active during radial motion were used for comparison with the areas that carried expectation signals and attentional modulations.

To verify that subjects were using the directional cue, we conducted a separate psychophysical session in which directional cue trials were randomly intermixed with neutral cue trials (in which a plus sign cued all eight possible directions of motion). Psychophysical models of motion selection suggest that a neutral cue does not instruct any particular direction but a general set for motion. Behaviorally, subjects were faster and more accurate when they used directional cues than neutral cues, indicating that the arrow cue was successful in generating an expectation for direction of motion that facilitated the perception of subsequently presented coherent motion.

The BOLD responses initiated during the cue and test periods were estimated with a linear regression model assuming that the MR signal on any frame is the linear sum of different components. No assumptions were made about the shape of the hemodynamic response function. Previous work using event-related fMRI design and rapid presentation rate has successfully estimated the BOLD response to different *trials* by randomly jittering the intertrial interval (e.g., Dale and Buckner, 1997). To estimate the response to different events *within a trial* (e.g., BOLD responses to the cue and to the test stimulus), it is also necessary to present a small percentage of "catch" trials in which only the first component

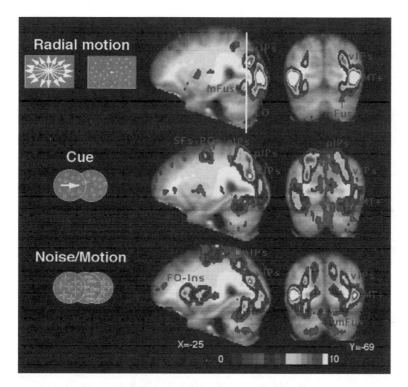

**Figure 1.3**
Group z-maps for activations during radial motion (*top row*), the cue period of trials involving a directional cue (*middle row*), and the noise/motion period of trials involving a directional cue (*bottom row*). A sagittal slice of the left hemisphere is shown in the left column, a coronal slice in the right column. The white line through the sagittal slice in the top left panel shows the location of the coronal slice. The color scale represents the z-score of the activation, and all displayed pixels have passed a multiple comparison procedure that includes a Bonferroni correction for the number of hemodynamic response functions used to generate the z-map. aIPs, anterior intraparietal sulcus; pIPs, posterior intraparietal sulcus; vIPs, ventral intraparietal sulcus; SFs-PCs, superior frontal-precentral sulcus; Lo, lateral occipital; FO-Ins, frontal operculum-insula; mFus, mid-fusiform gyrus. (See plate 1 for color version.)

is present (cue-only trials). A separate validation of this new method has been presented by Ollinger and colleagues (1998).

The top row of figure 1.3 (see also plate 1) shows areas active for radial sensory motion. They include the mid-fusiform gyrus (mFus), lateral occipital, middle temporal area (MT+), ventral and anterior intraparietal regions (vIPs, aIPs), and cortex near the precentral sulcus (PrCs).

Some of the same motion-sensitive regions were active during the cue period following the presentation of a (static) directional cue (figure 1.3, middle row). They included the anterior and ventral IPs region, the ventral portion of area MT+, lateral occipital, and the precentral region (at the intersection with the superior frontal sulcus on the left). This activity did not simply reflect the sensory response evoked by the onset of the cue stimulus, because it was significantly stronger during directional than passive cues. Other non-motion-sensitive regions were also active during the cue period. A region in the posterior portion of the IPs was uniquely active during the cue period. A region in the anterior fusiform gyrus (antFus), located more laterally, ventrally, and anteriorly to the one active for radial motion, strongly responded during the cue period for both directional and passive cues. The location of this region is near cortex previously found active during face and shape processing (Haxby et al., 1994; Wojciulik et al., 1998), and may be involved in the initial shape analysis of the static cue. This interpretation implies that some shape analysis is conducted on both directional and passive cue trials, that is, both when the cue is relevant and when it is irrelevant.

Figure 1.4 shows averaged (across subjects) time courses in motion-sensitive (aIPs and MT+) and non-motion-sensitive regions (pIPs, antFus) during the cue and test periods for directional and passive trials. Note that anterior IPs and MT+ show a separate response during both the cue and the noise/motion (or noise, not shown) periods, whereas posIPs is active only during the cue period. The magnitude of the response is significantly stronger during directional than during passive trials, indicating that these signals do not simply reflect the sensory onset of the cue. These time courses clearly demonstrate that this method can separate processes within a trial. They also provide information about the relative role of each region in the processing of the cue. For instance, activity in parietal cortex (anterior and posterior IPs) was more sustained than in MT+ or in other occipital regions (e.g., antFus). Also, activity in antFus was the strongest across all visual areas during directional and passive cues.

One possible model is that the static shape cue was initially encoded in the antFus region (active in both cue conditions), and transformed into a suitable motion signal via early motion regions (e.g., MT+) that showed an early response during the cue period. The expectation signal for motion was then maintained in regions of the intraparietal sulcus during the cue period. These parietal regions could also participate in the encoding phase. This model suggests that the intraparietal regions are the source of top-down signals which encode expectations about upcoming visual motion in this task. This result is evocative of recent results of Maunsell and colleagues, who found that neuronal modulations for motion discrimination within the intraparietal sulcus are strongly dependent on the information carried by the cue (see Maunsell and McAdams, chapter 6 in this volume). Surprisingly, no prefrontal activity was localized during the cue period (see below), as one might expect on the basis of reports of cue-related delay activity in prefrontal cortex during match-to-sample tasks (Funahashi et al., 1993; Miller et al., 1996), although a left precentral region (SFs-PrCs) showed cue-related activity. Therefore, any link between

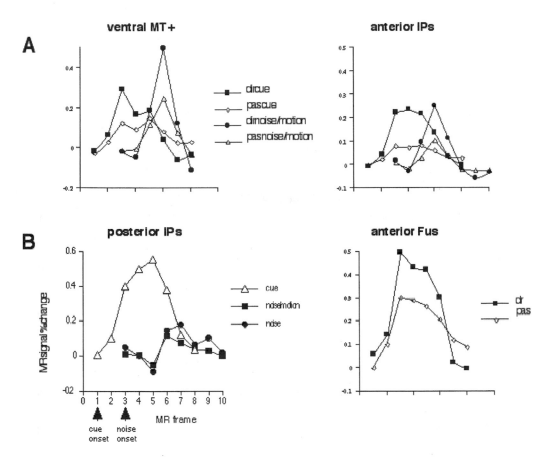

**Figure 1.4**
(*A*) Group time course of activations in two motion-sensitive regions (left vMT+, left antIPs) during the cue and test periods for directional and passive cues. Time courses are averaged over 3D regions of interest formed from voxels that were significantly activated during both periods. Both regions show a response during the cue period (after taking into account the hemodynamic delay), followed by a second response during the test period. Note difference in response magnitude between directional and passive trials, and sustained cue-related activity in antIPs but not vMT+. (*B*) Group time course of activation in non-motion-sensitive regions left posIPs during the cue and test periods, and right antFus during cue period only. posIPs was significantly active only during the cue period, and showed a sustained response. antFus showed strong responses both during directional and passive cues. Compare passive response in antFus with those recorded in vMT+ and antIPs. The antFus may be critical for the analysis of the shape of the cue during both trial types. AntIPs, anterior intraparietal sulcus; posIPs, posterior intraparietal sulcus; antFus, anterior fusiform gyrus; vMT+, ventral area MT complex.

posterior parietal and anterior regions during the cue period might have involved this precentral region. In any case, activity was still significantly more sustained in pIPs than in SFs-PrCs.

All motion-sensitive areas were activated at the presentation of the test stimulus (figure 1.3, bottom row, and time course in figure 1.4), and showed a stronger response to the test stimulus during directional than passive trials. This attentional modulation partly reflects the effect of the directional cue on the sensory processing of the test stimulus. Many other regions, more anterior in the brain, were also activated during the test period. Some regions, such as primary sensory-motor cortex (and the parietal operculum, or area SII), were related to the execution of the key-press response, and showed higher activity during response (hit and false alarm) than no response (misses and correct rejections) trials. Other regions, such as SMA, anterior cingulate, and basal ganglia, showed activations that began after the onset of the noise display, and were present for all trial types (hits, false alarms, misses, correct rejections). Activity in these regions may reflect preparatory motor signals initiated by the onset of the noise display, followed within a few hundred milliseconds by a target triggering a key-press response or by processes involved in searching a target in a noisy display.

A similar pattern was observed in dorsolateral prefrontal cortex (DLPFC) and frontal opercular regions. These regions have been activated during working-memory experiments, and are considered, on the basis of neuronal recordings, to be the source of biasing signals to the visual system. It is therefore important to consider the time course of activation in this region during cue and test periods. Figure 1.5 shows time courses in right and left DLPFC. The location of this region is analogous to the one reported in many working-memory experiments, and corresponds to Brodmann area 46. Note that DLPFC is silent during the cue period but strongly responds during the test period. The type of decision or execution of a response does not affect the magnitude of the response. These findings demonstrate that DLPFC is not universally involved in storing visual expectations which guide visual behavior, and that under certain circumstances this information can be stored in posterior visual regions. The absence of DLPFC activity during the cue period is consistent with a view in which prefrontal cortex is engaged only when stored information is actively manipulated or transformed. An alternative possibility is that DLPFC might be driven by more complex storage operations which perhaps involve a longer delay, linguistic information, or a more precise representation of the cue (e.g., during a match-to-sample task).

In conclusion, this experiment demonstrates that expectations about upcoming visual motion generated by a static symbolic cue preactivate motion pathways involved in the analysis of subsequently presented motion stimuli, as well as non-motion-sensitive regions. The intraparietal sulcus regions are the source of top-down signals, which interact

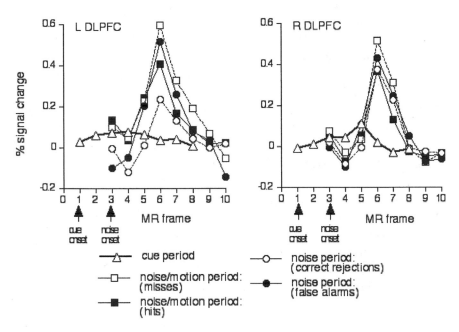

**Figure 1.5**
Group time courses in left and right dorsolateral prefrontal cortex (DLPFC) during the cue and test period. Test periods in which a motor response was executed (hits, false alarms) are indicated by filled symbols, and test periods in which a response was withheld (misses, correct rejections) are indicated by open symbols. No motor responses were made during cue periods. Time courses are based on a 3 × 3 voxel region of interest centered on the voxel yielding the maximum Z score in the region. BOLD responses are evident only during the test period, but are not contingent on whether a motion target was detected or a response was made.

in many motion-sensitive regions with incoming sensory stimulation, producing a stronger sensory response to incoming visual information. This (attentional) modulation leads, through unclear mechanisms, to a more accurate discrimination.

This experiment raises many new questions about visual expectations and top-down expectation signals. One would like to know more about the selectivity of such signals for direction of motion. In other experiments we found that the same regions were also active during the selection of target locations in the course of luminance detection tasks (Chelazzi et al., 2000; Corbetta et al, 2000). Other experiments have shown that attention to location and motion can have additive effects in modulating activity in the motion system (Beauchamp et al., 1997). Psychological results suggest that selection by a feature does not occur per se, but is mediated through location codes (Moore and Egeth,1998; Shih and Sperling, 1996). Another important question is whether the network that maintains expectation signals for motion will change, depending on the format in which the cue is presented. Is the posIPs activity reflecting some supramodal signal that will hold information independently of cue format, or will other regions come on-line by increasing the complexity of the transformation (e.g., DLPFC)? A final intriguing question is whether the level of top-down modulation will vary as a function of task demands. Is it possible to specifically preactivate different levels in the motion system, depending on whether the perceptual task relies on low- or high-level motion analysis (e.g., motion energy versus feature detection versus structure-from-motion; Sperling et al., chapter 10 in this volume)?

## 1.5   Relevance for Psychological and Neural Theories of Attention

The notion that top-down expectation signals preactivate sensory pathways is consistent with previously reviewed single-unit data during spatial attention (Luck et al., 1997) and match-to-sample tasks (Chelazzi et al., 1993). Tonic increases in the rate of baseline firing or delay activity related to the cue may represent putative neuronal correlates of the BOLD modulation described above. Pathway preactivation is also consistent with cognitive, computational, and neural models of higher vision. In Wolfe's guided search model (Wolfe et al., 1989), top-down expectation signals about the relevant feature bias activity in feature maps that represent the visual scene. In Tsotsos's model, a top-down biasing signal feeds back to feature-level maps, where it selectively activates winner-take-all competition circuits in order to emphasize relevant targets and deemphasize irrelevant distractors (Tsotsos et al., chapter 14 in this volume). In Desimone and Duncan's (1995) biased competition model, the bottom-up competition between objects in a visual scene is gradually resolved in favor of the object receiving a top-down biasing signal from frontal structures.

All these models implicitly assume that the top-down expectation signal has its primary effect on the relevant visual representation, that is, the one coding for the relevant object. The notion of pathway preactivation is also consistent with psychological theories previously discussed, although this experiment does not resolve between different accounts. The findings are certainly consistent with a signal enhancement mechanism, given the presence of preactivation in relevant pathways, and the fact that early levels in the motion system were modulated (MT+, lateral occipital). However, noise information was also coded in the same regions, so that we cannot rule out the possibility that expectation signals reflected noise suppression mechanisms. This issue could be solved by recording in the monkey from cortical columns that code for cued and uncued directions during the period of time following the symbolic cue. The cue's preactivation of irrelevant or relevant columns would be consistent, respectively, with a noise suppression or signal enhancement account.

Signal enhancement mechanisms are currently more strongly supported by the experimental evidence. Luck and colleagues (1997) observed in area V4 that the tonic increase in baseline firing rate, a correlate of a top-down biasing signal for location, is maximal at the attended location and falls off sharply as one moves away from the focus of attention, even within the same receptive field. In other words, the top-down signal is stronger at (attended) locations processing signal than at (unattended) locations processing noise. As reviewed earlier, most imaging studies show attentional modulations in areas coding for the relevant attribute, with little or no modulation in areas coding for the irrelevant attribute. It will be important to show with event-related fMRI methods that expectation signals coding for one particular visual attribute (among many potentially relevant attributes) preactivate only relevant sensory pathways. In a recent imagery experiment, Kanwisher and O'Craven demonstrated the feature selectivity of some top-down signals (Kanwisher and O'Craven, 1998). They measured BOLD signal simultaneously in two extrastriate visual regions, specialized respectively for face and place/building processing, while subjects formed mental images of famous faces (e.g., Bill Clinton) or buildings (e.g., Eiffel Tower) after verbal expectation. The BOLD signal increased specifically in each area as a function of the expectation, and presumably the mental image, being formed. In other words, the BOLD signal increased in the *face* area when a famous person was named. The expectation signal triggered by the verbal expectation was therefore stimulus-specific and modulated the relevant neural representation.

## 1.6   Conclusions

Neuroimaging research on attention since 1990 has convincingly demonstrated the importance of visual expectations for visual processing. Extensive modulations throughout visual cortex have been demonstrated, using a variety of selection criteria and paradigms. Modulations occur predominantly in task-relevant pathways, and represent an interaction effect between top-down signals that encode/maintain visual expectations, and incoming sensory information. Recent advances in functional imaging methods have begun to provide a glimpse of the temporal dynamics of the processes involved in attentional control.

## References

Ball, K., and Sekuler, R. (1981). Cues reduce direction uncertainty and enhance motion detection. *Percep. Psychophys.* 30: 119–128.

Beauchamp, M. S., Cox, R. W., and DeYoe, E. A. (1997). Graded effects of spatial and featural attention on human area MT and associated motion processing regions. *J. Neurophysiol.* 78: 516–520.

Boynton, G. M., Engel, S. A., Glover, G. H., and Heeger, D. J. (1996). Linear systems analysis of fMRI in human V1. *J. Neurosci.* 16: 4207–4221.

Brefczynski, J. A., and DeYoe, E. A. (1999). A physiological correlate of the "spotlight" of visual attention. *Nature Neurosci.* 2: 370–374.

Britten, K. H., Shadlen, M. N., Newsome, W. T., and Movshon, J. A. (1993). The analysis of visual motion: A comparison of neuronal and psychophysical performance. *J. Neurosci.* 12: 4745–4765.

Broadbent, D. (1982). Task combination and selective intake of information. *Acta Psychol.* 50: 253–290.

Bruce, C. J., and Goldberg, M. E. (1985). Primate frontal eye fields. I. Single neurons discharging before saccades. *J. Neurophysiol.* 53: 603–635.

Buchel, C., Josephs, O., Rees, G., Turner, R., Frith, C., and Friston, K. (1998). The functional anatomy of attention to visual motion. *Brain* 121: 1281–1294.

Buckner, R. L., Bandettini, P. A., O'Craven, K. M., Savoy, R. L., Petersen, S. E., Raichle, M. E., and Rosen, B. R. (1997). Detection of transient and distributed cortical activation during single trials of a cognitive task using fMRI. *Proc. Nat. Acad. Sci. USA* 93: 14878–14883.

Chelazzi, L., Miller, E. K., Duncan, J., and Desimone, R. (1993). A neural basis for visual search in inferior temporal cortex. *Nature* 363: 345–347.

Colby, C. L., Duhamel, J. R., and Goldberg, M. E. (1996). Visual, presaccadic, and cognitive activation of single neurons in monkey lateral intraparietal area. *J. Neurophysiol.* 76: 2841–2852.

Corbetta, M., Miezin, F. M., Dobmeyer, S., Shulman, G. L., and Petersen, S. E. (1991). Selective and divided attention during visual discriminations of shape, color, and speed: Functional anatomy by positron emission tomography. *J. Neurosci.* 11: 2383–2402.

Dale, A. M., and Buckner, R. L. (1997). Selective averaging of rapidly presented individual trials using fMRI. *Hum. Brain Mapping* 5: 329–340.

Desimone, R., and Duncan, J. (1995). Neural mechanisms of selective visual attention. *Annu. Rev. Neurosci.* 18: 193–222.

Deutsch, J., and Deutsch, D. (1963). Attention: Some theoretical considerations. *Psychol. Rev.* 70: 80–90.

Duncan, J. (1980). The locus of interference in the perception of simultaneous stimuli. *Psychol. Rev.* 87: 272–300.

Dupont, P., Orban, G. A., Vogels, R., Bormans, G., Nuyts, J., Schiepers, C., De Roo, M., and Mortelmans, L. (1993). Different perceptual tasks performed with the same visual stimulus attribute activate different regions of the human brain: A positron emission tomography study. *Proc. Nat. Acad. Sci. USA* 90: 10927–10931.

Engel, A. K., König, P., and Singer, W. (1991). Direct physiological evidence for scene segmentation by temporal coding. *Proc. Nat. Acad. Sci. USA* 88: 9136–9140.

Eriksen, C. W., and Hoffman, J. E. (1972). Temporal and spatial characteristics of selective encoding from visual displays. *Percep. Psychophys.* 12: 201–204.

Friston, K. J., Josephs, O., Rees, G., and Turner, R. (1998). Nonlinear event-related responses in fMRI. *Magn. Reson. Med.* 39: 41–52.

Funahashi, S., Chafee, M. V., and Goldman-Rakic, P. S. (1993). Prefrontal neuronal activity in rhesus monkeys performing a delayed anti-saccade task. *Nature* 365: 753–756.

Fuster, J. M. (1973). Unit activity in prefrontal cortex during delayed-response performance: Neuronal correlates of transient memory. *J. Neurophysiol.* 36: 61–78.

Gandhi, S. P., Heeger, D. J., and Boynton, G. M. (1999). Spatial attention affects brain activity in human primary visual cortex. *Proc. Nat. Acad. Sci. USA* 96: 3314–3319.

Gilbert, C. D. (1996). Plasticity in visual perception and physiology. *Curr. Opin. Neurobiol.* 6: 269–274.

Haenny, P. E., Maunsell, J. H. R., and Schiller, P. H. (1988). State dependent activity in monkey visual cortex. II. Retinal and extraretinal factors in V4. *Exp. Brain Res.* 69: 245–259.

Hawkins, H. L., Hillyard, S. A., Luck, S. J., Mouloua, M., Downing, C. J., and Woodward, D. P. (1990). Visual attention modulates signal detectability. *J. Exp. Psychol. Hum. Percep. Perf.* 16: 802–811.

Haxby, J. V., Horwitz, B., Ungerleider, L. G., Maisog, J. M., Pietrini, P., and Grady, C. L. (1994). The functional organization of human extrastriate cortex: A PET–rCBF study of selective attention to faces and locations. *J. Neurosci.* 14: 6336–6353.

Hillyard, S. A., and Picton, T. W. (1987). Electrophysiology of cognition. In F. Plum, V. B. Mountcastle, and S. T. Geiger (eds.), *The handbook of physiology*. Sect. 1, *The nervous system*, vol. 5, *Higher functions of the brain*, pt. 2 (pp. 519–584). Bethesda, MD: American Physiological Society.

Hillyard, S. A., Vogel, E. K., and Luck, S. J. (1998). Sensory gain control (amplification) as a mechanism of selective attention: Electrophysiological and neuroimaging evidence. *Philos. Trans. R. Soc. London* B 353: 1257–1270.

Ito, M., Westheimer, G., and Gilbert, C. D. (1998). Attention and perceptual learning modulate contextual influences on visual perception. *Neuron* 20: 1191–1197.

Kanwisher, N., and O'Craven, K. M. (1998). Extrastriate activity during visual imagery is stimulus specific. *Soc. Neurosci. Abstr.* 24: 530.

Karni, A., Meyer, G., Jezzard, P., Adams, M. M., Turner, R., and Ungerleider, L. G. (1995). Functional MRI evidence for adult motor cortex plasticity during motor skill learning. *Nature* 377: 155–158.

Kastner, S., De Weerd, P., Desimone, R., and Ungerleider, L. G. (1998). Mechanisms of directed attention in the human extrastriate cortex as revealed by functional MRI. *Science* 282: 108–111.

Knierim, J. J., and Van Essen, D. C. (1992). Neuronal responses to static texture patterns in area V1 of the alert macaque monkey. *J. Neurophysiol.* 67: 961–980.

Logothetis, N. K., Guggenberger, H., Peled, S., and Pauls, J. (1999). Functional imaging of the monkey brain. *Nature Neurosci.* 2: 555–562.

Luck, S. J., Chelazzi, L., Hillyard, S. A., and Desimone, R. (1997). Neuronal mechanisms of spatial selective attention in areas V1, V2, and V4 of macaque visual cortex. *J. Neurophysiol.* 77: 24–42.

Mangun, G. R., Hillyard, S. A., and Luck, S. J. (1993). Electrocortical substrates of visual selective attention. In D. Meyer and S. Kornblum (eds.), *Attention and performance XIV* (pp. 219–243). Cambridge, MA: MIT Press.

Martinez, A., Anllo-Vento, L., Sereno, M. I., Frank, L. R., Buxton, R. B., Dubowitz, D. J., Wong, E. C., Hinrichs, H., Heinze, H. J., and Hillyard, S. A. (1999). Involvement of striate and extrastriate visual cortical areas in spatial attention. *Nature Neurosci.* 2: 364–369.

Maunsell, J. H. R. (1995). The brain's visual world: Representation of visual targets in cerebral cortex. *Science* 270: 764–769.

Miller, E. K., Erickson, C. A., and Desimone, R. (1996). Neural mechanisms of visual working memory in prefrontal cortex of the macaque. *J. Neurosci.* 16: 5154–5167.

Moore, C. M., and Egeth, H. (1998). How does feature-based attention affect visual processing? *J. Exp. Psychol. Hum. Percep. Perf.* 24: 1296–1310.

Moran, A. J., and Desimone, R. (1985). Selective attention gates visual processing in the extrastriate cortex. *Science* 229: 782–784.

Motter, B. C. (1993). Focal attention produces spatially selective processing in visual cortical areas V1, V2, and V4 in the presence of competing stimuli. *J. Neurophysiol.* 70: 909–919.

Motter, B. C. (1994a). Neural correlates of attentive selection for color or luminance in extrastriate area V4. *J. Neurosci.* 14: 2178–2189.

Motter, B. C. (1994b). Neural correlates of feature selective memory and pop-out in extrastriate area V4. *J. Neurosci.* 14: 2190–2199.

Mountcastle, V. B., Motter, B. C., Steinmetz, M. A., and Sestokas, A. K. (1987). Common and differential effects of attentive fixation on the excitability of parietal and prestriate (V4) cortical visual neurons in the macaque monkey. *J. Neurosci.* 7: 2239–2255.

Nystrom, L. E., Delgado, M. R., Sabb, F. W., Noll, D. C., and Cohen, J. (1998). Dynamics of fMRI: Broca's area activation reflects independent effects of duration and intensity of working memory processes. *NeuroImage* 7: 7.

O'Craven, K. M., Savoy, R. L., and Rosen, B. R. (1995). Attention modulates fMRI activation in human MT/MST. *Soc. Neurosci. Abstr.* 21: 1988.

Ollinger, J. M., Corbetta, M., Petersen, S. E., and Shulman, G. L. (1998). Separating events within a trial with event-related fMRI. *Soc. Neurosci. Abstr.* 24: 1178.

Olshausen, B. A., Anderson, C. H., and Van Essen, D. C. (1993). A neurobiological model of visual attention and invariant pattern recognition based on dynamic routing of information. *J. Neurosci.* 13: 4700–4719.

Pashler, H. E. (1998). *The psychology of attention.* Cambridge, MA: MIT Press.

Posner, M. I. (1980). Orienting of attention. *Q. J. Exp. Psychol.* 32: 3–25.

Raichle, M. E. (1994). Visualizing the mind. *Sci. Am.* 270: 58–64.

Rosen, B. R., Buckner, R. L., and Dale, A. M. (1998). Event related fMRI: Past, present, and future. *Proc. Nat. Acad. Sci. USA* 95: 773–780.

Shih, S., and Sperling, G. (1996). Is there feature-based attentional selection in visual search? *J. Exp. Psychol. Hum. Percep. Perf.* 22: 758–779.

Shulman, G. L., Ollinger, J. M., Akbudak, E., Conturo, T. E., Snyder, A. Z., Petersen, S. E., and Corbetta, M. (1999). Areas involved in encoding and applying directional expectations to moving objects. *J. Neurosci.* 19: 9480–9496.

Somers, D. C., Dale, A. M., Seiffert, A. E., and Tootell, R. B. H. (1999). Functional MRI reveals spatially specific attentional modulation in human primary visual cortex. *Proc. Nat. Acad. Sci. USA* 16: 1663–1668.

Stefanacci, L., Reber, P., Costanza, J., Way, E., Buxton, R., Zola, S., Squire, L., and Albright, T. (1998). fMRI of monkey visual cortex. *Neuron* 20: 1051–1057.

Tootell, R. B. H., Dale, A. M., Sereno, M. I., and Malach, R. (1996). New images from human visual cortex. *Trends Neurosci.* 19: 481–489.

Tootell, R. B. H., Hadjikhani, N., Hall, E. K., Marrett, S., Vanduffel, W., Vaughan, J. T., and Dale, A. M. (1998). The retinotopy of visual spatial attention. *Neuron* 21: 1409–1422.

Treisman, A. M. (1969). Strategies and models of selective attention. *Psychol. Rev.* 76: 282–299.

Treue, S., and Maunsell, J. H. R. (1996). Attentional modulation of visual motion processing in cortical areas MT and MST. *Nature* 382: 539–541.

Ts'o, D. Y., Frostig, R. D., Lieke, E. E., and Grinvald, A. (1990). Functional organization of primate visual cortex revealed by high resolution optical imaging. *Science* 27: 417–420.

Van Essen, D. C., and DeYoe, E. A. (1995). Concurrent processing in the primate visual system. In M. S. Gazzaniga (ed.), *The cognitive neurosciences* (pp. 383–400). Cambridge, MA: MIT Press.

Vandenberghe, R., Duncan, J., Dupont, P., Ward, R., Poline, J. B., Bormans, G., Michiels, J., Mortelmans, L., and Orban, G. A. (1997). Attention to one or two features in left and right visual field: A positron emission tomography study. *J. Neurosci.* 17: 3739–3750.

Vandenberghe, R., Dupont, P., Debruyn, B., Bormans, G., Michiels, J., Mortelmans, L., and Orban, G. A. (1996). The influence of stimulus location on the brain activation pattern in detection and orientation discrimination: A PET study of visual attention. *Brain* 119: 1263–1276.

Wojciulik, E., Kanwisher, N., and Driver, J. (1998). Covert visual attention modulates face-specific activity in the human fusiform gyrus: fMRI study. *J. Neurophysiol.* 79: 1574–1578.

Woldorff, M. G., Fox, P. T., Matzke, M., Lancaster, J. L., Veeraswamy, S., Zamarripa, F., Seabolt, M., Glass, T., Gao, J. H., Martin, C. C., and Jerabek, P. (1997). Retinotopic organization of early visual spatial attention effects as revealed by PET and ERPs. *Hum. Brain Mapping* 5: 280–286.

Wolfe, J. M., Cave, K. R., and Franzel, S. L. (1989). Guided search: An alternative to the feature integration model for visual search. *J. Exp. Psychol. Hum. Percep. Perf.* 15: 419–433.

Wurtz, R. H., Goldberg, M. E., and Robinson, D. L. (1980). Behavioral modulation of visual responses in the monkey: Stimulus selection for attention and movement. *Prog. Psychobiol. Physiol. Psychol.* 9: 43–83.

Wurtz, R. H., Richmond, B. J., and Newsome, W. T. (1984). Modulation of cortical visual processing by attention, perception, and movement. In G. M. Edelman, W. E. Gall, and W. M. Cowan (eds.), *Dynamic aspects of neocortical functions* (pp. 195–217). New York: Wiley.

Zarahn, E., Aguirre, G. K., and D'Esposito, M. (1997). Empirical analyses of BOLD fMRI statistics. I. Spatially unsmoothed data collected under null-hypothesis conditions. *NeuroImage* 5: 179–197.

# 2 Neuronal Correlates of Attention in Human Visual Cortex

David J. Heeger, Sunil P. Gandhi, Alexander C. Huk, and Geoffrey M. Boynton

## 2.1 Introduction

Our ability to perform a visual discrimination task is improved when we are cued in advance toward the spatial location of the relevant stimulus (Graham, 1989; Pashler, 1998). Neural correlates of this phenomenon can be studied electrophysiologically in awake monkeys, by recording the responses of individual neurons in visual cortex while the monkeys perform various visual tasks. Neurons in several areas of the visual cortex respond differently when the animal attends to the stimulus in question (Bushnell et al., 1981; Moran and Desimone, 1985; Motter, 1993; Desimone and Duncan, 1995; Treue and Maunsell, 1996; Luck et al., 1997; Press, 1998; Ito and Gilbert, 1999, McAdams and Maunsell, 1999). Pooled across many neurons, this attentional modulation can be measured using event-related potentials (ERPs) (Mangun et al., 1993; Gomez-Gonzales et al., 1994; Clark and Hillyard, 1996; Mangun et al., 1997; Martinez et al., 1999), positron emission tomography (PET) (Corbetta et al., 1993; Heinze et al., 1994; Woldorff et al., 1997), optical imaging through the skull (Gratton, 1997), and functional magnetic resonance imaging (fMRI) (O'Craven et al., 1997; Beauchamp et al., 1997; Watanabe, Harner, et al., 1998; Watanabe, Sasaki, et al., 1998; Tootell et al., 1998; Buchel et al., 1998; Culham et al., 1998; Kastner et al., 1998; Somers et al., 1999; Brefczynski and DeYoe, 1999; Gandhi et al., 1999).

These results lead one to hypothesize that the observed modulation of brain activity directly causes the observed improvement in behavioral performance. However, the current body of data is not obviously consistent with this hypothesis (Maunsell, 1995). In monkey single-unit physiology experiments, attentional effects in extrastriate cortex are strongest when monkeys are cued to attend to one of two nearby stimuli, that is, with both placed within a neuron's receptive field (Desimone and Duncan, 1995; Treue and Maunsell, 1996; Luck et al., 1997). The behavioral consequences of attention, on the other hand, would appear to be just as strong for two stimuli in adjacent receptive fields.

Some theories suggest that attention is mediated entirely by selection very early in the visual pathways, for instance, in the lateral geniculate nucleus of the thalamus or in primary visual cortex (area V1) (Crick, 1984; Koch and Ullman, 1985). Indeed, area V1 is a natural place in the brain for spatial attention to impose its effects because (1) the retinotopic map in area V1 is precise and (2) V1 is a bottleneck in the flow of visual information to the secondary visual brain areas. However, until very recently the consensus was that attention has no effect in area V1.

It is only since 1998 that neuroimaging (Watanabe, Harner, et al., 1998; Tootell et al., 1998; Kastner et al., 1998; Somers et al., 1999; Brefczynski and DeYoe, 1999; Gandhi et al., 1999) and single-unit studies (Press, 1998; McAdams and Maunsell, 1999; Ito and Gilbert, 1999) have demonstrated unambiguously that attention does affect activity in area V1. However, the attentional modulation of neuronal responses in area V1 is notoriously difficult to measure with microelectrodes. Indeed, the attentional effects measured with fMRI in humans are considerably stronger (20–30% changes in brain activity) than those measured under similar conditions with single-unit recording in monkeys (5–10%).

This chapter presents the results of experiments using fMRI (Ogawa et al., 1990, 1992; Belliveau et al., 1991; Kwong et al., 1992) that reveal the effect of spatial attention on neuronal activity in identified visual areas of the human brain (including area V1). Our primary aim was to compare attentional changes in brain activity with attentional improvements in behavioral performance, and to ascertain whether or not the former are sufficiently large to explain the latter. Toward that end, we developed a simple model of behavioral performance based on signal-detection theory. We also demonstrated the importance of isolating the effect of spatial attention from the more general effects of performing a demanding visual task. Some of these results have been reported previously (Gandhi et al., 1998, 1999; Huk and Heeger, 2000).

## 2.2  Methods

### 2.2.1  General Paradigm

In some of our experiments, we used fMRI to measure modulations of cortical activity as the visual stimulation alternated between two different states. In localizing visual area MT+, for example, radially moving dots were presented for 18 s followed by 18 s of stationary dots. In other experiments, the stimulation remained constant throughout each scan but the subject alternated between two different visual tasks. In the spatial attention experiment, for example, subjects performed a series of speed discrimination trials while alternately attending to two peripheral stimulus apertures. Throughout the scan, stimuli were delivered simultaneously in both apertures, but subjects were cued to direct their attention alternately to one aperture or the other.

During all scans, subjects performed a visual motion discrimination task in a series of discrete trials. Each trial consisted of two brief stimulus intervals, followed by a response interval. The stimulus moved at a base speed in one interval and at a slightly faster test speed in the other interval; subjects pressed a button to indicate which interval contained the greater speed. Feedback was provided after each trial. Subjects practiced the tasks extensively (approximately 1000 trials) before scanning, until their performance reached asymptotic levels. The stimulus parameters were adjusted such that subjects performed approximately 80% of the trials correctly during the scan.

The fact that brief stimulus presentations were interspersed with blank intervals minimized contrast-dependent adaptation of visual responses during the long scanning sequence. In addition, the dynamic nature of the stimuli (moving gratings) helped to minimize light adaptation.

In the experiment on the effects of task performance, stimuli were displayed on an LCD flat panel positioned just beyond the end of the patient's bed. The display was viewed through binoculars specially modified for a high magnetic-field environment. Just beyond the objective lenses, two tilted mirrors were mounted to allow subjects to see the LCD display. In the experiment on the effects of spatial attention, stimuli were displayed on a rear-projection screen placed near the subjects' knees, at the opening of the bore of the MRI scanner. Subjects were lying on their backs and viewed the display through a mirror directly above their eyes. To stabilize eye position, subjects fixated a small mark of high contrast. The subjects' heads were immobilized by a bite bar.

### 2.2.2 Data Acquisition

Each subject participated in several fMRI scanning sessions: one to obtain a high-resolution anatomical scan; one to functionally define the early visual areas, including V1 and MT+ (see below); and several sessions to measure fMRI responses under various experimental conditions.

MR imaging was performed on a standard clinical GE 1.5 T Signa scanner with either a standard GE head (spatial attention experiment) or a custom-designed, dual-surface coil (task performance experiment). Functional MR images were recorded using a T2*-sensitive gradient recalled echo pulse sequence (1500 ms repetition time, 40 ms echo time, 90° flip angle, 2 interleaves, effective inplane resolution = 2 × 2 in., slice thickness = 4 mm) with a spiral readout (Noll et al., 1995; Glover and Lai, 1998). Eight adjacent planes of fMRI data were collected, with the most ventral slice positioned along the boundary between the occipital lobe and the cerebellum.

### 2.2.3 Registration

Each fMRI scanning session began by acquiring a set of low-resolution, sagittal anatomical images used for slice selection. A set of structural images was then acquired, using a T1-weighted spin echo pulse sequence (500 ms repetition time, minimum echo time, 90° flip angle) in the same slices and at the same resolution as the functional images. These inplane anatomical images were registered relative to a high-resolution anatomical scan of each subject's brain so that all MR images (across multiple scanning sessions) from a given subject could be aligned to a common three-dimensional coordinate grid.

### 2.2.4  fMRI Data Analysis

Each fMRI scan lasted 252 s. Data from the first 36 s cycle were discarded to minimize effects of magnetic saturation and visual adaptation. During the remaining 6 cycles of each scan, 72 functional images (1 every 3 s) were recorded for each slice. For a given fMRI voxel (corresponding to a $2 \times 2 \times 4$ mm brain volume), the image intensity changed over time and comprised a time series of data.

We computed the fMRI response amplitudes and phases by (1) removing the linear trend in the time series, (2) dividing each voxel's time series by its mean intensity, (3) averaging the resulting time series over the set of voxels corresponding to the stimulus representation within a previously defined visual area (see below), and (4) calculating the amplitude and phase of the best-fitting 36 s period sinusoid. The first step (removing the linear trend) is important because the fMRI signal tends to drift, for unknown reasons, very slowly over time. The second step is important because dividing by the mean intensity converts the data from arbitrary units of image intensity to units of fractional signal change.

The data were analyzed separately in each of four identifiable visual areas: left hemisphere V1, right hemisphere V1, left hemisphere MT+, and right hemisphere MT+. As mentioned in section 2.1, the effect of spatial attention on area V1 is of particular interest because of the precise retinotopic organization of area V1 and because of its unique position at the origin of visual cortical pathways. The effect on area MT+ is of particular interest because it is believed to play a central role in the kind of motion perception tasks performed by our subjects.

**Localizing V1**   Following well-established methods (Engel et al., 1994; Sereno et al., 1995; DeYoe et al., 1996; Engel et al., 1997), the organization of the retinotopic map with respect to polar angle of visual space was measured by recording fMRI responses while a radial stimulus rotated slowly around the center of the visual field (like the second hand of a clock). To visualize the results, a high-resolution MRI scan of each subject's brain was computationally flattened (Engel et al., 1997). In each cortical hemisphere, area V1 was identified as a large region of cortex in or near the calcarine sulcus with a retinotopic map corresponding to half of the contralateral visual field.

**Localizing MT+**   Human visual cortex contains an area in the lateral portion of the occipital lobe (MT+ or V5) that may be homologous to the complex of motion-sensitive areas MT, MST, and FST in the monkey (Zeki et al., 1991; Tootell and Taylor, 1995). The role of human MT+ in motion perception has been addressed previously, using a variety of techniques. Patients with lesions that include this brain area show deficits in motion perception (Zihl et al., 1983, 1991; Vaina et al., 1994, 1998). Transcranial magnetic stimulation (TMS) near MT+ in healthy volunteers interferes with motion perception

(Beckers and Hoemberg, 1992; Hotson et al., 1994; Beckers and Zeki, 1995). Functional neuroimaging studies have shown that MT+ is strongly activated when subjects view stimuli that appear to be moving, even illusory motion in stationary displays (Zeki et al., 1991, 1993; Watson et al., 1993; McCarthy et al., 1995; Tootell, Reppas, Dale, et al., 1995; Tootell, Reppas, Kwong, et al., 1995; Smith et al., 1998; Heeger et al., 1999). Activity in MT+ can be modulated by instructing subjects to selectively attend to moving stimuli (Corbetta et al., 1991; Beauchamp et al., 1997; O'Craven et al., 1997; Gandhi et al., 1999). In an fMRI study of dyslexia we observed a strong correlation between human MT+ activity and speed discrimination performance (Demb et al., 1997, 1998). Finally, MT+ responds selectively when subjects simply imagine visual motion stimuli (Goebel et al., 1998).

Following previous studies (Zeki et al., 1993; Watson et al., 1993; Tootell, Reppas, Kwong et al. 1995), we identified area MT+ based on fMRI responses to stimuli that alternated in time between moving and stationary dot patterns. The dots (small white dots on a black background) moved radially inward and outward, alternating direction once every second, for a total of 18 s (speed 10°/s). During the next 18 s, the dot pattern remained stationary. The entire cycle of moving and stationary dots was repeated 7 times. We computed the cross-correlation between each fMRI voxel's time series and a sinusoid with the same temporal period (36 s). We drew MT+ regions by hand around contiguous areas of strong activation, lateral to the junction between the calcarine sulcus and the parieto-occipital sulcus, and beyond the retinotopically organized visual areas.

Areas V1 and MT+ were defined only once per subject. Because the fMRI data recorded during successive scanning sessions in a given subject were all aligned to a common three-dimensional coordinate grid (see above), we could localize both areas reliably in all scanning sessions.

### 2.2.5  Eye Movements

Eye movements were recorded in a psychophysical setup (outside the scanner), with an infrared eye-tracking system (Ober2, Timra, Sweden).

### 2.3  Effect of Task Performance

In this experiment, we were interested in how the activity of visual cortex changes when the subject does not merely view a stimulus but performs a visual task. The stimulus consisted of concentric gratings moving radially inward and outward from fixation (inward and outward motion alternated to minimize motion aftereffects; figure 2.1). Subjects performed nine trials of a speed discrimination task during the first 18 s of each scan, and then passively viewed the next nine trials, without producing a response, and so on. Each

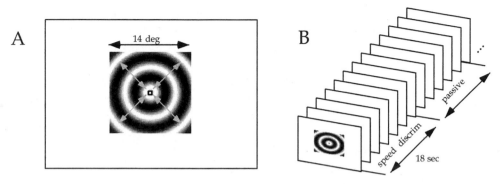

**Figure 2.1**
Design of task performance experiment. (*A*) The display consisted of a concentric sinusoidal grating moving radially inward or outward (diameter 14°). Inward and outward motion alternated to minimize motion aftereffects. (*B*) Every 18 s, the fixation mark changed color, cueing subjects either to perform a speed discrimination task or to view the stimulus passively. The task involved comparing the speed of two successive 1 s display periods.

fMRI scan consisted of 7 cycles, each 36 s, of the alternation between task performance and passive viewing. The fixation mark changed color every 18 s to instruct subjects either to perform the task (green) or to view the stimulus passively (red).

Each trial consisted of two stimulus intervals of 500 ms each, one in which the stimulus moved at base speed and another in which it moved at a slightly faster test speed (mean speed 8°/s). Following each trial, subjects indicated which interval contained the greater speed by pressing a button and received immediate feedback. As in previous studies of speed discrimination (McKee et al., 1986), we randomized irrelevant stimulus parameters so that subjects could base their response only on stimulus speed. In particular, stimulus contrast was randomized (16–24% contrast) so that subjects could not rely on apparent contrast, and stimulus duration was randomized (400–600 ms) so that subjects could not count the cycles of the stimulus. Spatial frequency was randomized (0.4–0.6 cycle/deg) so that subjects could not base their responses on temporal frequency.

During passive viewing, the stimuli were presented in a series of mock trials in which subjects did not make a response. Stimulus speed was the same during both intervals, preventing subjects from performing the task covertly (mean speed 8°/s). It is unlikely that removing the threshold-level velocity changes affected our fMRI measurements because (1) the average velocity per trial was the same during task performance and passive viewing trials; (2) the velocity changes were very small compared with the other stimulus attributes that were randomly varied from trial to trial; and (3) pilot experiments in which the increments were present showed the same pattern of results as scans with the increments removed.

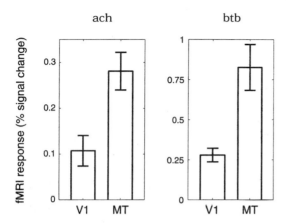

**Figure 2.2**
fMRI responses (percent MR signal modulation) evoked by alternating between task performance and passive viewing, in brain areas V1 and MT+ for two subjects. Height of each bar represents the mean of three to six measurements that were repeated in separate scans. Error bars represent ±1 standard error of the mean.

The results, shown in figure 2.2, demonstrate that brain activity in both brain areas (V1 and MT+) changed significantly as subjects alternated between task performance and passive viewing ($p < 0.02$, one-tailed t-test). Comparable modulations can be obtained with radially moving dot patterns instead of radially moving gratings (not shown).

Watanabe, Harner and colleagues (1998) had reported previously that activity in areas V1 and MT+ changes when subjects were instructed to alternately attend to and passively view a moving stimulus. The data in figure 2.2 essentially replicate that finding with task instructions which exert a clear control over the subject's behavioral state (i.e., using a two-interval forced-choice threshold-level discrimination task, as opposed to instructing subjects simply to attend).

## 2.4 Effect of Spatial Attention

We have just shown that activity in visual cortex is higher when a task is performed with respect to a stimulus than when a stimulus is viewed passively. However, the increase in cortical activity may be due to processes other than attention, for example, the heightened vigilance and arousal that probably accompany the performance of a task. To demonstrate that the increase in cortical activity is specifically due to attention, we need to demonstrate that it conforms to the known characteristics of attention, among which spatial selectivity ranks foremost. We therefore performed a second experiment to ascertain whether the increase in cortical activity is spatially selective, that is, whether the increase is restricted

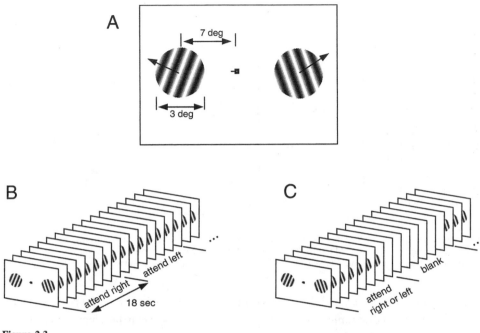

**Figure 2.3**
Design of spatial attention experiment. (*A*) Stimuli were moving sinusoidal gratings restricted to two peripheral, circular apertures (3° diameter, centered at 7° eccentricity). (*B*) In the spatial attention experiment, subjects performed a speed discrimination task in either the left or the right aperture (comparing two successive displays). Every 18 s the fixation mark changed, cueing subjects as to which aperture to attend. (*C*) Control experiment to help determine attentional modulation index. Subjects alternately performed the speed discrimination task (as in the spatial attention experiment) and passively viewed a blank display.

to task-relevant components of the stimulus rather than applying to relevant and irrelevant components alike.

In this experiment, two moving gratings (0.4 cycles/deg) were presented simultaneously within two apertures, one to the left and another to the right of fixation (figure 2.3A). Subjects were cued to attend to the right aperture during the first 7 trials (18 s), then to the left aperture during the next 7 trials (18 s), and so on (figure 2.3B). Each fMRI scan consisted of seven complete 36 s cycles of this right-left alternation. On each trial, subjects performed a speed discrimination task with respect to the cued aperture. Trials consisted of two stimulus intervals of 750 ms, separated by a blank interval of 250 ms (figure 2.3B). The mean speed varied randomly from trial to trial, in both the cued and (independently) the uncued apertures (7.5°/s to 12.5°/s). Following the two intervals, subjects were given a window of 820 ms to indicate during which interval the cued aperture had contained the greater speed. Feedback was provided immediately after pressing the button. During

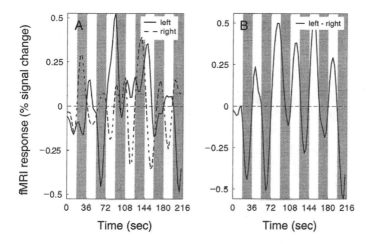

**Figure 2.4**
Time course of fMRI signal in area V1 while subject gmb alternated attention between the right and left stimulus
aperture. (A) Responses in the left (solid) and right (dashed) hemispheres. (B) Response in the left hemisphere
minus the response in the right hemisphere. Responses shown are averages taken over 8 repetitions.

the response period, the shape of the fixation mark changed to indicate which aperture
was to be attended during the next trial.

If the modulation of brain activity is spatially selective, as one would expect if it truly
reflects attention, fMRI responses in the *left* hemisphere should first increase and then
decrease when the right and left apertures are cued in that order. Conversely, fMRI responses in the *right* hemisphere should first decrease and then increase.

Figure 2.4 illustrates the results obtained from area V1 in the left and right hemispheres
of one subject. As expected, responses in area V1 of the left and right hemispheres tend
to be greater during the first (right-cued) and second (left-cued) half of each cycle, respectively (figure 2.4A). The effect is even more evident when we plot the difference between
the area V1 responses from the two hemispheres (figure 2.4B).

The results from two subjects are summarized in figure 2.5. The format used is a polar
plot, in which the amplitude of the fMRI response is represented by radial distance from
the origin, and the phase is represented by the angle from the positive x-axis. Phase angles
near 0° (right side of the plot) indicate that brain activity was greater when the *right*
aperture was cued. Phase angles near 180° (left side of the plot) indicate greater brain
activity when the *left* aperture was cued. The results for the *left* hemisphere (open symbols)
show that the peak of fMRI responses occurred during the right aperture cue. For the *right*
hemisphere (filled symbols), we find that peak fMRI responses coinicided with the left
aperture cue. For both subjects and in both V1 and MT+, the responses from the two

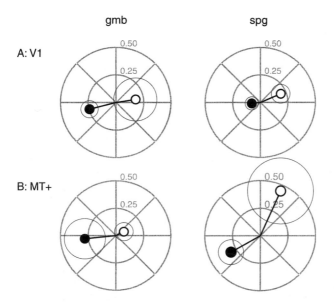

**Figure 2.5**
Polar plots of fMRI responses while the subjects alternated attention between the right and the left stimulus
aperture. (*A*) Attentional modulation in area V1. (*B*) Attentional modulation in MT+. Response amplitude (percent MR signal modulation) is indicated by radial distance from the origin, and response temporal phase is
indicated by the angle from the horizontal axis. Responses from the left hemisphere (open symbols) are near
0°, in phase with the cue to attend right. Responses from the right hemisphere (filled symbols) are near 180°,
in phase with the cue to attend left. Plot symbols represent the vector average of eight measurements that were
repeated in separate scans. Large circles represent 95% confidence intervals on the bivariate distributions of
response amplitudes and phases.

hemispheres were significantly different (p < 0.01, Hotelling t-test for significant difference between the two bivariate distributions). The slight counterclockwise phase shift of
peak fMRI responses is due to the 3–4 s time lag by which the hemodynamic changes
that give rise to the fMRI signal trail cortical activity (Boynton et al., 1996; Malonek and
Grinvald, 1996; Malonek et al., 1997).

The fMRI signals plotted in figure 2.5 indicate the difference in the cortical response
to attended and ignored stimulus apertures. However, the amplitudes of the fMRI signals
are difficult to interpret on their own. A small amplitude could result either when the
effect of attention is small or when the stimulus elicits only a small response to begin
with. To distinguish between these possibilities, we performed a control experiment. In
the control experiment, the grating stimuli were presented in both apertures for 18 s, and
then the subject viewed a uniform gray field for the next 18 s (figure 2.3C). In one series
of scans, subjects were cued to attend to the left aperture whenever the gratings were
presented. In a separate series of scans, subjects were cued to attend to the right aperture.

To compare the results of the control experiment with those of the attention experiment, we computed an attentional modulation index as the ratio of the mean signal amplitudes from both experiments. Specifically, the attentional modulation index (AMI) was computed as

$$AMI = 100 \times \frac{cued\ amplitude\ -\ uncued\ amplitude}{control\ amplitude}.$$

Similar indices are often used to quantify attentional effects in single-unit recording studies.

Figure 2.6 shows the means and standard errors of the AMI observed for two subjects and two cortical areas (V1 and MT+). A value of zero implies that there is no attentional modulation of the fMRI signal. A value of unity indicates that the attentional modulation of the fMRI signal is equivalent to switching the stimulus on and off.

The mean AMI values in V1 were 32% and 23% for subjects SPG and GMB, respectively. Comparing MT+ and and V1, we found essentially the same AMI value for GMB and a modestly increased AMI value for SPG. In single-unit recordings from monkey cortex, however, a much stronger attentional modulation is observed in area MT (Treue and Maunsell, 1996) than in area V1 (Press, 1998; McAdams and Maunsell, 1999). Also, more dramatic attentional modulations seem to have been observed in other fMRI studies of human area MT+ (Beauchamp et al., 1997; O'Craven et al., 1997).

It is conceivable that systematic, cue-correlated eye movements could have biased our measurements of attentional modulation, especially in V1, where cortical magnification

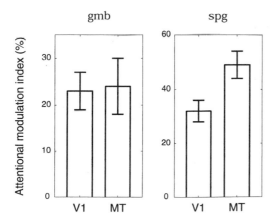

**Figure 2.6**
Mean and standard error of the spatial attentional modulation index for two subjects and for the brain areas V1 and MT+.

is substantially greater in the center than in the periphery of the visual field (Engel et al., 1997; Horton and Hoyt, 1991). Thus, if subjects were to consistently move their eyes toward the cued aperture, the cued stimulus would fall on more central parts of the visual field and evoke activity over a larger area of visual cortex. This would result in an overestimate of the attentional modulation in area V1.

To rule out this possibility, we recorded eye movements while subjects repeated the spatial attention experiment in a psychophysical laboratory (i.e., outside the scanner) because it was not possible to conduct these measurements during the scanning sessions themselves. We analyzed the time series of horizontal eye position at the periodicity corresponding to the alternation of the cue and the periodicity corresponding to stimulus presentation. In both subjects, the systematic (and potentially problematic) differences in eye position measured less than 0.15°. Since the cortical magnification factor in area V1 is known (Engel et al., 1997), we can estimate that this difference in eye position would change the cortical area stimulated by one of our stimulus apertures by less than 4%. Thus, eye movements can account for at most 4% of the 23% to 32% attentional modulation we have observed in V1.

## 2.5   Comparison with Behavioral Performance

To confirm that directing attention at the cued aperture had a positive effect on discrimination performance, we conducted a further control experiment. In this experiment, subjects were denied the benefit of the cue and had to monitor both apertures simultaneously (Verghese and Stone, 1995). The stimuli in this "spatial uncertainty" experiment were essentially the same as in the spatial attention experiment (see figure 2.3), the only difference being that a speed change occurred in only one (randomly chosen) aperture rather than in both. The size of the speed change was adjusted such that subjects achieved approximately 80% correct performance. Just as in the spatial attention experiment, subjects responded by indicating the interval with the greater speed.

In the spatial attention experiment, the chosen speed increments of 6% and 7% resulted in performance levels of 73% and 78% for subjects SPG and GMB, respectively. In the spatial uncertainty experiment, much larger speed increments were required to attain comparable levels of performance. Specifically, speed increments of 13% and 11.5% were needed for 78% and 74% performance, again for subjects SPG and GMB, respectively. Note that, by design, the performance of both subjects in both experiments was about the same ($p > 0.25$ and $p > 0.75$ for SPG and GMB, respectively). This shows that the cue in the spatial attention experiment is utilized to direct spatial attention, resulting in improved performance (or comparable performance with smaller speed increments).

We now turn to the relationship between brain activity and behavioral performance. Does the modulation of brain activity reported in the previous section *directly cause* the observed improvement of behavioral performance? To establish such a causal link would require consideration of a number of factors. At a minimum, there has to be a quantitative relationship between brain activity and behavioral performance. Here we test a specific model that predicts the quantitative relationship between our behavioral and neuroimaging data.

The basic idea of the model is that behavioral decisions depend on a sum of neuronal signals from both stimulus apertures. When attention is directed at the cued aperture, signals from this aperture are enhanced relative to signals from the other aperture. By enhancing task-relevant signals from the cued aperture and attenuating task-irrelevant signals from the uncued aperture, the effective signal-to-noise ratio improves and the frequency of correct decisions increases.

In constructing the model, we made assumptions about (1) the neuronal responses to stimulus speed, (2) the nature of the noise in the neuronal responses, and (3) the psychophysical decision rule. Specifically, we assumed that speed discrimination judgments are based on the responses of a population of neurons broadly tuned for stimulus speed. Substantial evidence supports the assumption that stimulus speed is computed and represented by neuronal populations in areas MT and MST. For example, lesion experiments with monkeys show that a lesion of areas MT/MST specifically impairs the animal's speed discrimination (Pasternak and Merigan, 1994; Orban et al., 1995). Figure 2.7A illustrates the speed tuning of our population of model neurons. This tuning is generally consistent with the speed tuning exhibited by neurons in the area MT of monkeys (Maunsell and Van Essen, 1983; Rodman and Albright, 1987; Simoncelli and Heeger, 1998).

Each stimulus presentation elicits a vector response, one response value per neuron. The expected, or most likely, value of the response follows directly from the speed tuning of each neuron. The actual response differs for each stimulus presentation because of noise. Specifically, we assume that the variance of the response is proportional to the expected value (mean), which approximates the situation for cortical neurons (Dean, 1981; Tolhurst et al., 1983; Bradley et al., 1987; Snowden et al., 1992; Britten et al., 1993):

$$\sigma_i^2(s) = \alpha \, r_i(s),$$

where $i$ is an index for neurons with different speed tuning, $s$ is stimulus speed, $r_i(s)$ is the mean response of the $i$th neuron, $\sigma_i^2(s)$ is the response variance, and $\alpha$ is a proportionality constant. This determines the joint probability distribution of the population response to a given stimulus speed.

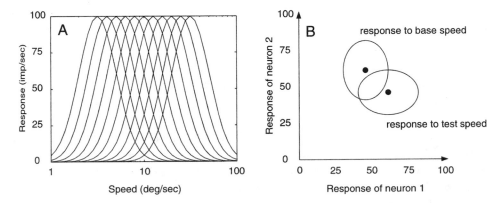

**Figure 2.7**
Speed discrimination model. (*A*) Speed tuning curves for a hypothetical population of model MT neurons. (*B*) Illustration of ideal observer decision rule for the case of two neurons. Neuronal responses are modeled as multivariate random variables. Plot symbols represent the mean responses of two neurons to each of two stimulus speeds. Ellipses represent one standard deviation of the noise in the responses. Responses to base speed and test speed are modeled as random draws from the upper-left and lower-right distributions, respectively. Performance (d′) depends on the amount of overlap between the two distributions (i.e., on the vector distance between the two means relative to the noise).

We further assume that the decision is optimal, that is, corresponds to an "ideal observer." An ideal observer has knowledge of the joint probability distribution of population responses to all possible stimuli, and adopts a maximum likelihood rule, to reach a decision about any particular stimulus. In the present context, the discriminability (d′) of two stimulus speeds depends on the vector distance between the response means $r_i(s)$ and also on the response variances $\sigma_i^2(s)$ (figure 2.7B) in the following way:

$$d' = \sqrt{\frac{2}{\beta} \sum_i \frac{[r_i(s_1) - r_i(s_2)]^2}{r_i(s_1) + r_i(s_2)}},$$

where $s_1$ and $s_2$ are the two stimulus speeds. The free parameter $\beta$ in this model corresponds essentially to the number of neurons. This was adjusted to match the performance of the subjects.

Finally, to predict performance in experiments with two stimulus apertures, we need to make some assumption as to how neuronal signals from the two apertures are combined. Here we follow previous psychophysical work on speed discrimination in multiple apertures (Verghese and Stone, 1995). Human performance on discriminating stimulus speed in one, two, four, or six apertures is explained by a model that sums noisy speed estimates from all apertures. As a result, performance decreases with the number of apertures. Such a model also agrees with subjects' verbal reports that their decision was based on the average speed perceived in both apertures during each stimulus interval.

Adopting the combination rule of Verghese and Stone (1995), we used two populations of speed-tuned neurons, one for each aperture. To predict performance in the spatial uncertainty experiment (when there was no cue), we summed responses from the two apertures for each pair of neurons with identical speed preference. As the speed changed in only one aperture, the addition of corresponding responses from the other aperture only increased the noise, thus yielding poorer performance. Figure 2.8A shows the predicted psychometric function for the spatial uncertainty experiment. To predict performance in the spatial attention experiment, we assumed that responses from the cued aperture were boosted by a factor of 2 prior to summation. This corresponds to an attentional modulation index of 50%, which is approximately what we observed in area MT+ for subject SPG. Figure 2.8B shows the predicted psychometric function for the spatial attention experiment.

The comparison of the psychometric functions in figures 2.8A and 2.8B reveals the different speed increments that are required for threshold performance in each experiment. The model predicts requisite speed increments of 7.25% and 12% for the spatial attention and spatial uncertainty experiments, respectively. This agrees almost exactly with the average speed increments of 6.5% and 12.25%, respectively, measured for both observers. An

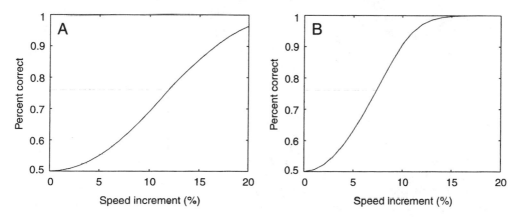

**Figure 2.8**
Simulated psychometric functions and speed increment thresholds. (A) Spatial uncertainty experiment: psychometric function when the signals from the two stimulus apertures are summed equally. Simulated threshold ($d' = 1$) corresponded to a 12% speed increment. (B) Spatial attention experiment: psychometric function when the signals from the cued aperture are given twice the weight as signals from the uncued aperture. Simulated threshold, 7.25% speed increment.

attentional modulation index of 50% is, therefore, sufficiently large to account for the measured improvement in behavioral performance.

## 2.6  Discussion

We found that visual responses in area V1 increase significantly when subjects perform a visual discrimination task (figures 2.1, 2.2) and, furthermore, that the increase is spatially selective and thus almost certainly a consequence of spatial attention (figures 2.3–2.6).

Our results contrast with a number of previous functional neuroimaging and ERP studies, which found no effect of attention in area V1 (Corbetta et al., 1993; Heinze et al., 1994; Woldorff et al., 1997; Beauchamp et al., 1997; Mangun et al., 1993; Gomez-Gonzalez et al., 1994; Clark and Hillyard, 1996; Mangun et al., 1997). There are several possible explanations for the discrepancy. First, it may be that the effect of attention in area V1 increases with the attentional demand of the behavioral task. If so, one expects to observe neural correlates of attention only when there are corresponding effects on behavioral performance. The spatial uncertainty experiment showed that our situation meets this condition, since the availability of a cue which can direct attention enhances performance. Second, our fMRI measurements offer superior spatial localization compared with other human neuroimaging techniques such as PET and ERP. Our analysis was restricted to a small part of area V1 that is responsive to the stimulus aperture. Third, attention may elevate background firing rates without increasing the stimulus-evoked response (Luck et al., 1997). In this case, the fMRI response would reflect both the elevated background and the increased stimulus-evoked response, whereas ERP would be sensitive only to the latter. Fourth, the fMRI measurements might reflect a delayed activation of area V1 due to feedback from extrastriate cortical areas (Aine et al., 1995; Martinez et al., 1999).

Although there have been previous claims of spatially selective effects of attention in area V1, in some of these studies the spatially selective effect of attention was confounded by the more general effects of performing a visual task. For example, Watanabe, Sasaki, and colleagues (1998) instructed subjects either to discriminate stimuli presented to the left or right of fixation, or to view them passively. Obviously, the two situations differ in two respects: whether or not a task is performed and (possibly) whether or not attention is directed to the left or right of fixation. In a study by Somers and colleagues (1999), subjects discriminated either a sequence of letters in the central visual field or the direction of motion of stimuli in the peripheral visual field. Once again the two situations differ in two respects: the nature of the task and the attended part of the visual field. In our spatial experiment, only the attended part of the visual field changed; the nature of the task remained the same. This paradigm allowed us to distinguish between the neural effects of spatial attention and the more general neural consequences of performing different visual tasks.

The presence of a cue that can direct attention to one spatial location or another changes brain activity in a consistent and systematic fashion. In area V1, the size of the attentional modulation reached approximately 25% of the response to the stimulus itself. This is considerably more than the 5–10% effects that have been reported for single-unit recordings in monkeys (Press, 1998; McAdams and Maunsell, 1999). However, there are numerous possible reasons for the discrepancy between functional imaging and single-unit recording results. First, little is known about the relationship between fMRI responses and the underlying neuronal firing rates (see below), and a sufficiently nonlinear relationship would complicate the comparison substantially. Second, small shifts in eye position, equal in size to the V1 receptive fields, present a difficulty for the electrophysiology experiments. If eye position is systematically correlated with shifts in spatial attention, then the responses of individual V1 neurons will modulate as the receptive fields are shifted toward and away from the stimulus (Maunsell, 1995). These potential biases can be avoided by carefully accounting for eye position (Press, 1998; McAdams and Maunsell, 1999), but perhaps at a cost of underestimating the magnitude of the attentional effects. Small shifts in eye position do not present a difficulty in the fMRI experiments because they have a negligible effect on measurements of pooled neuronal activity. Third, because of the difficulty of training monkeys on a demanding task, single-unit experiments tend to employ relatively undemanding behavioral situations that may involve attention only to a lesser extent, or not at all. For this reason it is critical to demonstrate that behavioral performance varies with attention (as we have done). A fourth and related reason is that monkeys may have been overtrained, with the result that task performance again does not involve attention. That training can have a critical impact on attentional effects at the level of single units is shown by Ito and colleagues (chapter 5 of this volume). Finally, there may be a genuine species difference so that the attentional effects we observe in area V1 of human subjects are simply not present in monkeys.

### 2.6.1 Assumptions for Comparing fMRI and Behavior

We interpreted the correlation between the magnitude of fMRI responses and levels of behavioral performance, given four assumptions. We now discuss each assumption in turn.

First, we assumed that the primary effect of attention is to increase the stimulus-evoked response of neurons (firing rates). This need not be the case. Attention may instead elevate background firing rates and/or increase neuronal firing at a time when the stimulus-evoked response has passed (via feedback from higher cortical areas). Presumably, fMRI responses would reflect all three kinds of changes: changes in stimulus-evoked firing, background firing, and delayed firing. Thus, further experiments will be necessary to vali-date this assumption.

Second, we assumed that fMRI responses are proportional to the average activity of a local population of neurons. The chain of events between neuronal firing and the meas-urement of an fMRI signal is complicated and poorly understood (Buxton et al., 1998; Malonek et al., 1996, 1997). It is unlikely that the complex interaction between neuronal firing, regional blood flow, and the MR scanner produces a precise numerical average of neuronal firing rates. Even so, it would appear that a numerical average is a reasonable approximation of these interactions. Indeed, we have tested this assumption in two ways (Boynton et al., 1996): (1) the dependence of fMRI responses on stimulus timing and that on stimulus contrast are *separable,* and (2) fMRI responses to brief stimuli predict re-sponses to long stimuli. Although this does not prove that fMRI responses are proportional to average firing rates (there could still be hidden nonlinearities), these results are certainly consistent with this possibility. In addition, in a study of motion perception, we found that fMRI signals recorded from the human brain are correlated with electrophysiological responses (average spiking activity) recorded in the monkey brain (Heeger et al., 1999). Hopefully, the recent advances in performing fMRI measurements on monkeys will soon provide far better information about the relationship between fMRI signals and neuronal activity.

Third, we made certain assumptions about the neuronal noise, specifically, that response variance increases in proportion to the response mean. This assumption is consistent with the preponderance of evidence (Dean, 1981; Tolhurst et al., 1983; Bradley et al., 1987; Snowden et al., 1992; Britten et al., 1993), but it ignores the modest degree of covariation in the firing patterns of neighboring neurons (Zohary et al., 1994).

Fourth, we made certain assumptions as to how neuronal signals from the two stimulus apertures are combined, and as to how the population response is analyzed in order to determine the faster of the two stimulus intervals in every trial. However, these assump-tions appear to be quite reasonable and have proven their value in psychophysical studies (e.g., Verghese and Stone, 1995).

## 2.7  Summary

Visual responses are modulated by top-down factors even at the very earliest levels of visual processing. Performing a task and directing attention to a particular location can alter visual responses in areas as early as V1. In the face of these observations, it is clear that fMRI studies of human vision need to control for behavioral states in general and for attentional states in particular. Stimulus-evoked responses cannot be properly assessed under conditions of passive viewing.

A simple model relates the behavioral effects of spatial attention to the magnitude of fMRI signal changes. According to this model, the role of attention is twofold. First, attention increases the signal-to-noise ratio of task-relevant signals at the cued location and, second, attention decreases the contribution from task-irrelevant signals elsewhere in the field of view (see Chapter 5 in this volume for a similar point of view). This makes it possible to account for the results with an extremely simple strategy (summing/averaging) for combining the relevant and irrelevant neuronal signals.

The model demonstrates that the measured modulations in brain activity are comparable with (although somewhat smaller than) those needed to explain the improvement of behavioral performance with attention. However, the details of the model are unlikely to withstand rigorous scrutiny. The simple rule for combining relevant and irrelevant signals, the statistically efficient decision, and the exclusive reliance on neuronal activity in one visual area (MT+) are all likely to oversimplify the true situation. Even so, the model provides a useful starting point for relating brain-imaging results to behavioral measures. It would certainly be useful to compare imaging and behavioral results for other visual tasks, such as contrast discrimination (see Boynton et al., 1999), contrast detection, and orientation discrimination. Other promising areas of application are the effects of task difficulty and of dividing attention on neuronal responses, both of which are poorly understood.

Finally, this study demonstrates that some questions may be more easily answered by functional imaging than by single-unit electrophysiology. Naturally, there are many questions that cannot be addressed with functional imaging. However, functional imaging is eminently suitable for the basic question of quantifying attentional effects in early visual cortex.

## Acknowledgments

Special thanks to G. H. Glover and the Richard M. Lucas Center for Magnetic Resonance Spectroscopy and Imaging, supported by an NIH National Center for Research Resources grant, for technical support. DJH was supported by an NEI grant (R01-EY11794) and an NIMH grant (R29-MH50228). SPG was supported by a Stanford University undergraduate research opportunities grant. ACH was supported by an NSF graduate student fellowship. GMB was supported by an NIMH postdoctoral research fellowship.

## References

Aine, C. J., Supek, S., and George, J. S. (1995). Temporal dynamics of visual-evoked neuromagnetic sources: Effects of stimulus parameters and selective attention. *Internat. J. Neurosci.* 80: 79–104.

Beauchamp, M. S., Cox, R. W., and DeYoe, E. A. (1997). Graded effects of spatial and featural attention on human area MT and associated motion processing area. *J. Neurophysiol.* 78: 516–520.

Beckers, G., and Hoemberg, V. (1992). Transitory akinetopsia induced by transcranial magnetic stimulation of human area V5. *Proc. R. Soc. London* B249: 173–178.

Beckers, G., and Zeki, S. (1995). The consequences of inactivating areas V1 and V5 on visual motion perception. *Brain* 118: 49–60.

Belliveau, J. W., Kennedy, D. N., McKinstry, R. C., Buchbinder, B. R., Weisskoff, R. M., Cohen, M. S., Vevea, J. M., Brady, T. J., and Rosen, B. R. (1991). Functional mapping of the human visual cortex by magnetic resonance imaging. *Science* 254: 716–719.

Boynton, G. M., Engel, S. A., Glover, G. H., and Heeger, D. J. (1996). Linear systems analysis of fMRI in human V1. *J Neurosci.* 16: 4207–4221.

Boynton, G. M., Demb, J. B., Glover, G. H., and Heeger, D. J. (1999). Neural basis of contrast discrimination. *Vis. Res.* 39: 257–269.

Bradley, A., Skottun, B., Ohzawa, I., Sclar, G., and Freeman, R. D. (1987). Visual orientation and spatial frequency discrimination: A comparison of single neurons and behavior. *J. Neurophysiol.* 57: 755–772.

Brefczynski, J. A., and DeYoe, E. A. (1999). A physiological correlate of the "spotlight" of visual attention. *Nature Neurosci.* 2: 370–374.

Britten, K. H., Shadlen, M. N., Newsome, W. T., and Movshon, J. A. (1993). Responses of neurons in macaque MT to stochastic motion signals. *Vis. Neurosci.* 10: 1157–1169.

Buchel, C., Josephs, O., Rees, G., Turner, R., Frith, C. D., and Friston, K. J. (1998). The functional anatomy of attention to visual motion. *Brain* 121: 1281–1294.

Bushnell, M. C., Goldberg, M. E., and Robinson, D. L. (1981). Behavioral enhancement of visual responses in monkey cerebral cortex. I. Modulation of posterior parietal cortex related to selective visual attention. *J.Neurophysiol.* 46: 755–772.

Buxton, R. B., Wong, E. C., and Frank, L. R. (1998). Dynamics of blood flow and oxygenation changes during brain activation: The balloon model. *Magn. Reson. Med.* 39: 855–864.

Clark, V. P., and Hillyard, S. A. (1996). Spatial selective attention affects early extrastriate but not striate components of the visual evoked potential. *J. Cog. Neurosci.* 8: 387–402.

Corbetta, M., Miezin, F. M., Dobmeyer, S., Shulman, G. L., and Petersen, S. E. (1991). Selective and divided attention during visual discriminations of shape, color, and speed: Functional anatomy by positron emission tomography. *J. Neurosci.* 11: 2383–2402.

Corbetta, M., Miezin, F. M., Shulman, G. L., and Petersen, S. E. (1993). A PET study of visuospatial attention. *J. Neurosci.* 13: 1202–1226.

Crick, F. (1984). Function of the thalamic reticular complex: The searchlight hypothesis. *Proc. Nat. Acad. Sci. USA* 81: 4586–4590.

Culham, J., Brandt, S., Cavanagh, P., Kanwisher, N., Dale, A., and Tootell, R. (1998). Cortical fMRI activation produced by attentive tracking of moving targets. *J. Neurophysiol.* 80: 2657–2670.

Dean, A. F. (1981). The variability of discharge of simple cells in the cat striate cortex. *Exp. Brain Res.* 44: 437–440.

Demb, J. B., Boynton, G. M., and Heeger, D. J. (1997). Brain activity in visual cortex predicts individual differences in reading performance. *Proc. Nat. Acad. Sci. USA* 94: 13363–13366.

Demb, J. B., Boynton, G. M., and Heeger, D. J. (1998). fMR imaging of early visual pathways in dyslexia. *J. Neurosci.* 18: 6939–6951.

Desimone, R., and Duncan, J. (1995). Neural mechanisms of selective visual attention. *Ann. Rev. Neurosci.* 18: 193–222.

DeYoe, E. A., Carman, G. J., Bandettini, P., Glickman, S., Wieser, J., Cox, R., Miller, D., and Neitz, J. (1996). Mapping striate and extrastriate visual areas in human cerebral cortex. *Proc. Nat. Acad. Sci. USA* 93: 2382–2386.

Engel, S. A., Glover, G. H., and Wandell, B. A. (1997). Retinotopic organization in human visual cortex and the spatial precision of functional MRI. *Cereb. Cortex* 7: 181–192.

Engel, S. A., Rumelhart, D. E., Wandell, B. A., Lee, A. T., Glover, G. H., Chichilnisky, E. J., and Shadlen, M. N. (1994). fMRI of human visual cortex. *Nature* 369: 525.

Gandhi, S. P., Heeger, D. J., and Boynton, G. M. (1998). Spatial attention in human primary visual cortex. *Invest. Ophthalmol. Vis. Sci.* suppl. 39: S1130.

Gandhi, S. P., Heeger, D. J., and Boynton, G. M. (1999). Spatial attention affects brain activity in human primary visual cortex. *Proc. Nat. Acad. Sci. USA* 96: 3314–3319.

Glover, G. H., and Lai, S. (1998). Self-navigating spiral fMRI: Interleaved versus single-shot. *Magn. Reson. Med.* 39: 361–368.

Goebel, R., Khorram-Sefat, D., Muckli, L., Hacker, H., and Singer, W. (1998). The constructive natures of vision: Direct evidence from functional magnetic resonance imaging studies of apparent motion and motion imagery. *Euro. J. Neurosci.* 10: 1563–1573.

Gomez-Gonzalez, C. M., Clark, V. P., Fan, S., Luck, S. J., and Hillyard, S. A. (1994). Sources of attention-sensitive visual event-related potentials. *Brain Topog.* 7: 41–51.

Graham, N. (1989). *Visual pattern analyzers*. New York: Oxford University Press.

Gratton, G. (1997). Attention and probability effects in the human occipital cortex: An optical imaging study. *Neuroreport* 8: 1749–1753.

Heeger, D. J., Boynton, G. M., Demb, J. B., Seidemann, E., and Newsome, W. T. (1999). Motion opponency in visual cortex. *J. Neurosci.* 19: 7162–7174.

Heinze, H. J., Mangun, G. R., Burchert, W., Hinrichs, H., Scholz, M., Munte, T. F., Gos, A., Scherg, M., Johannes, S., Hundeshagen, H., Gazzaniga, M. S., and Hillyard, S. A. (1994). Combined spatial and temporal imaging of brain activity during visual selective attention in humans. *Nature* 372: 543–546.

Horton, J. C., and Hoyt, W. F. (1991). The representation of the visual field in human striate cortex. *Arch. Ophthalmol.* 109: 816–824.

Hotson, J., Braun, D., Herzberg, W., and Boman, D. (1994). Transcranial magnetic stimulation of extrastriate cortex degrades human motion direction discrimination. *Vis. Res.* 34: 2115–2123.

Huk, A. C., and Heeger, D. J. (2000). Task-related modulation of visual cortex. *J. Neurophysiol.* 83: 3525–3536.

Ito, M., and Gilbert, C. D. (1999). Attention modulates contextual influences in the primary visual cortex of alert monkeys. *Neuron* 22: 593–604.

Kastner, S., De Weerd, P. D., Desimone, R., and Ungerleider, L. G. (1998). Mechanisms of directed attention in the human extrastriate cortex as revealed by functional MRI. *Science* 282: 108–111.

Koch, C., and Ullman, S. (1985). Shifts in selective visual attention: Towards the underlying neural circuitry. *Hum. Neurobiol.* 4: 219–227.

Kwong, K. K., Belliveau, J. W., Chesler, D. A., Goldberg, I. E., Weiskoff, R. M., Poncelet, B. P., Kennedy, D. N., Hoppel, B. E., Cohen, M. S., Turner, R., Cheng, H.-M., Brady, T. J., and Rosen, B. R. (1992). Dynamic magnetic resonance imaging of human brain activity during primary sensory stimulation. *Proc. Nat. Acad. Sci. USA* 89: 5675–5679.

Luck, S. J., Chelazzi, L., Hillyard, S. A., and Desimone, R. (1997). Neural mechanisms of spatial selective attention in areas V1, V2, and V4 of macaque visual cortex. *J. Neurophysiol.* 7: 24–42.

Malonek, D., Dirnagl, U., Lindauer, U., Yamada, K., Kanno, I., and Grinvald, A. (1997). Vascular imprints of neuronal activity: Relationships between the dynamics of cortical blood flow, oxygenation, and volume changes following sensory stimulation. *Proc. Nat. Acad. Sci. USA* 94: 14826–14831.

Malonek, D., and Grinvald, A. (1996). Interactions between electrical activity and cortical microcirculation revealed by imaging spectroscopy: Implications for functional brain mapping. *Nature* 272: 551–554.

Mangun, G. R., Hillyard, S. A., and Luck, S. J. (1993). Electrocortical substrates of visual selective attention. In D. Meyer and S. Kornblum (eds.), *Attention and performance XIV* (pp 219–243). Cambridge, MA: MIT Press.

Mangun, G. R., Hopfinger, J. B., Kussmaul, C. L., Fletcher, E. M., and Heinze, H. J. (1997). Covariations in ERP and PET measures of spatial selective attention in human extrastriate visual cortex. *Hum. Brain Mapping* 5: 273–279.

Martinez, A., Aullo-Vento, L., Sereno, M. I., Frank, L. R., Buxton, R. B., Dubowitz, D. J., Wong, E. C., Hinrichs, H. J., and Hillyard, S. A. (1999). Involvement of striate and extrastriate visual cortical areas in spatial attention. *Nature Neurosci.* 2: 364–369.

Maunsell, J. H. R. (1995). The brain's visual world: Representation of visual targets in cerebral cortex. *Science* 270: 764–769.

Maunsell, J. H. R., and Van Essen, D. C. (1983). Functional properties of neurons in middle temporal visual area of the macaque monkey. I. Selectivity for stimulus direction, speed, and orientation. *J. Neurophysiol.* 49: 1127–1147.

McAdams, C. J., and Maunsell, J. H. R. (1999). Effects of attention on orientation-tuning functions of single neurons in macaque cortical area V4. *J Neurosci.* 19: 431–441.

McCarthy, G., Spicer, M., Adrignolo, A., Luby, M., Gore, J., and Allison, T. (1995). Brain activation associated with visual motion studied by functional magnetic resonance imaging in humans. *Hum. Brain Mapping* 2: 234–243.

McKee, S. P., Silverman, G. H., and Nakayama, K. (1986). Precise velocity discrimination despite random variations in temporal frequency and contrast. *Vis. Res.* 26(4): 609–619.

Moran, A. J., and Desimone, R. (1985). Selective attention gates visual processing in the extrastriate cortex. *Science* 229: 782–784.

Motter, B. C. (1993). Focal attention produces spatially selective processing in visual cortical areas V1, V2, and V4 in the presence of competing stimuli. *J. Neurophysiol.* 70: 909–919.

Noll, D., Cohen, J., Meyer, C., and Schneider, W. (1995). Spiral k-space MR imaging of cortical activation. *JMRI* 5: 49–57.

O'Craven, K. M., Rosen, B. R., Kwong, K. K., Treisman, A., and Savoy, R. L. (1997). Voluntary attention modulates fMRI activity in human MT–MST. *Neuron* 18: 591–598.

Ogawa, S., Lee, T., Kay, A., and Tank, D. (1990). Brain magnetic resonance imaging with contrast dependent on blood oxygenation. *Proc. Nat. Acad. Sci. USA* 87: 9868–9872.

Ogawa, S., Tank, D., Menon, R., Ellermann, J., Kim, S., Merkle, H., and Ugurbil, K. (1992). Intrinsic signal changes accompanying sensory stimulation: Functional brain mapping using MRI. *Proc. Nat. Acad. Sci. USA* 89: 5951–5955.

Orban, G. A., Saunders, R. C., and Vandenbussche, E. (1995). Lesions of the superior temporal cortical motion areas impair speed discrimination in the macaque monkey. *Euro. J. Neurosci.* 7: 2261–2276.

Pashler, H. E. (1998). *The psychology of attention.* Cambridge, MA: MIT Press.

Pasternak, T., and Merigan, W. H. (1994). Motion perception following lesions of the superior temporal sulcus in the monkey. *Cereb. Cortex* 4: 247–259.

Press, B. (1998). Effects of spatial attention on macaque primary visual cortex. Ph.D. diss., California Institute of Technology.

Rodman, H. R., and Albright, T. D. (1987). Coding of visual stimulus velocity in area MT of the macaque. *Vis. Res.* 27: 2035–2048.

Sereno, M. I., Dale, A. M., Reppas, J. B., Kwong, K. K., Belliveau, J. W., Brady, T. J., Rosen, B. R., and Tootell, R. B. H. (1995). Borders of multiple visual areas in humans revealed by functional magnetic resonance imaging. *Science* 268: 889–893.

Simoncelli, E. P., and Heeger, D. J. (1998). A model of neural responses in visual area MT. *Vis. Res.* 38: 743–761.

Smith, A. T., Greenlee, M.W., Singh, K. D., Kraemer, F. M., and Hennig, J. (1998). The processing of first- and second-order motion in human visual cortex assessed by functional magnetic resonance imaging (fMRI). *J. Neurosci.* 18: 3816–3830.

Snowden, R. J., Treue, S., and Andersen, R. A. (1992). The response of neurons in areas V1 and MT of the alert rhesus monkey to moving random dot patterns. *Exp. Brain Res.* 88: 389–400.

Somers, D. C., Dale, A. M., Seiffert, A. E., and Tootell, R. B. H. (1999). Functional MRI reveals spatially specific attentional modulation in human primary visual cortex. *Proc. Nat. Acad. Sci. USA* 96: 1663–1668.

Tolhurst, D. J., Movshon, J. A., and Dean, A. F. (1983). The statistical reliability of single neurons in cat and monkey visual cortex. *Vis. Res.* 23: 775–785.

Tootell, R. B., and Taylor, J. B. (1995). Anatomical evidence for MT and additional cortical visual areas in humans. *Cereb. Cortex* 5: 39–55.

Tootell, R. B. H., Hadjikhani, N., Hall, E. K., Marrett, S., Vanduffel, W., Vaughan, J. T., and Dale, A. M. (1998). The retinotopy of visual spatial attention. *Neuron* 21: 1409–1422.

Tootell, R. B. H., Reppas, J. B., Dale, A. M., Look, R. B., Sereno, M. I., Malach, R., Brady, T. J., and Rosen, B. R. (1995). Visual motion aftereffect in human cortical area MT revealed by functional magnetic resonance imaging. *Nature* 375: 139–141.

Tootell, R. B. H., Reppas, J. B., Kwong, K. K., Malach, R., Born, R. T., Brady, T. J., Rosen, B. R., and Belliveau, J. W. (1995). Functional analysis of human MT and related visual cortical areas using magnetic resonance imaging. *J. Neurosci.* 15: 3215–3230.

Treue, S., and Maunsell, J. H. R. (1996). Attentional modulation of visual motion processing in cortical areas MT and MST. *Nature* 382: 539–541.

Vaina, L. M., Grzywacz, N. M., and Kikinis, R. (1994). Segregation of computations underlying perception of motion discontinuity and coherence. *NeuroReport* 5: 2289–2294.

Vaina, L. M., Makris, N., Kennedy, D., and Cowey, A. (1998). The selective impairment of the perception of first-order motion by unilateral cortical brain damage. *Vis. Neurosci.* 15: 333–348.

Verghese, P. and Stone, L. S. (1995). Combining speed information across space. *Vis. Res.* 35: 2811–2824.

Watanabe, T., Harner, A. M., Miyauchi, S., Sasaki, Y., Nielsen, M., Palomo, D., and Mukai, I. (1998). Task-dependent influences of attention on the activation of human primary visual cortex. *Proc. Nat. Acad. Sci. USA* 95:11489–11492.

Watanabe, T., Sasaki, Y., Miyauchi, S., Putz, B., Fujimaki, N., Nielsen, M., Takino, R., and Miyakawa, S. (1998). Attention-regulated activity in human primary visual cortex. *J. Neurophysiol.* 79: 2218–2221.

Watson, J. D. G., Myers, R., Frackowiak, R. S. J., Hajnal, J. V., Woods, R. P., Mazziotta, J. C., Shipp, S., and Zeki, S. (1993). Area V5 of the human brain: Evidence from a combined study using positron emission tomography and magnetic resonance imaging. *Cereb. Cortex* 3: 79–94.

Woldorff, M. G., Fox, P. T., Matzke, M., Lancaster, J. L., Veeraswamy, S., Zamarripa, F., Seabolt, M., Glass, T., Gao, J. H., Martin, C. C., and Jerabek, P. (1997). Retinotopic organization of early visual spatial attention effects as revealed by PET and ERPs. *Hum. Brain Mapping* 5: 280–286.

Zeki, S., Watson, J. D. G., and Frackowiak, R. S. J. (1993). Going beyond the information given: The relation of illusory visual motion to brain activity. *Proc. R. Soc. London* B252: 215–222.

Zeki, S., Watson, J. D. G., Lueck, C. J., Friston, K. J., Kennard, C., and Frackowiak, R. S. (1991). A direct demonstration of functional specialization in human visual cortex. *J. Neurosci.* 11: 641–649.

Zihl, J., von Cramon, D., and Mai, N. (1983). Selective disturbance of movement vision after bilateral brain damage. *Brain* 106: 313–340.

Zihl, J., von Cramon, D., Mai, N., and Schmid, C. H. (1991). Disturbance of movement vision after bilateral posterior brain damage: Further evidence and follow up observations. *Brain* 114: 2235–2252.

Zohary, E., Shadlen, M. N., and Newsome, W. T. (1994). Correlated neuronal discharge rate and its implications for psychophysical performance. *Nature* 370: 140–143.

# 3 Capacity Limits in Selective Attention: Behavioral Evidence and Implications for Neural Activity

Nilli Lavie

## 3.1 Introduction

Selective attention involves focusing on *relevant* stimuli and avoiding distraction by *irrelevant* stimuli. Although all theories of attention agree that relevant and irrelevant information are processed differently, there is no consensus as to exactly which processes are affected by withholding attention. In particular, it remains an open question whether withholding attention can exclude irrelevant stimuli from perception (early selection; Treisman, 1969) or whether attention affects primarily postperceptual processes such as memory or responses (late selection; Duncan, 1980). The debate between the early and late selection views concerning the extent to which irrelevant stimuli are or are not perceived has stimulated much psychological research in the last few decades. However, no resolution has been reached, because substantial evidence has accumulated to support both points of view (Lavie and Tsal, 1994). In other words, there is good evidence that irrelevant information can be ignored and prevented from affecting perception (e.g., Yantis and Johnston, 1990), and also that irrelevant information cannot be ignored, and does affect perception (e.g., Tipper and Driver, 1988).

The existence of both kinds of evidence has led to a theoretical impasse for many years. In spite of this difficulty, the question of whether attention gates perceptual or postperceptual processing remains central. More recently, a fresh element has entered the debate through functional neuroimaging, which has provided several demonstrations that attention can indeed attenuate the perceptual processing of irrelevant information (Corbetta and Shulman, chapter 1 in this volume; Corbetta et al., 1991; O'Craven et al., 1997; Beauchamp et al., 1997; Kastner et al., 1998). Single-unit studies in the awake monkey confirm that attention reduces neuronal responses to irrelevant stimuli in visual cortex, which presumably reflects perceptual processing (Desimone and Duncan, 1995; Treue and Maunsell, 1996; Luck et al., 1997; Reynolds and Desimone, chapter 7 in this volume; Maunsell and McAdams, chapter 6 in this volume). Although these recent results favor early selection views in that they show attentional effects on perceptual processing, they do not resolve the early versus late selection debate, because they do not explain why attention would fail to affect perception in some situations (i.e., the psychological studies supporting late selection). Given the ample evidence that attention sometimes results in selective and sometimes in nonselective perception, a hybrid model may provide a better account of the diverse data than either a strict early selection or a strict late selection view.

I have recently suggested such a hybrid model, which combines aspects from both views of attention (Lavie, 1995). According to this model, perception has limited capacity (early selection view) but, *within these limits,* proceeds automatically for all stimuli (late selection view). The critical point is that attention prevents perception beyond, but not within, the capacity limit. Thus, irrelevant information is processed as long as it falls within this limit, but fails to be processed as soon as it exceeds the limit. A logical consequence of this model is that the extent to which irrelevant information is processed should depend on the *perceptual load* in the processing of relevant information. Situations in which relevant processing imposes a high perceptual load will exhaust available capacity, and will prevent the processing of irrelevant information. Conversely, when relevant processing imposes only a low perceptual load, substantial capacity will remain available, and spill over into the processing of irrelevant information.

Thus, given a perceptual load model of attention, conditions of high load predict early selection (i.e., selective perception), whereas conditions of low load predict late selection (i.e., nonselective perception). This chapter presents behavioral evidence for a perceptual load model, describes experimental tests of its implications for neural activity in the brain, and offers further implications for neurological deficits due to normal aging or brain injury.

## 3.2   Empirical Support for a Perceptual Load Model

### 3.2.1   Response Competition

A review of psychological studies relevant to the early selection versus late selection debate lends broad support to a perceptual load model (Lavie and Tsal, 1994). Typically, evidence for selective perception has been obtained in situations of high perceptual load, whereas evidence for nonselective perception has been found in situations of low perceptual load. Further evidence for a perceptual load model comes from a series of new experiments, which assess the extent to which irrelevant information is processed while manipulating the perceptual load posed by relevant information. In a typical experiment of this series, task-relevant stimuli (targets) appear at the display center while task-irrelevant stimuli (distractors) are presented at peripheral positions. The subject's task is to discriminate as quickly as possible between two alternative targets, for example, the letters X and N, while ignoring any distractors. In this situation, the extent to which distractors are processed can be assessed through indirect effects on the target response (response competition; Eriksen and Eriksen, 1974). The principle of this method is to employ distractors that are either *incompatible* with the correct target response (e.g., distractor X with target N), *compatible* with the correct response (e.g., distractor X with target X), or *neutral* with respect to the correct response (e.g., distractor S with target X). If target responses are significantly slower in the presence of incompatible distractors than in the presence of either compatible or neutral distractors, then this indicates that distractors were perceived.

Perceptual load can be manipulated in several ways, for example, by varying the number of target stimuli (i.e., set size) or by altering the processing requirements (e.g., discriminating either a target feature or a conjunction of target features). In one such experiment, subjects searched several letters near the center of the display for one of two target letters while ignoring irrelevant distractors in the periphery of the display (Lavie and Cox, 1997). Search load was manipulated by varying the similarity between the targets and nontargets in the center. For example, subjects searched for X or N targets among similar nontargets (e.g., V, Z, or H) in the high load condition, and among dissimilar nontargets (e.g., O) in the low load condition. In another experiment of this kind, search load was manipulated by varying the number of nontarget letters. We consistently found that efficient searches (i.e., with flat search slopes) led to inefficient rejection of distractors (i.e., response times depended on the nature of the distractor), presumably because the perceptual load was low and additional capacity remained available. By contrast, inefficient searches (i.e., with steep search slopes) led to efficient rejection of distractors (i.e., response times were independent of distractor identity), as long as they involved more than four nontargets so that capacity was exhausted (for other evidence that capacity limits arise at about four to five items, see Fisher, 1982; Yantis and Jones, 1991; Kahneman et al., 1993; Pylyshyn et al., 1994).

A concern in the interpretation of these studies is that high and low load conditions differed with respect to the physical display (i.e., in the shape or number of nontargets), and this might have led to differences other than load in perceptual processing. However, similar results are obtained when high and low load conditions are created by varying processing requirements in identical displays (Lavie, 1995). Figure 3.1 illustrates the task used in this study. Subjects discriminated a central target letter as quickly as possible (X or N) while attempting to ignore a peripheral distractor. However, the task also involved an additional go/no-go component, which depended on the shape (circle or line) of another central stimulus adjacent to the target letter. In the low load condition, subjects responded to the target when the adjacent shape was present and withheld the response when it was absent. In the high load condition, the decision as to whether or not to respond to the target depended on the exact size of the line or the exact position of the circle. A line of "normal" length or circle of "normal" position meant that the subject was to go ahead with the target response, whereas a slightly longer line or slightly displaced circle meant that the subject was to withhold a response. The analysis of the results focused on the "go" trials, in which the displays for high and low load conditions were exactly the same (figure 3.1). Once again the outcome was as expected from a perceptual load model: response competition from distractors was observed under low load conditions (i.e., reaction times were longer with incompatible than with compatible or neutral distractors), but not under high load conditions. Similar results were obtained when the go/no-go decision required the processing of either a simple feature (low load) or of a conjunction of features (high load).

**LOW LOAD - DETECTION**

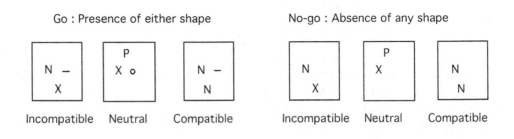

Go : Presence of either shape                    No-go : Absence of any shape

Incompatible   Neutral   Compatible        Incompatible   Neutral   Compatible

**HIGH LOAD - IDENTIFICATION**

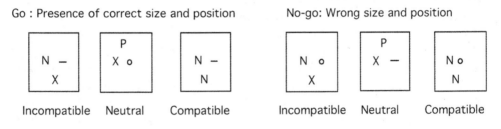

Go : Presence of correct size and position        No-go: Wrong size and position

Incompatible   Neutral   Compatible        Incompatible   Neutral   Compatible

**Figure 3.1**
Example displays for a ''response competition'' experiment with high and low perceptual load (Lavie, 1995). Subjects discriminate a central target letter (X or N) and ignore any distractors above or below. Perceptual load is manipulated by requiring the processing of another central shape (O or -). In the low load condition, subjects respond when a shape is present, otherwise not. In the high load condition, subjects respond when the shape has normal position (O) or length (-), otherwise not. The additional requirement to analyze exact position or length increases perceptual load dramatically. Although ignored, distractors may affect response times to targets, depending on whether they are incompatible, neutral, or compatible with the correct response. For example, a distractor N is incompatible with a target X because distractor and target call for different responses. The response delay caused by distractors reveals perceptual processing of task-irrelevant information.

### 3.2.2  Negative Priming

In all experiments mentioned so far, the extent to which irrelevant distractors are processed was assessed by measuring response competition (e.g., Eriksen and Eriksen, 1974). The fact that response competition is consistently seen to decrease under conditions of higher perceptual load clearly supports our claim that the perception of irrelevant distractors depends on the availability of attentional capacity.

However, an alternative account more consistent with late selection views is possible as well (e.g., Tipper and Milliken, 1996). On this alternative account irrelevant distractors are in fact perceived, but fail to enter into response competition because this is prevented by a process of "active inhibition." The existence of active inhibition is inferred from the phenomenon of "negative priming": the retardation of responses to relevant targets that previously appeared as irrelevant distractors (Tipper, 1985; Tipper and Milliken, 1996; for a noninhibitory account of negative priming, see Neill, 1997). If attentional selection is primarily the result of active inhibition (Driver and Tipper, 1989), then diminished response competition under high load does not necessarily reflect the *reduced perception* of distractors, but may instead reflect their *increased inhibition.* The critical prediction of this alternative account, then, is that negative priming should be greater with high perceptual load, because active inhibition is stronger with high than with low load. On the other hand, if perceptual load reduces distractor processing, as we claim, inhibition will be required only under conditions of low load to suppress responses to the perceived distributors, and negative priming should be greater with low perceptual load.

In collaboration with Elaine Fox, I tested these predictions for negative priming (Lavie and Fox, 2000). We presented subjects with pairs of displays (prime and probe) containing central target and nontarget stimuli and peripheral distractors (figure 3.2). Subjects discriminated three targets (x, n, and s) and indicated which of the three was present as quickly as possible. To manipulate priming, we varied the relation between the targets and distractors of prime and probe displays, as follows. In one condition, the distractor of the prime was the same as the target of the probe (*ignored repetition*); in another condition, it was not (*control*). In yet another condition, the targets of the prime and probe were the same (*attended repetition*). Perceptual load was manipulated by increasing the number of nontargets in the prime from one to six. The extent to which irrelevant distractors are actively inhibited is revealed through negative priming, that is, significantly slower responses under *ignored reptition* than under *control* conditions. (The *attended repetition* condition is not relevant here.) Presumably, active inhibition of a prime distractor persists over time and delays the response to it when it appears subsequently as the probe target.

The results were exactly as predicted by the perceptual load model. In several experiments, we always found negative priming (i.e., evidence for active inhibition) under low load conditions, but this was consistently eliminated under high load conditions (Lavie and Fox, 1998). We concluded that under high load conditions, irrelevant distractors do not interfere because they are simply not processed (early selection). Distractor responses need to be inhibited only in low load conditions, in which distractors are perceived (late selection).

In sum, experiments using both response competition and negative priming supported the perceptual load model. No matter how perceptual load was manipulated, a high load

## Low prime load

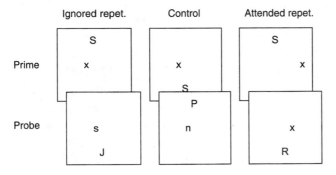

## High prime load

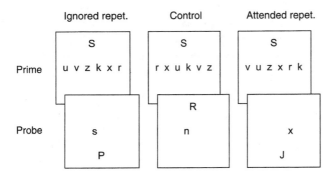

**Figure 3.2**
Example displays for a ''negative priming'' experiment with high and low perceptual load (Lavie and Fox, 2000). Subjects identified one of three possible targets (x, s, or n) in both the prime and the probe display, by pressing different keys, while ignoring distractors above or below. Perceptual load was manipulated by increasing the number of candidate targets from one to six. Distractors could affect target processing not only in the same display but also in the following display. In particular, processing tended to be slower if prime distractor and probe target were the same letter (ignored repetition) than if they were different letters (control). The third condition, in which prime target and probe target are the same letter (attended repetition) is less relevant in this context.

consistently eliminated perceptual processing of irrelevant information. Under conditions of low load, however, perceptual processing of irrelevant information continued. I conclude that early selection takes place under conditions of high load, and that late selection is found under conditions of low load.

One problem remains, however. Higher loads tend to require longer processing times, which might provide more time for distractor information to decay. Thus, it seems possible that distractors are processed after all, but that their effects have dissipated by the time a response is made. If this is the case, then any manipulation that prolongs target processing should be effective in reducing distractor effects. Thus it is important to dissociate the specific effects of perceptual load from the more general effects of slow processing speed. This is the purpose of the studies described in the next section.

### 3.2.3 Capacity Limits Versus Sensory Difficulty

Several experiments were carried out to dissociate the effects of perceptual load from the general effects of processing speed (Lavie, 1996). In this context it is important to distinguish perceptual load, which is defined in terms of the demand on attentional capacity, from other types of task difficulty, which affect processing speed but do not place additional demands on attention. For example, a type of task difficulty that is unrelated to attentional demand concerns the quality of sensory information provided by a stimulus (i.e., signal-to-noise ratio), and can be manipulated by reducing stimulus contrast, superimposing noise, or reducing presentation time.

Although degrading sensory information will increase task difficulty, it is important to realize that this will not necessarily increase the demand on attentional capacity. For example, if a target stimulus is degraded so severely that it becomes invisible, further allocation of attention will not improve its perception. This insight is behind the distinction between different kinds of processing limitations first suggested by Norman and Bobrow (1975): between ''data limits'' in the quality of sensory information and ''resource limits'' in the processing of that information. They further suggested that data limits cannot be compensated for by applying additional resources, and resource limits cannot be compensated for by improving sensory information. Thus, degrading sensory information should increase task difficulty and slow processing speed; however, it should not increase the demands on attentional capacity.

As a further test of the perceptual load model, we may therefore compare the effects on distractor processing of manipulations that increase attentional demand and manipulations that degrade sensory information. To assess distractor processing under these conditions, we once again employed a variant of the response competition paradigm. Subjects made a speeded choice between two central targets while ignoring an irrelevant distractor

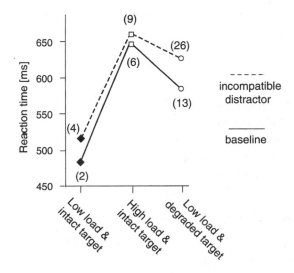

**Figure 3.3**
The effects on response competition of increasing attentional load versus degrading sensory information (Lavie, 1996). Both manipulations increase reaction time and error rates (percentages in parentheses). However, distractor effects (i.e., reaction time differences between incompatible and compatible distractors) diminish only with higher load, not with sensory degradation. Thus, the processing of task-irrelevant information depends specifically on attentional load.

in the periphery that was either *compatible* or *incompatible* with the correct response (i.e., the general design and display was similar to figure 3.1). Attentional demand was manipulated by increasing the number of relevant targets near the center of the display (see Lavie and Cox, 1997). That is, targets were presented either alone (low load) or accompanied by five nontargets (high load). Sensory information was degraded by either reducing target size, or decreasing target contrast and presentation time, or increasing the target's retinal eccentricity (Lavie, 1996).

Representative results from one experiment of this series are presented in figure 3.3. As shown in the figure, reaction times and error rates were increased similarly by high attentional load and by target degradation. However, response competition effects, which served to index distractor processing, were quite different. Response competition effects were weak under conditions of high load, but remained comparably strong under both conditions of low load (i.e., with either intact or degraded target) despite their substantial difference in task difficulty. The same pattern of results was obtained consistently in all experiments of the series. It is perhaps worth noting that the tendency for somewhat stronger response competition under low load/degraded target (compared with low load/ intact target) may be due to an increased frequency of distractor intrusions when target processing is slower because the task became more difficult. The important point is that under the high load/intact target condition, target processing was also difficult and slow, yet distractor intrusions were largely absent.

In conclusion, these experiments support the claim that irrelevant information is excluded from processing only when a high perceptual load exhausts attentional capacity. This has a number of interesting implications for the neural response to irrelevant distractors, discussed in the next section.

## 3.3  Neural Response to Distractors

Our perceptual load model makes several predictions regarding the neural response to distractors. The theory predicts that the neural response of sensory systems to behaviorally irrelevant stimuli should depend on the perceptual load imposed by a behaviorally relevant task. Specifically, a significant neural response to irrelevant stimuli should be found despite the subject's efforts to ignore them, provided the perceptual load of the relevant task is low. The response to irrelevant stimuli should be reduced only when relevant stimuli pose high perceptual load. We have recently tested these predictions using functional imaging (fMRI) to characterize neural responses to moving stimuli.

However, since our starting point is the perceptual load model, our study takes a different approach from previous studies of attention and motion perception (e.g., Chaudhuri, 1991; Corbetta et al., 1991; O'Craven et al., 1997; Shulman, 1991; Treue and Maunsell, 1996). All of these studies have compared explicit attention to motion with explicit ignoring of motion. Any difference between these two conditions can be attributed either to enhanced responses to attended motion or attenuated responses to ignored motion, so that the specific contribution of the latter condition cannot become clear. Thus, these studies do not answer the principal issue of selective attention theory: whether irrelevant stimuli can be successfully ignored and excluded from perceptual processing.

We tested the perceptual load model by comparing two situations in which motion is equally irrelevant and the only difference lies in the perceptual load of the subject's task. Moreover, we reasoned that the relevant load should determine distractor processing even when relevant and irrelevant stimuli are processed in entirely different areas of cortex (as long as distractor processing depends on attention and the relevant task consumes most of the available capacity). To test these predictions using fMRI, we employed the task illustrated in figure 3.4 (Rees et al., 1997).

We presented a stream of words at fixation (rate = one word per second) and, in the periphery, a field of numerous small dots. The dots were either stationary or moving radially outward from fixation, but subjects were instructed to concentrate on the words and to ignore the dots altogether. In the low load condition, subjects discriminated between

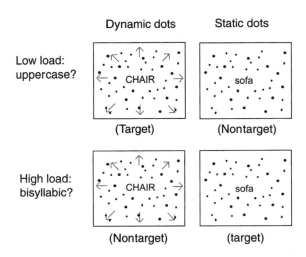

**Figure 3.4**
Example displays for fMRI experiment on neural responses to task-irrelevant motion. Subjects concentrate on the words at display center, and ignore the dots in the periphery, which are either moving or stationary. In the low load condition, subjects discriminate uppercase and lowercase words. In the high load condition, they distinguish between bisyllabic words and mono- or trisyllabic words. Comparing fMRI signals for moving versus stationary dots reveals neural responses to task-irrelevant motion. In the high load condition, such responses are eliminated (see table 3.1).

uppercase and lowercase letters in the words, whereas in the high load condition they discriminated bisyllabic words from mono- or trisyllabic words. The display itself was exactly the same under both load conditions.

In analyzing the results, we were mainly concerned with the brain activity produced by task-irrelevant motion as a function of relevant task load (table 3.1). The results agreed exactly with our predictions: motion-related activity in cortical area V5/MT, which was measured by comparing moving and stationary dots, varied as a function of load in the word task. Activity in V5/MT was significant under conditions of low load, but was eliminated under conditions of high load. The same interaction between relevant load and neural responses to irrelevant motion was found in other cortical areas responsive to moving stimuli, among them the V1/V2 border and the superior colliculus (Shipp and Zeki, 1985; Ungerleider et al., 1984). In sum, we found that a whole network of sensorimotor areas involved in motion processing responded to task-irrelevant motion, provided that the relevant task load was low, but that this activity was significantly reduced as relevant task load was increased.

In a further, psychophysical experiment we used the same task and displays to assess the processing of task-irrelevant motion by the duration of the induced motion aftereffect (Chaudhuri, 1991). The motion aftereffect is known to reflect both motion processing and

**Table 3.1**
Area where moving and stationary stimuli evoked significantly greater differential activity under conditions of low load than under conditions of high load

| Area | Tailarach coordinates | | | Z score |
|---|---|---|---|---|
| Left V5/MT complex | −44 | −64 | 4 | **6.69** |
| Right V5/MT complex | 42 | −66 | −8 | **3.40** |
| Right V1/V2 | 26 | −96 | −8 | **5.67** |
| Superior colliculus | −2 | −26 | −2 | **5.02** |
| Left fusiform | −40 | −74 | −14 | **5.52** |
| Left lingual gyrus | −8 | −80 | −12 | **5.14** |
| Right premotor cortex | 10 | 2 | 68 | **5.06** |
| Left superior parietal lobule | −26 | −64 | 32 | **4.79** |
| Right superior frontal gyrus | 8 | 58 | 26 | **5.62** |

Note: Only areas with significant responsiveness to motion are included ($p < .05$ after correction for multiple comparisons, except for area V5/MT, where $p < .001$ was used without correction).

activity in area V5/MT (Tootell et al., 1995). We found that the duration of motion after-effect induced by task-irrelevant motion was significantly reduced when the perceptual load of the word task was high. This purely behavioral measure provides converging evidence in accord with our functional imaging results, to show that perceptual load in a word discrimination task can decrease the perceptual processing of task-irrelevant motion.

Our consistent finding that the processing of irrelevant information can be prevented by sufficiently high load in a relevant task has some counterintuitive implications for individuals who might be described as suffering from a reduced processing capacity. According to the perceptual load model, such individuals should perform better than normal controls in the following restricted sense: a small increase in processing load should render their performance less susceptible to disruption by distractors. This is because for such individuals a small increase in load may be sufficient to exhaust capacity, and thus eliminate the processing of distractors. In normal controls, however, a small increase in load would have little or no effect on the processing of distractors.

In the next two sections, I examine the implications of this prediction for patients with unilateral neglect and for the normal consequences of aging.

## 3.4 Perceptual Load and Unilateral Neglect

In collaboration with Ian Robertson, I examined the implications of the perceptual load model for patients with a right hemisphere lesion centered on the parietal lobe (Lavie and Robertson, 1997). These patients suffer from "unilateral neglect" of visual information presented to the side opposite to the lesion (contralesional), especially if their attention is captured by a stimulus on the same side as the lesion (ipsilesional). Current theories of neglect typically postulate a spatial bias toward the ipsilesional field (Rafal, 1994), and several recent accounts have suggested that neglect may involve not merely reduced attention to the contralesional but hyperattention to the ipsilesional side (Kinsbourne, 1993; Ladavas, 1993).

In addition to the clear spatial bias, neglect may also involve a reduction in processing capacity, which is often overlooked (see also Duncan et al., in press). For example, after a *bilateral* parietal lesion, one of the most striking deficits is an inability to perceive more than one object at a time (Balint's syndrome; Balint, 1909). In addition, there is clinical evidence for deficits in recognizing objects (especially from unusual views) after lesions to the parietal lobe (Warrington and Taylor, 1973), and this may be another consequence of reduced processing capacity. Finally, arousal pathways are thought to be right lateralized (Oke et al., 1978; Pardo et al., 1991), and a general capacity reduction might result from a right lesion simply because arousal is an important component of mental capacity (Kahneman, 1973).

If neglect patients with right hemisphere lesions indeed suffer from a general loss of processing capacity in addition to a rightward bias, then it should be possible to moderate the disturbing effect of *ipsilesional* stimuli by a small increase in perceptual load. The reasoning is the same as for distractor effects in normals, which also can be reduced by increasing processing load. Except that here we predict that a *small* increase in load—just sufficient to exhaust the reduced processing capacity—should eliminate or reduce the effect of right (ipsilesional) distractors. If confirmed, such an outcome would qualify previous claims that pathological distraction by rightward events is fully automatic in left neglect.

We tested this prediction in three patients who had suffered a right hemisphere stroke leading to left neglect. These patients participated in a response competition task in which we manipulated perceptual load at fixation (figure 3.5). The patients were asked to make a speeded choice response as to whether an A or a B appeared in the center of the display while ignoring an irrelevant distractor letter that appeared on either the left or the right side. (Although we were interested mostly in right distractors, we also presented left distractors to discourage strategic shifts in eye position.) As in our previous response competition experiments, the distractor was either compatible or incompatible with the target response. As before, the manipulation of interest was the perceptual load of the central task. In the low load condition, the target letter appeared above or below a circle in the center of the screen. In the slightly higher load condition, the circle was replaced by the letter R. The presence of this additional letter increased the processing load because the target now had to be found among two central letters.

The results for these patients and for a control group of healthy volunteers are presented in figure 3.6, which shows distractor effects as a function of load for each group. As can

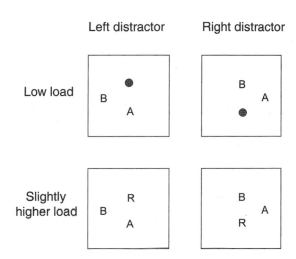

**Figure 3.5**
A response competition experiment for patients with left lateral neglect (Lavie and Robertson, 1996). Subjects discriminated a target letter (A or B) at the center, which was accompanied either by a blob (low load) or by another letter (slightly higher load). Irrelevant distractors appeared in the left (contralesional) or right (ispi-lesional) hemifield, and were either compatible or incompatible with the correct target response.

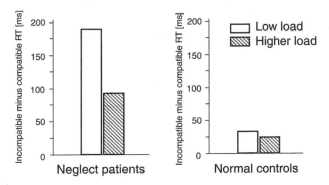

**Figure 3.6**
Results for patients with left lateral neglect and for a normal control group. Distractor effects in the low load and higher load conditions are greater for neglect patients than for normal subjects. However, a slight increase in load reduced distractor effects (response competition) far more in patients than in normal subjects. Thus, even the potent distractor effects observed in neglect depend on perceptual load.

be seen in the figure, the small increase of perceptual load was sufficient to significantly reduce distractor effects in the patient group, and this was true in all three patients (not shown). In the control group, the slight manipulation of load had no effect on distractor processing. Note that the differential outcome was not simply due to the fact that the patient group suffered from a much larger distractor effect than the control group: the difference remained significant even when it was expressed as a proportion of baseline reaction time for each group. Thus our results agree with the suggestion that left neglect involves a rightward bias, so that right stimuli are more distracting than left stimuli. However, the more important finding is that a slight increase in perceptual load can moderate the inordinate effects of right distractors.

We concluded that attention capture by ipsilesional events (Kinsbourne, 1993; Ladavas, 1993) is not fully automated and that unilateral neglect involves, in addition to the spatial bias, a general reduction in processing capacity. Interestingly, our study shows that one can take advantage of this reduction and reduce distractor effects by slightly increasing perceptual load.

## 3.5   Perceptual Load and the Aging Brain

A joint study with Elizabeth Maylor (Maylor and Lavie, 1998) tested some implications of the perceptual load model for the normal aging process, which is often thought to lead to some restriction of perceptual processing capacity (e.g., Ball et al., 1988). If this is correct, we may expect older adults to benefit more than younger adults from smaller increases in perceptual load, because these may be enough to exhaust their reduced capacity and eliminate distractor processing.

To test this prediction, we ran sixteen younger (ages nineteen to thirty) and sixteen older (ages sixty-five to seventy-nine) adults in a response competition task in which perceptual load increased in a graded fashion. Subjects made a speeded choice as to which of two target letters was present at the center of the display while attempting to ignore a peripheral distractor that was either response-incompatible or response-neutral. We manipulated perceptual load by varying the number of nontargets in the center (zero, one, three, or five).

Figure 3.7 shows the observed distractor effect (difference in reaction time between incompatible and neutral distractors) as a function of the set size and age group. The results show clearly that elderly subjects suffer significantly greater distractor effects at small relevant set sizes (i.e., one or two nontargets), consistent with a reduced capacity for perception. Moreover, a small increase in load (i.e., from one to two or from two to four nontargets) is sufficient to significantly reduce distractor effects in elderly but not in young subjects. In young subjects, only six nontargets constitute a sufficient load to elimi-

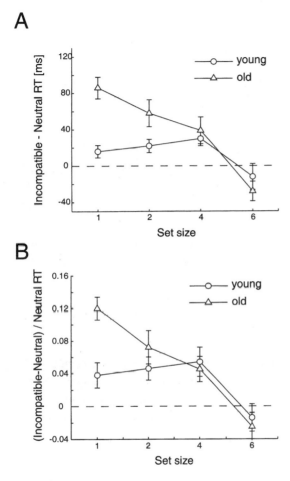

**Figure 3.7**
Response competition in young (ages nineteen to thirty) and elderly (ages sixty-five to seventy-nine) subjects. Absolute (*A*) and relative (*B*) differences in reaction time between incompatible and compatible distractors, as a function of perceptual load (set size). At very low load (set size 1), response competition is much larger for elderly than for young subjects. However, response competition decreases more rapidly with increasing load for elderly subjects. This suggests that ageing adversely affects attention both at the level of perceptual (early) selection and at the level of response (late) selection.

nate distractor effects. Thus, as we predicted, older subjects benefit more than younger subjects from smaller increases of load, which are sufficient to reduce distractor effects only for them. However, at very low load (e.g., one candidate target, figure 3.7) distractor effects are clearly greater than in younger subjects.

The large distractor effect at very low load is not predicted by the perceptual load hypothesis. This effect cannot be explained by a general slowing of reaction times with age, because the difference between elderly and young subjects persists even when the effect is calculated as the proportion of the absolute reaction time for each group (figure 3.7B). However, the large distractor effects at low load are consistent with previous reports, which show age-related impairments in the ability to focus on relevant stimuli in the presence of competing inputs (Hartley, 1992; McDowd and Birren, 1990; Farkas and Hoyer, 1980; Shaw, 1991). These studies typically employed situations of low perceptual load (i.e., only one relevant object).

This inability to focus on targets in the presence of distractors seems, therefore, to reflect an additional age-related deficit in the ability to suppress irrelevant response tendencies to distractors that are perceived. The hypothesis that aging involves a specific decline in inhibitory control mechanisms (Hasher and Zacks, 1989) has received support from a number of previous studies. For example, it is often found that negative priming is reduced with age (Hasher et al., 1991; Kane et al., 1994; McDowd and Oseas-Kreger, 1991).

Thus, we conclude that normal aging involves (at least) two changes with respect to attention. First, an age-related decrease in the capacity for perception, which can actually lead to some counterintuitive improvement in the mechanisms of *early selection* (albeit from a poor base). Second, an additional age-related decline in the *late selection* mechanisms that allow us to suppress responses to irrelevant stimuli which are nevertheless perceived at a low perceptual load.

## 3.6   Conclusions

This chapter has presented various types of evidence for a perceptual load model of attention. I have discussed evidence from several studies, all of which demonstrate that selective attention can result in either selective perception (early selection) or just in selective behavior (late selection), depending on perceptual load. At low perceptual load, early selection fails and irrelevant information continues to be processed, in which case late selection becomes necessary. At high perceptual load, early selection takes place, irrelevant information is not processed, and there is no longer a need for late selection. Evidence in support of this model was found with several measures for the processing of irrelevant distractors: response competition, negative priming, aftereffects from ignored motion, and neural responses to ignored motion (as revealed by fMRI in cortical area V5/MT). Taken together, these studies show that distractor processing ceases when perceptual capacity is exhausted. Moreover, the differential effects of increasing processing load versus degrading sensory information showed that distractor processing depends specifically on resource limits rather than data limits (Norman and Bobrow, 1975). In other words, only those aspects of task difficulty which draw on attentional capacity are most crucial for distractor processing.

The reviewed studies also showed that subjects consistently processed task-irrelevant distractors, despite their peripheral location and clear instructions to ignore them, whenever perceptual load was low. This demonstrates that late selection (i.e., perceptual processing of irrelevant stimuli) does indeed occur, although invariably in situations of low perceptual load. Any complete account of selective attention must therefore consider both early and late selection mechanisms. Indeed, when both task-relevant and -irrelevant stimuli have been processed, late selection is indispensable to guarantee that behavior is controlled only by task-relevant stimuli.

Our aging study sheds further light on late selection mechanisms. Young subjects typically succeeded in making appropriate responses (i.e., both response accuracy and speed were high) even when both relevant and irrelevant stimuli had been processed. With older subjects, however, this was not always the case. The presence of distractors was far more harmful to performance of older subjects, and response competition (measured in terms of slowing of reaction time) was three times as large as for young subjects. On the other hand, distractor interference diminished much more rapidly for older than for young subjects when perceptual load was increased. Our results thus demonstrate that early and late selection mechanisms are differentially affected by aging.

Capacity limits played an important role even in patients with left neglect after a right parietal lesion. In addition to their strong rightward bias, we suggested that such patients may also suffer from decreased processing capacity (see also Duncan et al., 1999). Consistent with this, we found that even the pathologically strong distractor effects from right stimuli decreased significantly when processing load was increased slightly, in order to exhaust the diminished processing capacity. Thus, even distractor effects in unilateral neglect patients conform to the predictions of the perceptual load model.

I conclude that capacity limits play a major role in selective attention, and that even purely psychological concepts of capacity can lead to clear and testable predictions for neural activity in the brain when considered in terms of a perceptual load model. Thus, although it is currently still hard to define precisely what leads to capacity limits in the brain, further work with the capacity concept may yet prove very useful for our understanding of the brain mechanisms of selective attention.

## Acknowledgment

This work was supported by BBSRC grant number 31/S09509, MRC grant number G9805400, and a Human Frontiers Science Program grant.

## References

Balint, R. (1909). Die Seelenlahmung des schauens, optische ataxie, raumliche storung der ausmerksamkeit. *Monatsscherift psychiat. neurol.* 25: 51–81.

Ball, K. K., Beard, B. L., Roenker, D. L., Miller, R. L., and Griggs, D. S. (1988). Age and visual search: Expanding the useful field of view. *J. Optical Soc. America* 5: 2210–2219.

Chaudhuri, A. (1991). Modulation of the motion aftereffect by selective attention. *Nature* 344: 60–62.

Corbetta, M., Miezin, F. M., Dobmeyer, S., Shulman, G. L., and Petersen, S. E. (1991). Selective and divided attention during visual discriminations of shape, color, and speed: Functional anatomy by positron emission tomography. *J. Neurosci.* 11: 2383–2402.

Desimone, R., and Duncan, J. (1995). Neural mechanisms of selective visual attention. *Annu. Rev. Neurosci.* 18: 193–222.

Driver, J., and Tipper, S. P. (1989). On the nonselectivity of "selective" seeing: Contrasts between interference and priming in selective attention. *J. Exp. Psychol. Hum. Percep. Perf.* 15: 304–314.

Duncan, J. (1980). The locus of interference in the perception of simultaneous stimuli. *Psychol. Rev.* 87: 272–300.

Duncan, J., Bundesen, C., Olson, A., Humphreys, G., Chavda, S., and Shibuya, H. (1999). Systematic analysis of deficits in visual attention. *J. Exp. Psychol. Gen.* 128: 450–478.

Eriksen, B. A., and Eriksen, C. W. (1974). Effects of noise letters upon the identification of a target letter in a non search task. *Percep. Psychophys.* 16: 143–149.

Farkas, M., and Hoyer, W. (1980). Processing consequences of perceptual grouping in selective attention. *J. Gerontol.* 35: 207–216.

Fisher, D. L. (1982). Limited-channel models of automatic detection: Capacity and scanning in visual search. *Psychol. Rev.* 89: 662–692.

Hartley, A. A. (1992). Attention. In F. I. M. Craik and T. A. Salthouse (eds.), *The handbook of aging and cognition* (pp. 3–49). Hillsdale, NJ: Lawrence Erlbaum Associates.

Hasher, L., and Zacks, R. T. (1988). Working memory, comprehension, and aging: A review and a new view. In G. H. Bower (ed.), *The psychology of learning and motivation,* vol. 22 (pp. 193–225). New York: Academic Press.

Hasher, L., Stoltzfus, E. R., Zacks, R. T., and Rypma, B. (1991). Age and inhibition. *J. Exp. Psychol. Learn. Mem. Cog.* 17: 163–169.

Kahneman, D. (1973). *Attention and effort.* Englewood Cliffs, N.J.: Prentice Hall.

Kahneman, D., and Treisman, A. (1984). Changing views of attention and automaticity. In R. Parasuraman and D. R. Davies (eds.), *Varieties of attention* (pp. 29–61). New York: Academic Press.

Kahneman, D., Treisman, A., & Gibbs, B. (1992). The reviewing of object files: Object-specific integration of information. *Cog. Psychol.* 24: 175–219.

Kane, M. J., Hasher, L., Stoltzfus, E. R., Zacks, R. T., and Connelly, S. L. (1994). Inhibitory attentional mechanisms and aging. *Psychol. Aging* 9: 103–112.

Kastner, S., De Weerd, P., Desimone, R., and Ungerleider, L. G. (1998). Mechanisms of directed attention in the human extrastriate cortex as revealed by functional MRI. *Science* 282: 108–111.

Kinsbourne, M. (1993). Orientational bias model of unilateral neglect: Evidence from attentional gradients within hemispace. In I. H. Robertson and J. C. Marshall (eds.), *Unilateral neglect: Clinical and experimental studies* (pp. 63–86). Hove, UK: Lawrence Erlbaum Associates.

Ladavas, E. (1993). Spatial dimensions of automatic and voluntary orienting components of attention. In I. H. Robertson and J. C. Marshall (eds.), *Unilateral neglect: Clinical and experimental studies* (pp. 193–210). Hove, UK: Lawrence Erlbaum Associates.

Lavie, N. (1995). Perceptual load as a necessary condition for selective attention. *J. Exp. Psychol. Hum. Percep. Perf.,* 21: 451–468.

Lavie, N. (1996). The roles of data versus resource limits in selective visual attention. Presented at XXVI International Congress of Psychology, Montreal (August).

Lavie, N., and Cox, S. (1997). On the efficiency of attentional selection: Efficient visual search results in inefficient rejection of distraction. *Psychol. Sci.,* 8: 395–398.

Lavie, N., and Fox, E. (2000). The role of perceptual load in negative priming. *J. Exp. Psychol. Hum. Percep. Perf.* 26: 1038–1052.

Lavie, N., and Robertson, I. (1997). The role of perceptual load in neglect: Rejection of ipsilesional distractors is facilitated with higher central load. Presented to the Fourth Meeting of the Cognitive Neuroscience Society, Boston (March).

Lavie, N., and Tsal, Y. (1994). Perceptual load as a major determinant of the locus of selection in visual attention. *Percep. Psychophys.* 56: 183–197.

Luck, S. J., Chelazzi, L., Hillyard, S. A., and Desimone, R. (1997). Neural mechanisms of spatial selective attention in areas V1, V2, and V4 of macaque visual cortex. *J. Neurophysiol.* 77: 24–42.

Maylor, E., and Lavie, N. (1998). The influence of perceptual load on age differences in selective attention. *Psychol. Aging* 13: 563–573.

McDowd, J. M., and Birren, J. E. (1990). Aging and attentional processes. In J. E. Birren and K. W. Schaie (eds.), *Handbook of the psychology of aging,* 3rd ed. (pp. 222–233). San Diego: Academic Press.

McDowd, J. M., and Oseas-Kreger, D. M. (1991). Aging, inhibitory processes, and negative priming. *J. Gerontol. Psychol. Sci.* 46: 340–345.

Motter, B. C. (1994). Neural correlates of attentive selection for color or luminance in extrastriate area V4. *J. Neurosci.* 14: 2178–2189.

Neill, W. T. (1997). Episodic retrieval in negative priming and repetition priming. *J. Exp. Psychol. Learn. Mem. Cog.* 23: 1291–1305.

Norman, D. A., and Bobrow, D. G. (1975). On data-limited and resource-limited processes. *Cog. Psychol.* 7: 44–64.

O'Craven, K. M., Rosen, B. R., Kwong, K. K., Treisman, A., and Savoy, R. L (1997). Voluntary attention modulates fMRI activity in human MT–MST. *Neuron* 18: 591–598.

Oke, A., Keller, R., Mefford, I., and Adams, R. N. (1978). Lateralization of norepinephrine in human thalamus. *Science* 200: 1411–1413.

Pardo, J. V., Fox, P. T., and Raichle, M. E. (1991). Localization of a human system for sustained attention by positron emission tomography. *Nature* 349: 61–64.

Pylyshyn, Z., Burkell, J., Fisher, B., and Sears, C. (1994). Multiple parallel access in visual attention. *Can. J. Exp. Psychol.* 48: 260–283.

Rafal, R. D. (1994). Neglect. *Curr. Opin. Neurobiol.* 4: 231–236.

Rees, G., Frith, C., and Lavie, N. (1997). Modulating irrelevant motion perception by varying attentional load in an unrelated task. *Science* 278: 1616–1619.

Shaw, R. (1991). Age-related increases in the effects of automatic semantic activation. *Psychol. Aging* 6: 855–862.

Shipp, S., and Zeki, S. (1985). Segregation of pathways leading from area V2 to areas V4 and V5 of macaque monkey visual cortex. *Nature* 315: 322–325.

Shulman, G. L. (1991). Attentional modulation of mechanisms that analyze rotation in depth. *J. Exp. Psychol. Hum. Percep. Perf.* 17: 726–737.

Tipper, S. P. (1985). The negative priming effect: Inhibitory effects of ignored primes. *Quart. J. Exp. Psychol.* 37A: 571–590.

Tipper, S. P., and Driver, J. (1988). Negative priming between pictures and words: Evidence for semantic analysis of ignored stimuli. *Mem. Cog.* 16: 64–70.

Tipper, S. P., and Milliken, B. (1996). Distinguishing between inhibition-based and episodic retrieval-based accounts of negative priming. In A. F. Kramer, M. G. H. Coles, and G. D. Logan (eds.), *Converging operations in the study of visual selective attention* (pp. 77–106). Washington, DC: American Psychological Association.

Tootell, R. B., Reppas, J. B., Kwong, K. K., Malach, R., Born, R. T., Brady, T. J., Rosen, B. R., and Belliveau, J. W. (1995). Functional analysis of human MT and related visual cortical areas using magnetic resonance imaging. *J. Neurosci.* 15: 3215–3230.

Treisman, A. M. (1969). Strategies and models of selective attention. *Psychol. Rev.* 76: 282–299.

Treue, S., and Maunsell, J. H. R. (1996). Attentional modulation of visual motion processing in cortical areas MT and MST. *Nature* 382: 539–541.

Ungerleider, L. G., Desimone, R., Galkin, T. W., and Mishkin, M. (1984). Subcortical projections of area MT in the macaque. *J. Comp. Neurol.* 223: 368–386.

Warrington, E. K., and Taylor, A. M. (1973). Contribution of the right parietal lobe to object recognition. *Cortex* 9: 152–164.

Yantis, S., and Johnston, J. C. (1990). On the locus of visual selection: Evidence from focused attention tasks. *J. Exp. Psychol. Hum. Percep. Perf.* 16: 135–149.

Yantis, S., and Jones, E. (1991). Mechanisms of attentional selection: Temporally modulated priority tags. *Percep. Psychophys.* 50: 166–178.

# 4 Frontal Lobe Function and the Control of Visual Attention

John Duncan

## 4.1 Introduction

In this chapter I shall describe three projects concerned in different ways with the role of the frontal lobe in visual attention. Undoubtedly this is a field in which research is extremely preliminary, and our early results give no more than a hint of how it may develop. Already, however, I hope to indicate both important questions and some means by which they may be investigated.

A general thought directing our work is that frontal systems should play some role in *control* of visual attention (Desimone and Duncan, 1995), in line with their broader role in control and organization of many different aspects of behavior (e.g., Luria, 1966; Norman and Shallice, 1980). How, then, should the control of visual attention be conceptualized? Because processing capacity is limited, selective attention to one part of the visual input comes at the cost of neglecting other parts. In this sense we may say that inputs *compete* to be processed. But which inputs should be selected and which should be ignored? Effective control implies selective focus on objects of *relevance* to current behavior. In a competitive system, it is useful to think of each competitor as having a strength or weight, such that strong competitors are processed well and weak competitors less well (e.g., Rumelhart, 1970). Thus attentional control may be seen as a process of using task context to guide or *bias* competition by appropriate weight setting. Competing objects in the visual input must be given weights reflecting how relevant they are to current behavioral concerns. The general thought, therefore, is that frontal systems may be important in this process of visual weight setting.

A striking property of frontal neurons is the diversity and flexibility of their responses. In the monkey, cells of the lateral frontal convexity show selective activity during the broadest possible range of tasks, including many variants of short-term memory for locations or objects, learning and use of stimulus–response mapping rules, and retrieval from long-term memory (e.g., di Pellegrino and Wise, 1993; Fuster et al., 1985; Funahashi et al., 1989; Miller, 1999). Within a task, selective responses can be seen during stimulus input, short-term memory delays, response preparation or execution, or other trial periods. Indeed, it is perhaps not too speculative to conclude that, whatever the task a monkey is set to carry out, a good proportion of prefrontal neurons will show selective activity related to some aspect or another of this task's events. A likely implication is that the properties of frontal neurons must be somewhat dynamic, adapting themselves to reflect distinctions relevant to current behavior (Rao et al., 1997; Rainer et al., 1998b). Thus any role for frontal systems in control of visual attention must be considered in this context of diverse, adaptable function.

The first set of experiments I shall describe uses positron emission tomography (PET) to measure regional cerebral activity during spatially directed attention. Unexpectedly, the results show a region of frontal activity *ipsilateral* to the attended visual field. We suggest that one main role of frontal cortex in this task may be *inhibiting* processing of the contralateral field. The second line of work addresses relations between specific and general functions of frontal cortex. In line with the monkey data mentioned above, a synthesis of neuroimaging results from many different laboratories suggests that relatively well-defined regions of frontal cortex have rather general functions, adapting themselves to the solution of diverse cognitive problems. Since these are much the same regions as those activated in our own studies, our results may reflect adaptation of rather general systems to the specific problem of attentional control. In the third section of the chapter, a method is presented for measuring impairments in attentional control. The method is illustrated with the first data we have started to collect from patients with focal frontal lobe lesions.

## 4.2   Attention to Left and Right

Displays from one of our first PET studies of directed attention (Vandenberghe et al., 1997) are illustrated in figure 4.1. Each display in this experiment contained two circular patches of grating, one in the upper left visual field and the other in the lower right visual field. Each grating was presented inside a frame of four dots; a central dot marked fixation, which was continuously monitored by electro-oculogram. From one trial to the next, each grating varied randomly in two attributes, orientation (clockwise or counterclockwise from

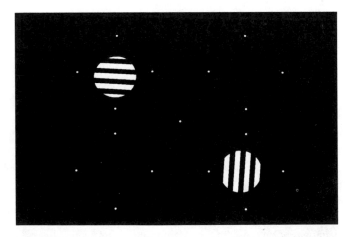

**Figure 4.1**
Example display from Vandenberghe et al. (1997).

the horizontal for the left patch, clockwise or counterclockwise from the vertical for the right patch) and exact location within the surrounding frame (above or below center for the left patch, left or right of center for the right patch). In different conditions, therefore, subjects could be instructed to identify orientation of the left patch, location of the left patch, orientation of the right patch, location of the right patch, or any combination of these. The instruction remained fixed throughout the 106 s period of a single scan, with different instructions in different scans. Within one scan, trials followed one another at a rate of 36/min. For each trial, the display was presented for 495 ms, and the subject made an immediate verbal report indicating the value of whichever attribute(s) he or she had been asked to identify.

The data to be discussed here come only from focused attention conditions, in which, for a whole block of trials, subjects focused on either the left or the right patch, and on each trial identified just a single attribute (orientation or location) of that patch. As it turned out, results for orientation and location blocks were rather similar. Accordingly, we may consider only mean differences between attention to left and right fields, collapsing across these two types of discrimination. Significant differences are shown in figure 4.2, the upper row showing regions of higher cerebral activity (regional cerebral blood

### A. Leftward minus rightward attention
| -8mm | 4mm | 16mm | 28mm | 40mm |

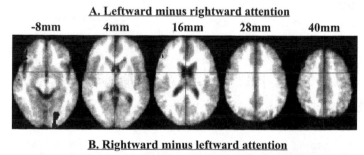

### B. Rightward minus leftward attention

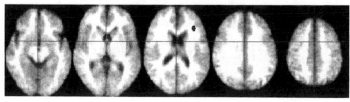

**Figure 4.2**
Results from Vandenberghe et al. (1997). Regions of significant activation are shown on averaged magnetic resonance image (MRI) of fourteen subjects, separately for (A) leftward minus rightward attention and (B) rightward minus leftward attention. Within each row, brain is shown in five horizontal slices, running from bottom (leftmost) to top (rightmost); z-levels at top of figure are from standard space of Talairach and Tournoux (1988). Within each slice, left of the brain is to the left. Analyses performed with SPM software (Wellcome Department of Cognitive Neurology, London). Reproduced with permission from Duncan (1998).

flow, or rCBF) for attend-left conditions, and the lower row showing higher activity for attend-right. In each row the brain is shown in five horizontal sections running from bottom (leftmost section) to top (rightmost).

Three results may be noted. First, a region of the right occipital lobe was more active when attention was devoted to the left (figure 4.2, upper row, first slice). Very much as expected, this suggests attentional enhancement of early visual areas, with their predominantly crossed representation of the visual field (see also Heeger et al., chapter 2 in this volume; Martínez et al., 1999; Van Voorhis and Hillyard, 1977). Though our first studies showed a significant attentional modulation only in the right hemisphere, the result is commonly symmetrical, as we too have observed in subsequent work (Vandenberghe et al., 2000).

The second finding concerns the conventional view that attention is largely controlled by lateralized activity of the parietal lobe. According to a simple version of this view, each parietal lobe is largely responsible for directing attention to the opposite hemifield (for more complex possibilities, see Mesulam, 1981; Posner et al., 1984). In our studies, however, parietal lobe activity was unaffected by the direction of attention. As shown by comparison with a sensorimotor control condition, our tasks were indeed associated with a substantial activation of the superior parietal lobule and intraparietal sulcus, especially in the right hemisphere. Such activations have now been observed in a wide array of visual tasks, involving verbal, manual, and oculomotor responses, and either foveal or peripheral stimuli (e.g., Corbetta and Shulman, 1998; Wojciulik and Kanwisher, 1999). As parietal activity in our experiment was not modulated by the direction of attention, however, it is not apparent in figure 4.2. Though other work hints at higher parietal activity contralateral to the attended side (e.g., Corbetta et al., 1993; Nobre et al., 1997), this seems to be a weak effect superimposed on generally stronger activity in the right hemisphere.

The third finding is most relevant to the theme of this chapter. Very unexpectedly, lateral prefrontal activity was greater on the side *ipsilateral* to attention. In the left hemisphere, there was a broad band of activation associated with attention to the left (figure 4.2, upper row, slices 1 and 3–5). In the right hemisphere, a smaller activation was associated with attention to the right (figure 4.2, lower row, slice 3). In a second experiment, this right hemisphere activation was also seen more ventrally.

How should such frontal lobe activity be interpreted? The hypothesis we suggested is that, in this task, one major role of the frontal lobe is inhibition of processing in the *ignored* visual field. Thus left frontal activity is associated not so much with attention to a target object on the left as with inhibition of the concurrent *nontarget* on the right; and vice versa for right frontal activity. Here, then, is one proposed role for frontal systems in attentional weight setting, specifically in decreasing the weights of unwanted inputs on the contralateral side.

The hypothesis is supported by a number of considerations. The tendency of sudden stimulus onsets to capture attention is well documented at both behavioral and neural levels (see Jonides and Yantis, 1988; Gottlieb et al., 1998). Inhibiting attentional capture by nontargets is thus a plausible component of the tasks we have used; indeed, lateralized frontal activity has in general not been observed in tasks requiring focused attention to left or right in the absence of contralateral distractors (Corbetta et al., 1993; Nobre et al., 1997). Frontal lesions, furthermore, can certainly result in disinhibition of unwanted activity directed to the opposite side of space, including reflexive eye movements (Butter et al., 1988; Paus et al., 1991).

At the same time, it does not seem plausible that large regions of frontal cortex are devoted *exclusively* to inhibition of the contralateral visual field, or indeed that this is the only frontal function in our tasks. As we have seen, the diverse activity patterns of different frontal neurons will commonly capture many different aspects of task events. Almost certainly, either direction of attention will be associated with active cells of many kinds in both hemispheres. Indeed, if a monkey is instructed to hold a certain location in working memory, an activity doubtless closely related to attending to that location, prefrontal neurons coding this target location are somewhat more common in the contralateral hemisphere (Rainer et al., 1998a). Such results seem inconsistent with the view that frontal activity in these tasks is exclusively concerned with contralateral nontarget inhibition.

In PET, of course, we measure only net activity of a whole brain area. Though greater net activation ipsilateral to the attended field may show that one important neural population is involved in nontarget inhibition, doubtless different cell types will show different patterns of modulation as the direction of attention changes. Untangling this complex state of affairs is a problem beyond the resolution of current neuroimaging methods. In the next section, this theme of diversity in frontal activity is taken up from a different perspective.

## 4.3 Frontal Response to Diverse Cognitive Demands

The second project I wish to discuss concerns regional specialization within prefrontal cortex. Undoubtedly there is some degree of specialization. In the monkey, for example, a few studies have shown clear double dissociations between impairments following large lesions of the orbital and lateral frontal cortex (Butter, 1969; Dias et al., 1996). At the same time, extreme specialization is questioned by the sheer diversity of neural properties found in any one frontal area, and by the suggestion that even individual neurons adapt their properties on the basis of current task demands. A good example concerns the influential proposal that dorsolateral and ventrolateral frontal cortex are respectively specialized for processing spatial (where) and object (what) information (Goldman-Rakic, 1988). In an examination of this distinction, Rao and colleagues (1997) found that many single neurons, scattered throughout a large region of both dorsolateral and ventrolateral cortex, carry not just ''what'' or ''where'' information separately, but both together. Importantly, exactly the same neuron could carry ''what'' information when this was relevant to the task, but switch to ''where'' when it no longer mattered which object had been seen, only where it had occurred.

At first sight, many recent neuroimaging results suggest regional specialization within human frontal cortex. In one experiment, manipulation of one cognitive demand may produce significant activation in frontal area X, whereas in another experiment, manipulation of a second demand produces activation in a different area Y. Both experiments, however, will have limited statistical power, meaning that only a part of the truly activated region will achieve significance by a conventional criterion. Through statistical noise alone, it is inevitable that any two studies—even those whose truly active regions are exactly the same—will give nonidentical results. To give a clearer indication of the overall brain activation associated with any one cognitive demand, it should be useful to combine data from multiple studies. Recently, Adrian Owen and I have attempted this for several distinct demands. For each one, we have combined the reported foci of frontal activation from a number of separate studies, allowing the spread of activations from different demands to be compared. Illustrative analyses are presented here; a fuller treatment appears in Duncan and Owen (2000).

One demand we considered was response conflict, manifest in the need to suppress a strong response tendency that is inappropriate to the current task. We combined results from four studies of the Stroop effect (conflict between a required spoken response and a written stimulus word) (Bench et al., 1993; Carter et al., 1995; George et al., 1994; Pardo et al., 1990), one study of reversing previously learned stimulus–response associations (Paus et al., 1993), and two studies of incompatible stimulus–response mappings (Sweeney et al., 1996; Taylor et al., 1994). In line with the view that frontal systems organize novel but not automatic behavior, a second demand we considered was task novelty. We combined data from four studies comparing the initial learning of an unfamiliar cognitive task with later, well-practiced performance (Jenkins et al., 1994; Jueptner et al., 1997; Klingberg and Roland, 1998; Raichle et al., 1994). In line with the role of frontal systems in working memory, a third demand was the number of elements to be stored and organized in a standard working-memory task, the $N$-back task. In this task, a sequence of stimuli is presented one after the other, and the subject must respond when the current stimulus matches the one preceding it by $N$ steps. Working memory must be constantly updated and reorganized as the sequence progresses; we combined data from three studies (Braver et al., 1997; Carlson et al., 1998; Cohen et al., 1997). Still in the realm of working memory, a fourth demand was memory delay in tasks requiring simply that one to four stimuli be remembered across a few seconds for subsequent test; again there were data from three studies (Barch et al., 1997; Goldberg et al., 1996; Smith et al., 1995). Finally, we wished to include a demand factor less conventionally associated with frontal lobe functions. Thus a fifth demand was perceptual difficulty, including two studies of stimulus degradation (Barch et al., 1997; Grady et al., 1996) and one study addressing object recognition from an unconventional viewpoint (Kosslyn et al., 1994). For each demand, we included only studies that had manipulated the specified factor (e.g., presence of response conflict, length of delay) in the context of an otherwise identical task.

Combined results from all studies listed above are shown in figure 4.3 (and plate 2). All reported activation foci within the frontal lobe, excluding only those falling within primary motor (Brodmann area 4) or premotor (Brodmann area 6) cortex according to the Talairach and Tournoux (1988) atlas, have been plotted together on a standard brain. Different colors distinguish our five demand factors. Six brain views are shown, including lateral and medial views of each hemisphere, and views of the whole brain from above and below.

The results suggest two equally striking conclusions. First, activations cluster in several rather tightly defined regions. On the medial surface, activations are restricted entirely to the dorsal part of the anterior cingulate. Though activity on the lateral surface is more diffuse, it shows clear concentrations in mid-dorsolateral and mid-ventrolateral regions, with (especially in the right hemisphere) a possible silent area between the two (Owen, 1997). Beyond scattered points toward the frontal pole, activation is absent from much of the remainder of the lateral surface (see especially dorsal brain view), and from the whole orbitomedial region (ventral view).

Second, there is substantial overlap between activations associated with different demand factors. Although a possible specialization is the preponderance of right hemisphere activations associated with the perceptual difficulty factor (blue), the major conclusion is that all five demand factors similarly activate the dorsal anterior cingulate, the mid-dorsolateral, and the mid-ventrolateral regions.

Of course, there are important restrictions to the conclusions that can be drawn from an exercise of this sort. Though certainly there is substantial overlap in the gross regions recruited by different cognitive demands, important differences could exist at a finer scale. Certainly it is plausible that, at increasingly fine scale, one will increasingly find clusters of neurons with similar response properties. At the same time, the monkey data also suggest that neurons with a range of different properties will sometimes be closely mingled together within any one frontal region, and, as we have seen, that the properties even of single neurons will vary from one task context to another.

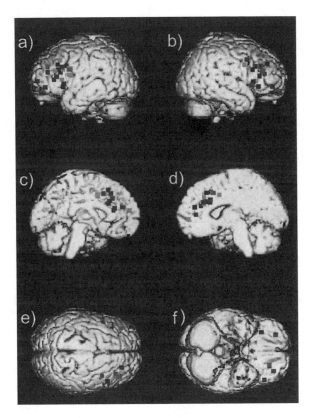

**Figure 4.3**
Frontal activations associated with 5 different manipulations of cognitive demand, rendered together onto a standard brain using modified SPM software (Wellcome Department of Cognitive Neurology, London): lateral (*a* and *b*) and medial (*c* and *d*) views of each hemisphere, and views of whole brain from above (*e*) and below (*f*). Cognitive demands: green, response conflict; purple, novelty; orange, number of elements; red, delay; blue, perceptual difficulty. (See plate 2 for color version.)

What, then, may we conclude about the broad regions of frontal activation seen in our studies of lateralized visual attention? In figure 4.4 (also plate 3), activation foci from the study of Vandenberghe and colleagues (1997) have been plotted together with the results from the Duncan and Owen analysis. The left hemisphere points from Vandenberghe and colleagues are those showing higher activity for attention to the left, and the right hemisphere points are those showing higher activity for attention to the right. Once again, we observe substantial overlap between activations related to attention and those related to other cognitive demands. Thus, the data do not support the (unlikely) hypothesis that large

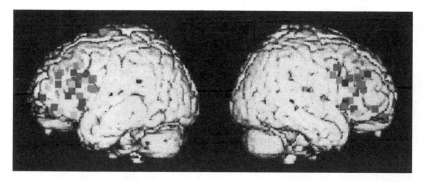

**Figure 4.4**
Lateral views from figure 4.3, with additional foci (yellow) associated with selective attention to left field (left hemisphere) and right field (right hemisphere). (See plate 3 for color version.)

regions of frontal cortex are specifically devoted to control of the attentional focus. Instead, the results hint at the existence of a general frontal system that adapts processing to the specific requirements of any given task context.

## 4.4   Measurement of Attentional Control

The third project to be described is a collaboration recently begun with Claus Bundesen in Copenhagen, Jon Driver in London, and Casimir Ludwig, Claudia Bonfiglioli, Chris Rorden, Alice Parr, and Nagui Antoun in Cambridge. In this project we use a behavioral measurement of top-down control to investigate possible control deficits in frontal lobe patients. Though the work is just beginning, I hope to show the general merits of the method, as well as to indicate the preliminary direction of our data. Once more, the conceptual context for this work is control of a competitive process by appropriate weight setting. Specifically, we use a variant of a classical experiment—the "partial report" task of Sperling (1960) and von Wright (1970)—to investigate selective processing of targets and rejection of nontargets in a brief visual display.

Experimental displays are illustrated in figure 4.5. On each trial, the display contains one or two letters, briefly presented (100–150 ms) and immediately followed by a backward mask of jumbled contours. Visual noise (a random dot field) is added to each display to bring performance into a suitable range (50–80% correct). A red cross marks the point of fixation. In different sessions, the subject is instructed either to identify white letters, ignoring black, or the reverse. Thus letters of one color are designated *targets* to be attended, and letters of the other color are designated *nontargets* to be ignored. The response

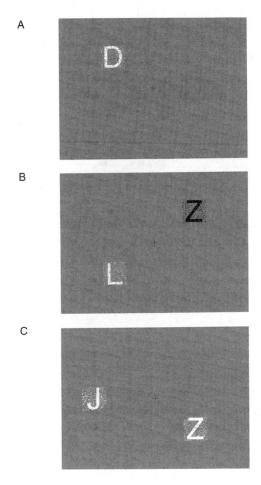

**Figure 4.5**
Sample partial report stimuli for three types of display: (*a*) target alone; (*b*) target + nontarget; (*c*) target + target.

is simply to name targets that are confidently identified. In the displays of figure 4.5, white letters are targets and black letters are nontargets. Thus correct responses for the three displays would be respectively "D," "L," and "J, Z" (or equivalently "Z, J").

For the data to be presented here, there were three types of display, randomly mixed in each block of trials. First, a target could appear alone, in either left or right visual hemifield (figure 4.5A). Second, a single target in either hemifield could be accompanied by a single nontarget, always in the opposite hemifield (figure 4.5B). Third, there could be one target in each hemifield, without nontargets (figure 4.5C). For each hemifield, accordingly, data are available for a target presented alone, accompanied by a nontarget (target + nontarget), or accompanied by a second target (target + target); accompanying letters always appearing in the opposite hemifield. In the target + target case, the two targets were always scored independently, giving separate accuracy measures for left and right visual fields.

What will the data look like in this task? The general expectation is illustrated in the top part of figure 4.6, as a schematic plot of proportion correct for the three different types

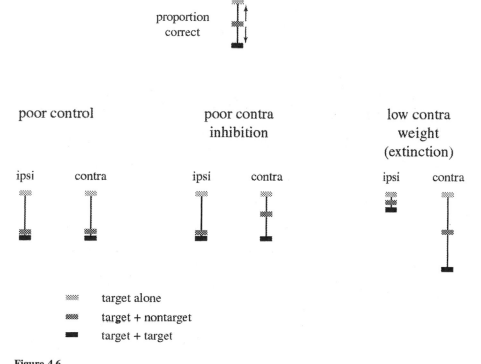

**Figure 4.6**
Schematic diagrams indicating partial report measure of attentional control. As shown in upper part of figure, target + nontarget performance must move between best possible attentional control (equivalent to target alone) and worst possible attentional control (equivalent to target + target). Below are three possible varieties of control impairment, as these affect performance in ipsilesional (ipsi) and contralesional (contra) visual fields.

of display. Obviously, we expect the best performance for a target presented alone (figure 4.6, light). Equally obviously, we expect worse performance for a target accompanied by a second, simultaneous target (target + target). Here, there are two letters relevant to the task and competing to be processed (figure 4.6, dark). This is the standard "divided attention decrement" measured in innumerable studies of limited attentional capacity (Broadbent, 1958; Treisman, 1969). But what should happen in a target + nontarget display? At one extreme, attentional control could be perfect. Competitive weights could be set high for targets but negligible for nontargets. In this case, the presence of a nontarget would have no impact on target processing; performance would be as good as performance for a single target presented alone. Subjectively, this would correspond to a state of exclusive attention to targets. At the opposite extreme, there could be no attentional control. Weights could be equal for targets and nontargets, meaning that a target accompanied by an additional item would be processed no better when that additional item was a nontarget than when it was a second target. Subjectively, attention would be devoted equally to targets and nontargets. Overall, therefore, target + nontarget performance is expected to lie somewhere between performance for target alone and for target + target. Exactly where it lies along this scale (figure 4.6, intermediate) provides a natural measure for the efficiency of attentional control under different conditions (e.g., selection based on color, location, or other stimulus features; see von Wright, 1970) or for different individuals (e.g., different patient groups; see Duncan et al., 1999). Elsewhere, we have developed methods for translating performance into direct estimates of competitive weights for targets and nontargets, based on the quantitative approach of Bundesen's Theory of Visual Attention or TVA (Bundesen, 1990; Duncan et al., 1999). The intuitive treatment presented above, however, is sufficient for present purposes.

It is instructive to compare partial report with another standard task in the literature, visual search (Neisser, 1963; Treisman and Gelade, 1980). In the usual visual search experiment, the time to detect or identify a single target is plotted as a function of the number of nontargets in the display. Again, therefore, the experiment concerns the impact of nontargets on target processing. In the easiest cases, the search function is flat. Added nontargets have no effect on performance, corresponding to the best possible case in partial report. In harder cases, the slope of the search function can increase to 100 ms/item or more, indicating increased attentional demand of nontargets. Here, however, there is no natural bound to the scale; because processing of $N$ nontargets is not compared with processing of $N$ targets, there is no way of knowing what search slope would correspond to zero control, or to equal attentional demand for targets and nontargets. As we have argued before (Bundesen et al., 1985; Duncan, 1980, 1985), including multiple targets as well as multiple nontargets in a display allows direct comparison of their attentional demands, and thus a bounded scale for measurement of attentional control.

What deficits might be expected in a group of frontal patients? Three possibilities are illustrated in the lower part of figure 4.6. On the left is a global impairment in control; performance is much the same for target + nontarget and target + target displays, whether target identification is measured in the ipsilesional (ipsi) or contralesional (contra) hemifield. Though this is one interesting possibility, the method can also distinguish a variety of other, more specific control impairments. In the middle is a model derived from the PET data reviewed in the first part of this chapter: nontarget inhibition is weak on the side opposite to the lesion, meaning that *ipsilesional* targets are identified similarly whether the accompanying contralesional letter is target or nontarget. On the right is a third model, global attentional bias toward the ipsilesional field, conceptualized as strong ipsilesional and weak contralesional competitive weights (see, e.g., Duncan, 1996; Ward et al., 1994). When letters appear in both visual fields, performance is well preserved on the ipsilesional side but strongly impaired on the contralesional side, in line with the clinical phenomenon of "extinction" following a wide range of cortical and subcortical lesions (Bender, 1952; Vallar et al., 1994).

Actual data appear in figure 4.7. In the left panel are mean results for our first ten normal control subjects, selected from the volunteer subject panel of the Cognition and Brain Sciences Unit (age range of thirty-nine to sixty-four). Proportion correct target identification is shown for each display type, separately for targets in left and right visual fields. The data follow roughly the expected pattern, with best performance for target alone, intermediate for target + nontarget, and worst for target + target. The substantial difference between target alone and target + nontarget cases indicates that, even in these normal subjects, attentional control is far from perfect in this task. Despite a conspicuous feature difference between targets and nontargets, the competitive influence of nontargets is far from negligible. At the same time, there is some successful modulation of competitive weight by task relevance, indicated by the advantage of target + nontarget over target + target displays.

Corresponding data from seven frontal lobe patients appear in the middle panel of figure 4.7. In this group the age range is thirty-eight to sixty-four. Each patient has a long-standing focal lesion entirely restricted to either left or right frontal lobe. Following the format of figure 4.6, data are shown separately for targets in ipsilesional (ipsi) and contralesional (contra) visual fields.

The most conspicuous result is complete absence of attentional control in this group. In neither visual field is there an advantage for target + nontarget over target + target displays. Certainly these are very preliminary data, and indeed, a convincing impairment is hard to demonstrate against the baseline of rather poor control even in normal subjects. Still, these data, in line with the "poor control" model in figure 4.6, provide suggestive support for some overall role of frontal cortex in attentional weight setting.

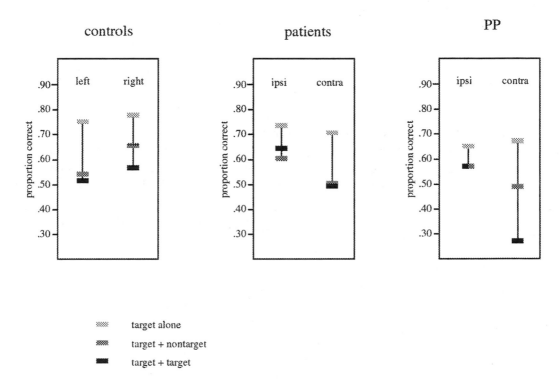

**Figure 4.7**
Partial report results for control subjects (*left*), frontal patients (*center*), and single patient PP (*right*). Conventions as in figure 4.6.

A second finding is also suggestive. In line with the "low contralesional weight" model of figure 4.6, it is contralesional targets that suffer the greatest loss of accuracy in target + target displays. This finding was highly variable from one patient to another; it was a conspicuous result for three patients but not for the remainder. Still, the data show that extinction-like results can be seen after focal prefrontal lesions, just as they can following damage to many other cortical and subcortical structures.

Clearly it is too soon to draw strong conclusions from these data. In the future, an important task will be analysis of individual patients, allowing us to ask how deficits of attentional control relate to specific areas of damage. An attractive possibility is cross-reference between patient and functional imaging studies, as illustrated in figure 4.8 (and plate 4). In the top row is the MRI of one representative patient (PP) from the current study, resliced in alignment with standard sections (bottom row) from the atlas of Talairach and Tournoux (1988). Superimposed on the scan are the lesion tracing for this patient (red) and peak activations from our PET study (Vandenberghe et al., 1997) of directed

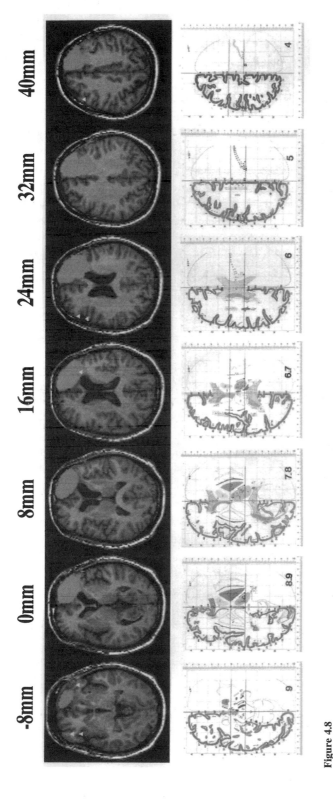

**Figure 4.8**
Horizontal slices (*upper row*) from MRI of a single frontal patient, PP. Using SPM software (Wellcome Department of Cognitive Neurology, London), MRI has been linearly transformed into standard space, and resliced in horizontal sections corresponding to matched sections (*lower row*) from atlas of Talairach and Tournoux (1988; reproduced by permission). Numbers at top indicate z-levels in the space of the atlas; within each section, the left of the brain appears to the left. Red region is lesion as traced by the consultant neuroradiologist. Yellow triangles indicate peak activations from Vandenberghe et al. (1997), associated in that experiment with attention to left (left hemisphere) or right (right hemisphere). (See plate 4 for color version.)

attention in normal subjects (yellow triangles: left hemisphere—greater activation for attend-left; right hemisphere—greater activation for attend-right). For this patient, the lesion shows some overlap with those right hemisphere regions associated in normal subjects with attention to the right. It also includes much of the right hemisphere region homologous to the left hemisphere activations associated with attention to the left. In partial report, this patient showed a strong extinction tendency, or reduced competitive weight for a target on the left or contralesional side (figure 4.7, rightmost panel). As shown by performance on target + nontarget displays, however, attentional control was relatively good, at least for targets on the left. (In related tests, indeed, this patient showed adequate control on both sides.) Though preliminary, such results show the potential for dissociating distinct aspects of attentional impairment, and for detailed investigation of relations between normal and impaired frontal function.

## 4.5   Conclusion

Perhaps more than anything else, the work reviewed here points up the uncertainties in our knowledge of frontal lobe function. Three examples may be considered.

In the specific domain of visual attention, an immediate puzzle is the relation between inhibitory and facilitatory effects in the contralateral visual field. As we have already seen, prefrontal lesions can lead to unwanted behavior directed to contralateral space, presumably through the relaxation of contralateral inhibition. The prefrontal activation we have observed contralateral to the unattended hemifield is also consistent with contralateral inhibition. Equally, however, prefrontal lesions can produce contralateral neglect and extinction, implying not relaxation of contralateral inhibition but a reduction of competitive weights in the contralateral hemifield (Heilman and Valenstein, 1972). This indeed is the picture suggested by our own lesion data, which suggest reduced competitive weights of contralesional targets, and arguably also by single-unit data (Rainer et al., 1998a). Very plausibly, prefrontal neurons combine both inhibitory and facilitatory influences in contralateral space, but as yet we can say little about how these work together, or when one or the other may predominate.

Our review of imaging work shows joint activity in three distinct regions of frontal cortex—mid-dorsolateral, mid-ventrolateral, and dorsal anterior cingulate—in association with many different aspects of cognitive demand. Indeed, once this pattern has been seen, it is truly extraordinary to see how often it reoccurs in one imaging study after another, suggesting a tightly integrated functional system. At the same time, there are hints of dissociation, for example, between mid-dorsolateral and mid-ventrolateral regions (Owen, 1997; Fletcher et al., 1998). Can separate functions be assigned to the subcomponents of this frontal system, or are neurons in each region so flexible and/or interactive that the whole system is better considered as one integrated unit?

Indeed, perhaps the major question raised by our work concerns specificity of frontal lobe functions at the cognitive or information-processing level. The dominant theme in current work is proposal of particular cognitive processes supported by the frontal lobe: plan formation (Shallice and Burgess, 1991), error management (Shallice and Burgess, 1991), working memory (Goldman-Rakic, 1988), goal selection (Duncan et al., 1996) and so on. There is, however, the unsettling possibility that no answer to the question of frontal function exists at this level. Given dynamic neural function, frontal systems may freely adapt to support whatever cognitive distinctions are relevant to a current task. As our imaging data suggest, frontal involvement in the control of visual attention may reflect not a specific attentional "module," but adaptation of a rather general system to this particular cognitive domain.

## Acknowledgments

Parts of this work were supported by grants from the Human Frontier Science Program (principal investigator G. Humphreys) and the Wellcome Trust (principal investigator J. Driver).

## References

Barch, D. M., Braver, T. S., Nystrom, L. E., Forman, S. D., Noll, D. C., and Cohen, J. D. (1997). Dissociating working memory from task difficulty in human prefrontal cortex. *Neuropsychologia* 35: 1373–1380.

Bench, C. J., Frith, C. D., Grasby, P. M., Friston, K. J., Paulesu, E., Frackowiak, R. S. J., and Dolan, R. J. (1993). Investigations of the functional anatomy of attention using the Stroop test. *Neuropsychologia* 31: 907–922.

Bender, M. B. (1952). *Disorders in perception.* Springfield, IL: Charles C. Thomas.

Braver, T. S., Cohen, J. D., Nystrom, L. E., Jonides, J., Smith, E. E., and Noll, D. C. (1997). A parametric study of prefrontal cortex involvement in human working memory. *NeuroImage* 5: 49–62.

Broadbent, D. E. (1958). *Perception and communication.* London: Pergamon.

Bundesen, C. (1990). A theory of visual attention. *Psycholog. Rev.* 97: 523–547.

Bundesen, C., Shibuya, H., and Larsen, A. (1985). Visual selection from multielement displays: A model for partial report. In M. I. Posner and O. S. M. Marin (eds.), *Attention and performance XI* (pp. 631–649). Hillsdale, NJ: Erlbaum.

Butter, C. M. (1969). Perseveration in extinction and in discrimination reversal tasks following selective frontal ablations in *Macaca mulatta. Physiol. Behav.* 4: 163–171.

Butter, C. M., Rapcsak, S., Watson, R. J., and Heilman, K. M. (1988). Changes in sensory inattention, directional motor neglect and "release" of the fixation reflex following a unilateral frontal lesion: A case report. *Neuropsychologia* 26: 533–545.

Carlson, S., Martinkauppi, S., Rämä, P., Salli, E., Korvenoja, A., and Aronen, H. J. (1998). Distribution of cortical activation during visuospatial $n$-back tasks as revealed by functional magnetic resonance imaging. *Cereb. Cortex* 8: 743–752.

Carter, C. S., Mintun, M., and Cohen, J. D. (1995). Interference and facilitation effects during selective attention: An $H_2^{15}O$ PET study of Stroop task performance. *NeuroImage* 2: 264–272.

Cohen, J. D., Peristein, W. M., Braver, T. S., Nystrom, L. E., Noll, D. C., Jonides, J., and Smith, E. E. (1997). Temporal dynamics of brain activation during a working memory task. *Nature* 386: 604–608.

Corbetta, M., Miezin, F. M., Shulman, G. L., and Petersen, S. E. (1993). A PET study of visuospatial attention. *J. Neurosci.* 13: 1202–1226.

Corbetta, M., and Shulman, G. L. (1998). Human cortical mechanisms of visual attention during orienting and search. *Phil. Trans. R. Soc. London* B353: 1353–1362.

Desimone, R., and Duncan, J. (1995). Neural mechanisms of selective visual attention. *Ann. Rev. Neurosci.* 18: 193–222.

Dias, R., Robbins, T. W., and Roberts, A. C. (1996). Dissociation in prefrontal cortex of affective and attentional shifts. *Nature* 380: 69–72.

di Pellegrino, G., and Wise, S. P. (1993). Visuospatial versus visuomotor activity in the premotor and prefrontal cortex of a primate. *J. Neurosci.* 13: 1227–1243.

Duncan, J. (1980). The locus of interference in the perception of simultaneous stimuli. *Psychol. Rev.* 87: 272–300.

Duncan, J. (1985). Visual search and visual attention. In M. I. Posner and O. S. M. Marin (eds.), *Attention and performance XI* (pp. 85–104). Hillsdale, NJ: Erlbaum.

Duncan, J. (1996). Cooperating brain systems in selective perception and action. In T. Inui and J. L. McClelland (eds.), *Attention and performance XVI* (pp. 549–578). Cambridge, MA: MIT Press.

Duncan, J. (1998). Converging levels of analysis in the cognitive neuroscience of visual attention. *Phil. Trans. R. Soc. London* B353: 1307–1317.

Duncan, J., Bundesen, C., Olson, A., Humphreys, G., Chavda, S., and Shibuya, H. (1999). Systematic analysis of deficits in visual attention. *J. Exp. Psychol. Gen.* 128: 450–478.

Duncan, J., Emslie, H., Williams, P., Johnson, R., and Freer, C. (1996). Intelligence and the frontal lobe: The organization of goal-directed behavior. *Cog. Psychol.* 30: 257–303.

Duncan, J., and Owen, A. M. (2000). Common regions of the human frontal lobe recruited by diverse cognitive demands. *Trends Neurosci.* 23: 475–483.

Fletcher, P. C., Shallice, T., Frith, C. D., Frackowiak, R. S. J., and Dolan, R. J. (1998). The functional roles of prefrontal cortex in episodic memory. II. Retrieval. *Brain* 121: 1249–1256.

Funahashi, S., Bruce, C. J., and Goldman-Rakic, P. S. (1989). Mnemonic coding of visual space in the monkey's dorsolateral prefrontal cortex. *J. Neurophysiol.* 61: 331–349.

Fuster, J. M., Bauer, R. H., and Jervey, J. P. (1985). Functional interactions between inferotemporal and prefrontal cortex in a cognitive task. *Brain Res.* 330: 299–307.

George, M. S., Ketter, T. A., Parekh, P. I., Rosinsky, N., Ring, H., Casey, B. J., Trimble, M. R., Horwitz, B., Herscovitch, P., and Post, R. M. (1994). Regional brain activity when selecting a response despite interference: An $H_2^{15}O$ PET study of the Stroop and an emotional Stroop. *Hum. Brain Mapping* 1: 194–209.

Goldberg, T. E., Berman, K. F., Randolph, C., Gold, J. M., and Weinberger, D. R. (1996). Isolating the mnemonic component in spatial delayed response: A controlled PET $^{15}O$-labeled water regional cerebral blood flow study in normal humans. *NeuroImage* 3: 69–78.

Goldman-Rakic, P. (1988). Topography of cognition: Parallel distributed networks in primate association cortex. *Ann. Rev. Neurosci.* 11: 137–156.

Gottlieb, J. P., Kusunoki, M., and Goldberg, M. E. (1998). The representation of visual salience in monkey parietal cortex. *Nature* 391: 481–484.

Grady, C. L., Horwitz, B., Pietrini, P., Mentis, M. J., Ungerleider, L. G., Rapoport, S. I., and Haxby, J. V. (1996). Effect of task difficulty on cerebral blood flow during perceptual matching of faces. *Hum. Brain Mapping* 4: 227–239.

Heilman, K. M., and Valenstein, E. (1972). Frontal lobe neglect in man. *Neurology* 22: 660–664.

Jenkins, I. H., Brooks, D. J., Nixon, P. D., Frackowiak, R. S. J., and Passingham, R. E. (1994). Motor sequence learning: A study with positron emission tomography. *J. Neurosci.* 14: 3775–3790.

Jonides, J., and Yantis, S. (1988). Uniqueness of abrupt visual onset in capturing attention. *Percep. Psychophys.* 43: 346–354.

Jueptner, M., Stephan, K. M., Frith, C. D., Brooks, D. J., Frackowiak, R. S. J., and Passingham, R. E. (1997). Anatomy of motor learning. I. Frontal cortex and attention to action. *J. Neurophysiol.* 77: 1313–1324.

Klingberg, T., and Roland, P. E. (1998). Right prefrontal activation during encoding, but not during retrieval, in a non-verbal paired-associates task. *Cereb. Cortex* 8: 73–79.

Kosslyn, S. M., Alpert, N. M., Thompson, W. L., Chabris, C. F., Rauch, S. L., and Anderson, A. K. (1994). Identifying objects seen from different viewpoints: A PET investigation. *Brain* 117: 1055–1071.

Luria, A. R. (1966). *Higher cortical functions in man.* London: Tavistock.

Martínez, A., Anllo-Vento, L., Sereno, M. I., Frank, L. R., Buxton, R. B., Dubowitz, D. J., Wong, E. C., Hinrichs, H., Heinze, H. J., and Hillyard, S. A. (1999). Involvement of striate and extrastriate visual cortical areas in spatial attention. *Nature Neurosci.* 2: 364–369.

Mesulam, M.-M, (1981). A cortical network for directed attention and unilateral neglect. *Ann. Neurol.* 10: 309–325.

Miller, E. K. (1999). Prefrontal cortex and the neural basis of executive functions. In G. Humphreys, J. Duncan, and A. Treisman (eds.), *Attention, space, and action: Studies in cognitive neuroscience* (pp. 251–272). Oxford: Oxford University Press.

Neisser, U. (1963). Decision-time without reaction-time: Experiments in visual scanning. *Am. J. Psychol.* 76: 376–385.

Nobre, A. C., Sebestyen, G. N., Gitelman, D. R., Mesulam, M.-M., Frackowiak, R. S. J., and Frith, C. D. (1997). Functional localization of the system for visuospatial attention using positron emission tomography. *Brain* 120: 515–533.

Norman, D. A., and Shallice, T. (1980). *Attention to action: Willed and automatic control of behavior* (report no. 8006). San Diego: University of California, Center for Human Information Processing.

Owen, A. M. (1997). The functional organization of working memory processes within human lateral frontal cortex: The contribution of functional neuroimaging. *Euro. J. Neurosci.* 9: 1329–1339.

Pardo, J. V., Pardo, P. J., Janer, K. W., and Raichle, M. E. (1990). The anterior cingulate cortex mediates processing selection in the Stroop attentional conflict paradigm. *Proc. Nat. Acad. Sci. USA* 87: 256–259.

Paus, T., Kalina, M., Patockova, L., Angerova, Y., Cerny, R., Mecir, P., Bauer, J., and Krabec, P. (1991). Medial vs. lateral frontal lobe lesions and differential impairment of central-gaze fixation maintenance in man. *Brain* 114: 2051–2068.

Paus, T., Petrides, M., Evans, A. C., and Meyer, E. (1993). Role of the human anterior cingulate cortex in the control of oculomotor, manual, and speech responses: A positron emission tomography study. *J. Neurophysiol.* 70: 453–469.

Posner, M. I., Walker, J. A., Friedrich, F., and Rafal, R. D. (1984). Effects of parietal injury on covert orienting of attention. *J. Neurosci.* 4: 1863–1874.

Raichle, M. E., Fiez, J. A., Videen, T. O., MacLeod, A. K., Pardo, J. V., Fox, P. T., and Petersen, S. E. (1994). Practice-related changes in human brain functional anatomy during non-motor learning. *Cereb. Cortex* 4: 8–26.

Rainer, G., Asaad, W. F., and Miller, E. K. (1998a). Memory fields of neurons in the primate prefrontal cortex. *Proc. Nat. Acad. Sci. USA* 95: 15008–15013.

Rainer, G., Asaad, W. F., and Miller, E. K. (1998b). Selective representation of relevant information by neurons in the primate prefrontal cortex. *Nature* 393: 577–579.

Rao, S. R., Rainer, G., and Miller, E. K. (1997). Integration of what and where in the primate prefrontal cortex. *Science* 276: 821–824.

Rumelhart, D. E. (1970). A multicomponent theory of the perception of briefly exposed visual displays. *J. Math. Psychol.* 7: 191–218.

Shallice, T., and Burgess, P. W. (1991). Deficits in strategy application following frontal lobe damage in man. *Brain* 114: 727–741.

Smith, E. E., Jonides, J., Koeppe, R. A., Awh, E., Schumacher, E., and Minoshima, S. (1995). Spatial vs object working memory: PET investigations. *J. Cog. Neurosci.* 7: 337–358.

Sperling, G. (1960). The information available in brief visual presentations. *Psychol. Monog.* 74, no. 11 (whole no. 498).

Sweeney, J. A., Mintun, M. A., Kwee, S., Wiseman, M. B., Brown, D. L., Rosenberg, D. R., and Carl, J. R. (1996). Positron emission tomography study of voluntary saccadic eye movements and spatial working memory. *J. Neurophysiol.* 75: 454–468.

Talairach, J., and Tournoux, P. (1988). *Co-planar stereotaxic atlas of the human brain.* New York: Thieme.

Taylor, S. F., Kornblum, S., Minoshima, S., Oliver, L. M., and Koeppe, R. A. (1994). Changes in medial cortical blood flow with a stimulus–response compatibility task. *Neuropsychologia* 32: 249–255.

Treisman, A. M. (1969). Strategies and models of selective attention. *Psychol. Rev.* 76: 282–299.

Treisman, A. M., and Gelade, G. (1980). A feature integration theory of attention. *Cog. Psychol.* 12: 97–136.

Vallar, G., Rusconi, M. L., Bignamini, L., Geminiani, G., and Perani, D. (1994). Anatomical correlates of visual and tactile extinction in humans: A clinical CT scan study. *J. Neurol. Neurosurg. Psychiat.* 57: 464–470.

Van Voorhis, S., and Hillyard, S. A. (1977). Visual evoked potentials and selective attention to points in space. *Percep. Psychophys.* 22: 54–62.

Vandenberghe, R., Duncan, J., Arnell, K. M., Bishop, S. J., Herrod, N. J., Owen, A. M., Minhas, P. S., Dupont, P., Pickard, J. D., and Orban, G. A. (2000). Maintaining and shifting attention within left or right hemifield. *Cereb. Cortex.* 10: 706–713.

Vandenberghe, R., Duncan, J., Dupont, P., Ward, R., Poline, J. B., Bormans, G., Michiels, J., Mortelmans, L., and Orban, G. A. (1997). Attention to one or two features in left or right visual field: A positron emission tomography study. *J. Neurosci.* 17: 3739–3750.

von Wright, J. M. (1970). On selection in visual immediate memory. In A. F. Sanders (ed.), *Attention and performance III* (pp. 280–292). Amsterdam: North-Holland.

Ward, R., Goodrich, S. J., and Driver, J. (1994). Grouping reduces visual extinction: Neuropsychological evidence for weight linkage in visual selection. *Vis. Cog.* 1: 101–129.

Wojciulik, E., and Kanwisher, N. (1999). The generality of parietal involvement in visual attention. *Neuron* 23: 1–18.

# 5 Attentional Modulation of Contextual Influences

**Minami Ito, Gerald Westheimer, and Charles D. Gilbert**

## 5.1 Introduction

To explore the role of attention in modulating responses of neurons in any cortical area, one must take into account the nature of the operations that the cortical area performs. Thus, the character of the stimulus plays an important role in determining the strength and nature of attentional effects. Attention itself, moreover, is not an all-or-none phenomenon. The nature and difficulty of the behavioral task influence the perceptual effects of attention and any consequent modulation of neuronal responses. Finally, attentional influences on task performance may not be constant over time, but may change with practice and experience. One must therefore also take into account possible nonstationarities in the effect of attention as measured psychophysically and physiologically.

## 5.2 Contextual Influences in Primary Visual Cortex

Before considering the potential role of attention in primary visual cortex, it is worthwhile reviewing some of the recent developments on the higher order properties of cells in primary visual cortex, or area V1. The early work on the stimulus specificity of cell responses in area V1 indicated that these cells analyze simple attributes such as orientation, direction of movement, depth, and color. More complex features were supposed to be encoded at higher stages in the visual pathway, as exemplified by face cells in inferotemporal cortex. Between the encoding of simple stimulus attributes and the most complex objects lie intermediate stages of visual processing, involving contour integration, surface segmentation, and grouping operations. The cortical areas responsible for these operations were supposed at one time to include those at the highest levels in visual cortical processing. The current view, however, is that many aspects of intermediate level vision are reflected in the properties of cells in area V1 (Kapadia et al., 1995; Sillito et al., 1995; Zipser et al., 1996; Roelfsema et al., 1998).

The higher order properties encountered in area V1 extend the traditional concept of the receptive field. The region of visual space over which a simple stimulus, such a line segment, will elicit a discharge, is only the core of a much larger region over which multiple stimuli, placed in certain geometric configurations, will modulate the response of a cell. This contextual modulation can be very strong, as is shown in figure 5.1A, which is adapted from Ito and Gilbert (1999). If one places line A within the receptive field center, one gets a response of a certain level. A line B placed just beyond the receptive field boundary elicits no response, as expected, given the mapping procedure that operationally

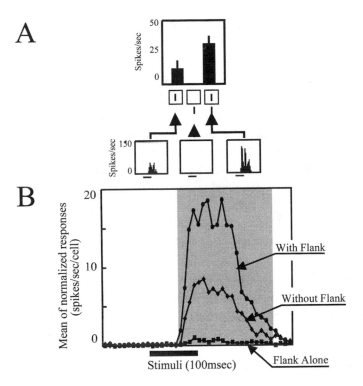

**Figure 5.1**
Effect of contextual stimuli on responses in primary visual cortex (area V1). (*A*) Responses of a cell in the superficial layers. An appropriately oriented stimulus inside the receptive field elicits a brisk response, a similar stimulus outside the receptive field gives no response, and together the two stimuli produce a response far larger than the sum of the responses to each stimulus alone. This nonlinear interaction is an instance of "contextual facilitation." (*B*) The time course of contextual facilitation matches that of the target response itself. Adapted from Ito and Gilbert (1999).

defines the receptive field. However, when lines A and B are presented simultaneously and in alignment with one another, the response can be as much as three times greater relative to that elicited by line A alone (figure 5.1A). A similar effect is seen in psychophysical studies, where the perceived brightness of a target line is increased by the presence of an aligned, flanking line. The psychophysical effect and the physiological response facilitation depend in similar ways on the spatial configuration of the target line and the flanking line. Both effects decrease as the distance between lines increases, as the lines move out of alignment, or as lines are rotated such that their orientations are no longer the same (Polat and Sagi, 1993; Kapadia et al., 1995; Polat et al., 1998). If one considers a population of cells, each of which shows facilitation for an optimal target–flanker configuration (chosen individually for each cell), the total amount of facilitation is substantial (figure 5.1B). As far as the neural circuits mediating this facilitation are concerned, it is of interest to note that the time course of facilitation matches that of the response itself (figure 5.1B).

The facilitation of responses by certain stimulus configurations outside the classical receptive field is likely to play an important role in contour integration. Stimuli that disrupt the perceptual continuity of a sequence of aligned line elements—an orthogonal bar placed between two aligned elements, for example—also block the physiological facilitation. Surrounding the receptive field with an array of randomly oriented and positioned lines inhibits the response to a target line inside the receptive field. Shifting line segments within this array into alignment with the target line, so that the target line forms part of a contour extending well beyond the receptive field, not only removes this inhibition but also facilitates the responses to a level higher than to that seen with the target line alone (Kapadia et al., 1995).

Several lessons can be drawn from these observations. First, the response of a cell to a complex visual stimulus cannot be predicted from its response to a simple stimulus placed in different positions around the visual field. Second, the responses of cells, even in primary visual cortex, are as dependent on global characteristics of contours extending well beyond the classical receptive field as they are on attributes of the stimulus lying within the classical receptive field. Third, the dependence of facilitatory influences on the precise geometric relationship between stimuli inside and outside the classical receptive field highlights the remarkable stimulus specificity of contextual influences. As we will show, any attempt to understand the effect of attention on responses in area V1 must take into account the specificity of such responses to complex stimulus configurations.

## 5.3 Attentional Modulation of Contextual Influences: Psychophysics

To examine how visual attention alters contextual influences, we created a stimulus array consisting of four *target lines* placed symmetrically around the fixation point (eccentricity approximately 4°), as illustrated in figure 5.2. Next to each target line and at an even greater eccentricity, we placed an aligned *flanking line* (figure 5.2B). Target and flanking lines did not always point directly at the fixation point; their orientation matched that of the recorded cells. Finally, we placed a single *reference line* next to the fixation point (figure 5.2A). We have shown previously that the presence of flanking lines not only lowers the contrast needed to detect a target line, but also increases the perceived brightness of target lines (Kapadia et al., 1995; Ito et al., 1998). Here we investigate how these two flanker effects—lower threshold and increased brightness—are modulated by attention.

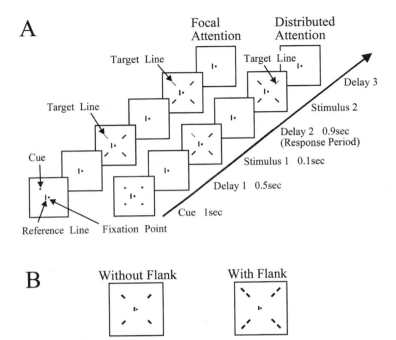

**Figure 5.2**
Experiment on contextual facilitation and its modulation by attention. (*A*) Stimuli and presentation sequence (schematic). Observers (human volunteers or macaque monkeys) fixated the central spot and reported whether one of four peripheral lines (target line) was brighter or dimmer than a reference line near the fixation. In focal attention trials, a cue indicated the future position of the target line, allowing observers to focus attention there. In distributed attention trials, all possible positions were cued, forcing observers to attend to all four peripheral lines. The diagram illustrates the sequence of events during a trial. Each cue presentation was followed by several stimulus presentations, each of which required a response by the observer. The number of stimulus presentations varied randomly; here only two presentations are shown. (*B*) In some trials, the stimulus contained only the basic pattern of four peripheral lines (without flank). In others, the stimulus contained four additional, somewhat brighter, flanking lines (with flank). The flanker lines tested contextual influences on the target line.

We manipulated the distribution of attention by spatial pre-cueing of one or more target positions. In each trial, one of the four target lines was either brighter or dimmer than the reference line (the other three target lines were equally bright). The observer indicated whether the "odd" target had been brighter or dimmer than the reference (the position of the "odd" target was not asked). In some trials, a small dot appeared at the future position of the "odd" target line, permitting the observer to focus attention on the cued location (*focal attention trials,* figure 5.2A, left). In other trials, small dots cued all four target positions, requiring the observer to distribute attention over all locations (*distributed attention trials,* figure 5.2A, right). The observer's ability to discriminate the brightness

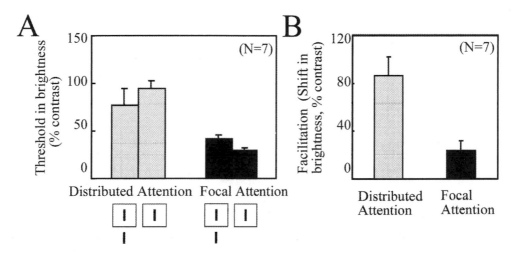

**Figure 5.3**
Effect of attention on contextual facilitation. (*A*) Thresholds for discriminating target brightness were lower with focal attention than with distributed attention, and this was true both with and without flanking lines. (*B*) The presence of flanking lines increased the perceived brightness of target lines (flanker facilitation). To measure this effect, we reduced physical target brightness until its perceived brightness matched that of the reference line. Flanker facilitation was substantially greater under distributed attention than under focal attention. Adapted from Ito and colleagues (1998).

of the "odd" target was significantly better with focal than with distributed attention (figure 5.3A). Similar results have been reported previously for contrast detection (Cohn and Lasley, 1974), orientation discrimination (Lindblom and Westheimer, 1992b), and stereoacuity (Lindblom and Westheimer, 1992a).

The most interesting aspect of these findings is how attention alters contextual influences from flanking lines. The increase in perceived target brightness can be measured by adjusting reference brightness until both are perceived to be the same (i.e., until the observer equally often reports a brighter and a dimmer target). In this way, the change in perceived brightness induced by the flanking line can be measured under different attentional states. The increase in perceived brightness is initially far larger with distributed than with focal attention (figure 5.3B). When observers had not been cued, and hence had to distribute attention over all four targets, the increase in perceived brightness was almost four times as large as when attention was focused. To compare, brightness discrimination thresholds differ approximately twofold between focal and distributed attention (figure 5.3A). Thus, the increase in perceived brightness is a particularly sensitive measure of contextual influences.

One way to interpret these findings is in terms of contour saliency. In natural visual scenes, saliency derives from certain geometric relationships between scene components that enhance the perceived difference between foreground and background. If attention is already directed toward a contour, no greater saliency is derived from contextual relationships. In effect, the saliency derived from focal attention appears to be interchangeable with the saliency derived from the physical characteristics of the stimulus. However, a degree of contextual facilitation remains even under focal attention, so that contour integration may take place even for attended stimuli.

## 5.4 Perceptual Learning and Attention

In addition to choosing the appropriate visual stimulus and task to bring out the effects of visual attention (e.g., a stimulus with flanking lines and a task measuring increased brightness), one must also take into account the strong contribution of experience and learning. The difference in behavioral performance between distributed and focal attention changes markedly with growing task experience. Although perceptual learning is well known in visual discrimination tasks, the observation of attentional changes with experience goes beyond earlier findings, and suggests that subjects can improve in their ability to attend to multiple sites.

In the visual discrimination task described above, the difference between distributed and focal attention gradually disappears over a period of approximately fifteen to twenty weeks (figure 5.4). This is due mostly to improved performance under distributed attention, because performance under focal attention remains fairly constant. The improvement under distributed attention is evident both in terms of reduced thresholds for brightness discrimination (figure 5.4A) and in terms of a notable decrease of contextual facilitation (figure 5.4B). This learning was observed in both humans and nonhuman primates, although in nonhuman primates it is difficult to measure the full effect of learning, because the initial measurement requires considerable training.

Interestingly, the learning shows considerable specificity for the stimulus configuration. When observers practice on displays with four targets, and then the number of targets is increased to eight, performance decreases and once again approaches the levels observed at the beginning. The improved performance holds, however, for the original four positions, suggesting that this learning is spatially specific. But matters are not so simple. If one presents four targets at the ''new'' positions (i.e., rotates the array), performance is also high. One has the impression that observers generate an attentional template matching the four-target array and that they are able to mentally rotate this template as long as the display does not contain additional targets.

These learning effects with distributed attention suggest that observers can increase the number of attentional foci maintained in parallel. The implication is that distributed atten-

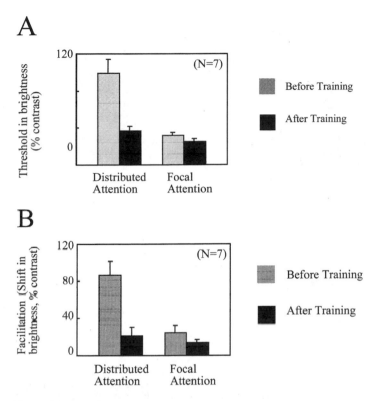

**Figure 5.4**
Perceptual learning with distributed attention. (*A*) Over several weeks of practice, brightness thresholds with distributed attention decreased, but those with focal attention did not. (*B*) Over the same period, flanker facilitation with distributed attention decreased toward the level observed with focal attention. Adapted from Ito and colleagues (1998).

tion is not necessarily diffused over a continuous region, but may involve multiple foci at discrete locations.

## 5.5   Attentional Modulation of Contextual Influences: Physiology

Our psychophysical results suggest that in order to bring out the effects of attention in any cortical area, it is important to choose a suitable stimulus configuration and behavioral task, and to take into account possible effects of training. With this in mind, we trained two macaque monkeys to perform the attentional task described above. Because of the extensive training needed for the animals to perform such a complex task, one cannot be

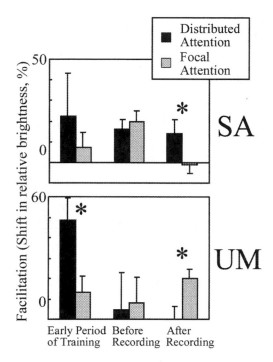

**Figure 5.5**
Effect of overtraining on brightness discrimination in two macaque monkeys. During the early training period, flanker facilitation was similar with distributed and focal attention. However, substantial differences developed over the subsequent period of single-unit recording. Animal SA exhibited greater flanker facilitation with distributed attention than with focal attention, whereas animal UM showed the reverse relationship. Adapted from Ito and Gilbert (1999).

certain that different attentional conditions have an effect on visual processing unless one verifies these effects through psychophysical measurements.

In fact, the two animals of this study performed quite differently during the recording period. Figure 5.5 illustrates contextual facilitation for animals SA and UM in the early training stage and at the beginning and end of the recording stage. At the end of the recording stage, one animal (SA) exhibited greater contextual facilitation under distributed attention, whereas the other animal (UM) showed greater contextual facilitation under focal attention. This difference probably results from the degree of overtraining the animals received during the recording stage. Note that the "after training" condition in figure 5.4 (for human and macaque observers) corresponds to the "before recording" condition in figure 5.5. The difference may also reflect the fact that one animal worked with somewhat different displays (containing different numbers of targets) after the initial training period. To interpret the physiological results properly, it is therefore critical to keep in mind that focal and distributed attention had large effects on contextual facilitation, and that these effects were opposite in the two animals.

In our analysis of physiological results, we distinguish between responses recorded during *distributed* and *focal* attention trials. Among focal attention trials, we distinguish further between trials where attention focused on the recorded receptive field (*focal-on* trials) and trials where attention focused at some distance from the recorded receptive field (*focal-away* trials). To assess contextual facilitation physiologically, we measured the response to a target line inside the receptive field, with and without a flanking line outside the receptive field.

Examples of the effect of attention in area V1 are shown in figure 5.6. The first cell is from animal SA, in which contextual facilitation was larger under distributed attention, as shown by the psychophysical measurements of perceived brightness described

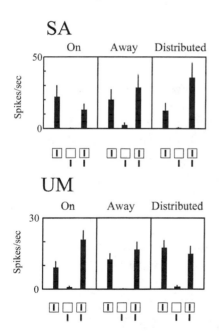

**Figure 5.6**
Two cells with attentional effects. Responses are compared for three attentional states: attention focused on the receptive field (on), attention focused away from the receptive field (away), and distributed attention (distributed). The cell from animal SA exhibited approximately threefold flanker facilitation with distributed attention, but none with focal attention on the receptive field. In contrast, the cell from animal UM showed flanker facilitation with focal attention on the receptive field, but none with either distributed attention or focal attention away from the receptive field. Adapted from Ito and Gilbert (1999).

above. This was confirmed by the physiological results, which showed large contextual facilitation with distributed attention (i.e., a nearly threefold increase in response due to the presence of a flanking line), but no contextual facilitation (possible even a contextual inhibition) with focal attention to the receptive field. The second cell is from animal UM, in which contextual facilitation as measured psychophysically was larger under focal attention. The physiological results were again consistent, in that contextual facilitation was large with focal attention to the receptive field (i.e., more than twofold increase of response), substantially reduced with focal attention away from the receptive field, and completely lacking with distributed attention. These examples show clearly that attention can dramatically increase responses in area V1, in some cases as much as threefold.

It is important to compare the average effect of attention on all recorded cells: though individual cells may show large modulations, this may simply reflect random variabilty in the recorded population. We analyzed the population data in two ways. First, for each recorded cell we computed contextual facilitation, based on the respective responses to target line alone and to target line plus flanking line, expressed as a percentage of the response to the target line. Average results for the 86 cells with significant facilitation are shown in figure 5.7. Although attention had no significant effect on responses to the target line alone (figure 5.7A and B), it had a very marked effect on facilitation (i.e., when a flanking line was present; figure 5.7C and D). In both animals, facilitation changed roughly twofold between distributed attention and focal attention to the receptive field, but in opposite directions. In animal SA, facilitation was larger with distributed attention, whereas in animal UM, it was larger with focal attention to the receptive field, exactly mirroring the different psychophysical results obtained with each animal. In contrast to the strong modulation of contextual facilitation, we found no attentional effect on contextual inhibition (Ito and Gilbert, 1999).

Our second analysis of the population data involved calculating the significance of attentional modulations on a trial-by-trial basis. Specifically, we used a Monte Carlo technique to compare the effect of attention with the effect one would expect simply on the basis of random variability in the responses. For each cell, we computed a "modulation index" for the effect of attention on flanker facilitation according to the following formula:

$$M = \frac{\max(F_{\text{distributed}}, F_{\text{focal on}}, F_{\text{focal away}}) - \min(F_{\text{distributed}}, F_{\text{focal on}}, F_{\text{focal away}})}{F_{\text{distributed}} + F_{\text{focal on}} + F_{\text{focal away}}},$$

where $F_{\text{focal on}}$, $F_{\text{focal away}}$, and $F_{\text{distributed}}$ are the flanker facilitations observed with focal attention on the receptive field, with focal attention away from the receptive field, and with distributed attention, respectively. To assess the significance of this modulation, we randomly assigned the responses from each trial to one of the three attentional states and

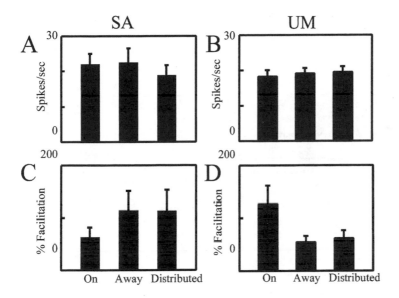

**Figure 5.7**
Average effect of attention in recorded population (86 cells showing significant flanker facilitation). (*A, B*)
Attentional state (focal on, focal away, or distributed, see figure 5.6) had no significant effect on responses to
target alone. (*C, D*) In contrast, attentional state significantly modulated flanker facilitation, with the greatest
difference between distributed attention and focal attention on the receptive field. Consistent with the difference
between their respective psychophysical results (figure 5.5), animal SA showed greater flanker facilitation with
distributed attention, whereas animal UM showed greater flanker facilitation with focal attention on the receptive
field. Adapted from Ito and Gilbert (1999).

computed a second set of modulation indices on the basis of the shuffled data. The population histograms of the modulation indices based on actual and shuffled data are compared
in figure 5.8 (top). The average modulation index was 0.34 ± 0.02 (N = 86) for actual
data, and 0.21 ± 0.02 for shuffled data, a difference that is significant at the level p <
.01 (t-test, t = 5.76). However, when this procedure is applied not to flanker facilitation
but to the response to target line alone, no significant difference between actual and shuffled data is found (figure 5.8 bottom). The fact that the two histograms are comparable
in this case demonstrates that responses to target line alone are not modulated by attention,
but simply exhibit random variability.

Since receptive fields are very small in area V1, neuronal responses depend critically
on eye position. Thus it is conceivable that observed dependence on attentional condition
could have been due to systematic differences in eye position. However, when we compared mean positions of fixation for different attentional conditions, we found the difference to be less than 0.1°, which was not a significant difference. Furthermore, when we

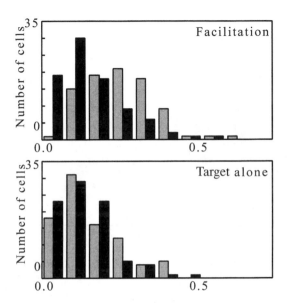

**Figure 5.8**
Distribution of the attentional modulation index in the recorded population. Each histogram was computed for actual data (gray bars) and for shuffled data (black bars) generated in a Monte Carlo simulation. See text for details. (*Top*) histogram, modulation index of flanker facilitation. Actual and shuffled data produce significantly different histograms, demonstrating that the observed modulation by attention cannot be explained by random variations in responses. (*Bottom*) histogram, modulation index for responses to target alone. Actual and shuffled data produce essentially identical histograms. In this case, the modulation is due to random response variations. Adapted from Ito and Gilbert (1999).

sorted trials into two groups with diametrically opposite eye fixation (within the permissible window), average responses were indistinguishable between the two groups of trials. This demonstrates—together with the fact that attention did not modulate responses to target alone—that differences in eye position were not responsible for the modulation of flanker facilitation by attention.

## 5.6   Conclusions

If one uses stimuli and examines properties appropriate to area V1, one finds that attention modulates contextual facilitation in area V1 approximately twofold. These substantial effects show that attention plays a pivotal role even at the earliest stages of cortical visual processing. Previous work showing little or no effect of attention in area V1 used simpler displays, and may not have placed sufficient attentional demand on the task. It has been pointed out that attention is not an all-or-none phenomenon, and that it is difficult to reduce attention to any given stimulus to zero (Nakayama and Joseph, 1997). The simple displays used in previous studies bear some similarity to our target alone condition, in which attentional effects were also lacking. Indeed, even in previous studies there were indications that attentional effects increase with the number of distractors (Haenny and Schiller, 1988; Motter, 1993; Luck et al., 1997; Vidyasagar, 1998). Thus, the salient difference between previous work and the current study seems to concern the nature of the visual display and, more specifically, the position of various stimuli relative to the receptive field boundary. Our results emphasize the importance of the specific juxtaposition of stimuli with respect to the receptive field boundary, and the interaction between stimuli lying inside and outside the receptive field, as critical factors for obtaining maximal attentional effects.

Our previous work on contextual interactions has shown how their characteristics coincide with the extent and specificity of the long-range horizontal connections that are intrinsic to area V1 (Gilbert and Wiesel, 1979, 1983, 1989, 1990; Kapadia et al., 1995). The interaction between the excitatory core of the receptive field and the modulatory surround changes according to stimulus contrast and foreground/background relationships, and the size of the receptive field itself changes as a consequence (Kapadia et al., 1998). Because attention does not modulate responses to a single target element, its primary effect may be exerted on the long-range horizontal connections between cells in area V1, perhaps by gating these connections via a feedback signal from higher cortical areas. This would account for the profound influence of attention on contextual interactions. It appears that attention has a specific effect on contextual influences, which are thought to be mediated by interactions between cells with widely separated receptive fields, involving horizontal connections intrinsic to area V1 (Kapadia et al., 1995). However, attention appears to affect only cells with receptive fields at or near its focus. This is suggested by the fact that contextual facilitation tends to be the same for distributed attention and for focal attention away from the receptive field. Finally, because contextual facilitation may play a role in contour integration, top-down influences such as attention may provide a mechanism for testing internally generated hypotheses about stimulus configuration against inputs reflecting physical reality.

There are several lines of evidence that support a dynamic nature of receptive field properties in primary visual cortex. The responses are context dependent, can be changed by altered visual experience and training, and, as shown here, are substantially modified by behavioral context and the state of attention. All of these sources of receptive field mutability are highly interdependent, and one cannot consider the role of any one of these influences without taking the others into account. The emerging picture is that response characteristics are modulated or gated by a nested and interactive set of internal influences, and that the response of cells, even in the primary visual cortex, are not exclusively a reflection of the immediate physical environment.

# References

Cohn, T. E., and Lasley, D. J. (1974). Detectability of a luminance increment: Effect of spatial uncertainty. *J. Optical Soc. America* 64: 1715–1718.

Gilbert, C. D., and Wiesel, T. N. (1979). Morphological and intracortical projections of functionally characterized neurons in the cat visual cortex. *Nature* 280: 120–125.

Gilbert, C. D., and Wiesel, T. N. (1983). Clustered intrinsic connections in cat visual cortex. *J. Neurosci.* 3: 1116–1133.

Gilbert, C. D., and Wiesel, T. N. (1989). Columnar specificity of intrinsic horizontal and corticocortical connections in cat visual cortex. *J. Neurosci.* 9: 2432–2442.

Gilbert, C. D., and Wiesel, T. N. (1990). The influence of contextual stimuli on the orientation selectivity of cells in primary visual cortex. *Vis. Res.* 30: 1689–1701.

Haenny, P. E., and Schiller, P. H. (1988). State dependent activity in monkey visual cortex. I. Single cell activity in V1 and V4 on visual tasks. *Exp. Brain Res.* 69: 225–244.

Ito, M., and Gilbert, C. D. (1999). Attention modulates contextual influences in the primary visual cortex of alert monkeys. *Neuron* 22: 593–604.

Ito, M., Westheimer, G., and Gilbert, C. D. (1998). Attention and perceptual learning modulate contextual influences on visual perception. *Neuron* 20: 1191–1197.

Kapadia, M. K., Ito, M., Gilbert, C. D., and Westheimer, G. (1995). Improvement in visual sensitivity by changes in local context: Parallel studies in human observers and in V1 of alert monkeys. *Neuron* 15: 843–856.

Kapadia, M. K., Westheimer, G., and Gilbert, C. D. (1998). Spatial distribution and dynamics of contextual interactions in cortical area V1. *Soc. Neurosci. Abstr.* 24: 1980.

Lindblom, B., and Westheimer, G. (1992a). Spatial uncertainty in stereoacuity tests: Implications for clinical vision test design. *Acta Ophthalmol.* 70: 60–65.

Lindblom, B., and Westheimer, G. (1992b). Uncertainty effects in orientation discrimination of foveally seen lines in human observers. *J. Physiol.* (London) 454: 1–8.

Luck, S. J., Chelazzi, L., Hillyard, S. A., and Desimone, R. (1997). Neural mechanisms of spatial attention in areas V1, V2, and V4 of macaque visual cortex. *J. Neurophysiol.* 77: 24–42.

Motter, B. C. (1993). Focal attention produces spatially selective processing in visual cortical areas V1, V2, and V4 in the presence of competing stimuli. *J. Neurophysiol.* 70: 909–919.

Nakayama, K., and Joseph, J. S. (1997). Attention, pattern recognition, and popout in visual search. In R. Parasuraman (ed.), *The attentive brain* (pp. 279–298). Cambridge, Mass.: MIT Press.

Polat, U., Mizopbe, K., Pettet, M. W., Kasamatsu, T., and Norcia, N. M. (1998). Collinear stimuli regulate visual responses depending on cell's contrast threshold. *Nature* 391: 580–584.

Polat, U., and Sagi, D. (1993). Lateral interactions between spatial channels: suppression and facilitation revealed by lateral masking experiments. *Vision Res.* 33: 993–999.

Roelfsema, P. R., Lamme, V. A. F., Spekreijse, H. (1998). Object-based attention in the primary visual cortex of the macaque monkey. *Nature* 395: 376–381.

Sillito, A. M., Griev, K. L., Jones, H. E., Cudeiro, J., and Davis, J. (1995). Visual cortical mechanisms detecting focal orientation discontinuities. *Nature* 378: 492–496.

Vidyasagar, T. R. (1998). Gating of neuronal responses in macaque primary visual cortex by an attentional spotlight. *NeuroReport* 9: 1947–1952.

Zipser, K., Lamme, V. A. F., and Schiller, P. H. (1996). Contextual modulation in primary visual cortex. *J. Neurosci.* 16: 7376–7389.

# 6 Effects of Attention on the Responsiveness and Selectivity of Individual Neurons in Visual Cerebral Cortex

John H. R. Maunsell and Carrie J. McAdams

## 6.1 Introduction

What we perceive depends critically on where we direct our attention. At any moment we fully attend to only a tiny fraction of the available sensory information. In a laboratory setting, attending to a particular location improves discrimination thresholds and accelerates reaction times for stimuli at that location. Indeed, in some situations attending or not attending makes the difference between seeing a stimulus clearly and not seeing it at all (Rensink et al., 1997; Simons and Levin, 1997; Mack and Rock, 1998; O'Regan et al., 1999; Braun et al., chapter 11 in this volume).

Neurophysiological studies have shown that the behavioral advantages associated with attention are accompanied by changes in the way the brain processes sensory information. Many of these studies have examined neuronal representations in the visual cerebral cortex. Functional imaging experiments in humans have shown that neuronal responses throughout visual cortex tend to be stronger when subjects are actively attending to a stimulus than when the same stimulus is ignored (Heinze et al., 1994; O'Craven and Savoy, 1995; Kastner et al., 1998; Mangun et al., 1998; Tootell et al., 1998; Watanabe et al., 1998; Brefczynski and DeYoe, 1999; Martinez et al., 1999; Corbetta and Shulman, chapter 1 this volume; Heeger et al., chapter 2 in this volume).

The effects of attention on neuronal responses can be examined at the level of individual neurons in studies using behaving monkeys. These experiments involve recording from neurons in animals while they do tasks that require them to either attend to or to ignore a stimulus placed in the receptive field of the recorded neuron. Using this approach, many laboratories have found that neurons often respond more strongly when the animal is attending to the stimulus that drives their response (see Goldberg et al., 1994; Desimone and Duncan, 1995; Maunsell, 1995; Reynolds and Desimone, chapter 7 in this volume). Attentional modulation of individual neuronal responses has been observed in all cortical visual areas examined, including primary visual cortex or area V1 (Haenny and Schiller, 1988; Motter, 1993; Luck et al., 1997; McAdams and Maunsell, 1999), although large attentional effects have been found in relatively few studies (Moran and Desimone, 1985; Mountcastle et al., 1987; Treue and Maunsell, 1996; Ito et al., chapter 5 in this volume).

Although many studies have documented that attention can affect the size of neuronal responses, less is known about the extent to which attention may alter more fundamental receptive field properties. One possibility is that attention may cause sweeping changes in the stimulus selectivity of cortical neurons. In this case, attending to a particular stimulus location or stimulus feature might increase the number of neurons responding to the attended location or feature. Naturally, a larger neuronal representation of behaviorally relevant stimuli could substantially improve performance in detecting or discriminating such stimuli. Consistent with this notion, some studies have suggested that attention may sharpen selectivity for stimulus orientation (Haenny and Schiller, 1988; Spitzer et al., 1988). Alternatively, attention might strengthen neuronal responses across the board, without altering the underlying stimulus selectivities. In line with this, some psychophysical studies have suggested that the primary effect of attention may be to boost neuronal signals, with little change in underlying selectivities (Lu and Dosher, 1998; see also Braun et al., chapter 11 in this volume). The question of whether attention alters neuronal response is important not only in the narrow context of attention, but also for understanding more generally how patterns of neuronal activity across cerebral cortex relate to sensory perceptions.

## 6.2    Attention and Orientation Tuning

We have explored this issue by examining the effect of attention on the orientation tuning of individual neurons in visual cerebral cortex. Macaque monkeys were trained to perform a visual task that caused stimuli to be either attended or ignored, and we measured the dependence of neuronal responses to the orientation of such stimuli. Specifically, animals performed the delayed match-to-sample task illustrated in figure 6.1 (McAdams and Maunsell, 1999). Two successive pairs of stimuli, one sample and one test, were presented on a video display. One stimulus in each pair was a Gabor pattern temporally modulated in counterphase, and the other was a patch of color with Gaussian saturation profile. Both stimuli had the same average luminance as the gray background. From trial to trial, the Gabor pattern varied in orientation and (independently) the Gaussian patch varied in color hue. The animal paid attention to the stimuli on one side (ignoring stimuli on the other side) and used a lever to report whether or not sample and test stimuli at the attended location had been the same. Depending on which type of stimulus—Gabor patterns or Gaussian patches—was on the attended side, the task required the discrimination of either stimulus orientation or stimulus color. Instructions as to which side was to be attended and which ignored were provided by means of instruction trials in which stimuli were present only on one side of the display. The animal learned to maintain attention on this side until a new instruction trial was given. Performance was high for each task, so that we could be sure the animal was attending to and reporting about the appropriate location (if it had reported about the wrong location, performance would have fallen to chance, that is, to approximately 50% correct).

Throughout the trial, the animal was required to gaze directly at a fixation spot at display center. Eye position was monitored using a scleral search coil, and trials were terminated

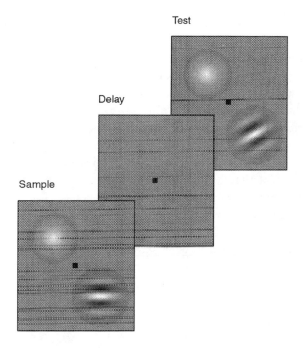

**Figure 6.1**
Delayed match-to-sample task. Two successive pairs of stimuli were presented for 500 ms each (sample and test), with a 500 ms delay in between. In each pair, one stimulus was a Gabor pattern time-modulated in counterphase at 4 Hz, and the other was a patch of color with a Gaussian intensity profile. Averaged over time, both were isoluminant with the gray background. The Gabor pattern varied in orientation from trial to trial and, independently, the color patch varied in color saturation. Animals were instructed to attend to stimuli on one side (ignoring stimuli on the other side) and to report whether sample stimulus and test stimulus on the attended side had been the same. Depending on which type of stimulus—Gabor pattern or color patch—appeared at the attended side, the task required discrimination of either stimulus orientation or color. The animal was required to hold its gaze on the fixation spot throughout all trials, and the stimuli on one side were positioned to fall on the receptive field of the recorded neuron. The spatial frequency and size of the Gabor pattern were optimized for each cell. This paradigm allowed us to measure the response to Gabor patterns of different orientations when these were either attended to or ignored by the animal.

if gaze drifted more than 0.7° of visual angle from the center of the fixation spot. This fixation requirement ensured that retinal stimulation was the same no matter which location the animal was attending. Gabor patterns were placed in the receptive field center of the recorded neuron, and their size and spatial frequency were optimized to elicit maximal responses. Color patches were placed in the other visual hemifield, diametrically opposite from the Gabor patterns. Gabor orientation varied from trial to trial, so that orientation tuning curves could be established. By instructing the animal to discriminate different locations, we could determine orientation tuning both when the animal was attending inside the receptive field (during orientation discrimination) and when it was attending outside the receptive field (during color discrimination). In this way we could examine the effect of attention on the orientation tuning of visual cortical neurons.

We recorded from 262 individual neurons in visual cortical area V4 of two macaque monkeys. Area V4 was selected in part because it represents a level of processing that is high enough to be substantially modulated by attention, yet also low enough to respond well to simple stimuli of different orientation. Responses from a representative neuron in area V4 are shown in figure 6.2. The average rate of firing during the presentation of the sample display is plotted as a function of stimulus orientation. For each orientation, filled circles represent the response during orientation discrimination when the Gabor pattern was attended and open circles the response during color discrimination when the Gabor pattern was ignored. The dotted line represents spontaneous activity, measured immediately before each stimulus presentation. As expected from earlier studies of area V4 (e.g., Moran and Desimone, 1985; Haenny et al., 1988; Maunsell et al., 1991; Motter, 1994a,b; Connor et al., 1996), responses were stronger when the animal was attending to the Gabor

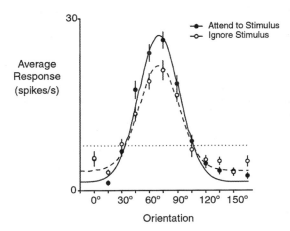

**Figure 6.2**
Effects of attention on the orientation tuning of a representative area V4 neuron. Closed circles represent the average response to attended Gabor patterns, that is, when the animal actively discriminated the Gabor pattern in the receptive field. Open circles reflect the average response to ignored Gabor patterns, that is, when the animal discriminated the color patch in the opposite visual hemifield. Vertical bars indicate the standard errors of the mean. The solid and dashed lines are the best-fitting Gaussian functions for each data set, which were used to assess the effects of attention. The dotted line is the level of spontaneous activity. In this cell, attention increased the magnitude of the responses but not its selectivity for orientation: the amplitude of the Gaussian fit to the response to attended stimuli was 26 spikes/s, whereas that for the ignored stimuli was 19 spikes/s. At the same time, the standard deviation of the Gaussian fit to the response to attended stimuli was 30 spikes/s, whereas that for ignored stimuli was 31 spikes/s. An increase in response amplitude without a change in response selectivity was typical for neurons in area V4.

pattern in the receptive field than when it was ignored. However, the modulation was not restricted to Gabor patterns of the preferred orientation and responses to Gabor patterns of all orientations appeared amplified.

To quantify the effects of attention on orientation tuning, we fitted a Gaussian function to each of the two data sets for each cell. We chose Gaussian functions because they are known to provide good fits for the tuning functions of visual cortical neurons (Henry et al., 1973; Geisler and Albrecht, 1997). To assess the effects of attention, we compared the functions fitted to data from the attended and ignored conditions. A different amplitude indicated a change in response strength, whereas a different width (standard deviation) implied a change in the sharpness of tuning.

For the representative neuron shown in figure 6.2, attention clearly increased the strength of responses. The peak response to an attended stimulus in the receptive field was approximately 26 spikes/s, whereas to an ignored stimulus it was only approximately 19 spikes/s. At the same time, there was no significant change in the sharpness of orientation tuning. The standard deviation of the Gaussian fitted to attended responses was 30°, and that for ignored responses was 31°. This outcome was typical for area V4 neurons. Averaging over all neurons for which both attended and ignored responses were fit well by a Gaussian (197/262), the median effect of attention was a 22% increase in the strength of the response but no change at all (0%) in the sharpness of tuning.

It should be noted that the behavioral task of the animal may not have resulted in a completely one-sided distribution of attention. Although the animal was motivated to direct attention at the task-relevant location, it might have been possible for the animal to pay attention to both locations but to report only about the relevant one. Also, the animal presumably had to devote some attention to the fixation spot, in order to maintain a stable gaze. However, the fact that neuronal responses differed between task conditions leaves no doubt that the animal did shift attention, at least to some extent. Because we cannot know how complete or incomplete this shift was, the observed difference between responses should be taken as a lower limit of the modulations that may result from shifting attention.

The overall effect of attention on orientation tuning in area V4 is summarized in figure 6.3, which plots the population tuning for both attended and ignored stimuli. The population tuning was computed by normalizing the peak response of each cell to unity (i.e., the response to an attended stimulus of the preferred orientation), by measuring orientation relative to the preferred orientation (so that the peak response occurs at 0° relative orientation), and by averaging the responses of all cells to attended and ignored stimuli. The curves in figure 6.3 are the best-fitting Gaussians to each data set, and the dotted line represents the average spontaneous activity.

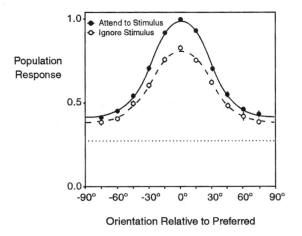

**Figure 6.3**
Overall effect of attention on orientation selectivity in area V4. The responses of 262 neurons recorded in V4 are averaged in this figure. Before averaging, the peak response of each neuron was normalized to unity (i.e., the response to an attended stimulus of preferred orientation), and orientation was measured relative to the preferred orientation (so that the peak response of each neuron occurs at 0°). The dotted line is the average normalized level of spontaneous activity. The solid and dashed lines are Gaussian functions fitted to the result, and show the average effect of attention on orientation selectivity in area V4. Attention increases the strength of the average response by 32%, but has no effect on average orientation tuning (both Gaussian functions have a standard deviation of 38°).

The population tuning curve is based on all 262 neurons in area V4 that were tested, and gives an impression of the average effect of attention on orientation tuning in that area. In the population average, the peak response increased by a factor 1.32. This value is somewhat larger than the median increase for the 197 cells with responses that were well fit by Gaussians, because some of the cells in the larger group did not respond at all to stimuli that the animal ignored. Even so, the population tuning also provided no evidence for a change in the sharpness of tuning, and the standard deviation of both tuning curves in figure 6.3 was 38°.

The data in figure 6.3 reveal further that attention had no effect on the level of spontaneous activity. Spontaneous activity was measured *after* the animal had been instructed to either attend to or ignore the receptive field location, but *before* any stimulus actually appeared in the gray background. Because attention changed neither spontaneous activity nor sharpness of tuning, the only effect of attention was to increase response to any orientation by the same factor. Thus, the effect of attention can be described as a multiplicative scaling of the *driven response* (i.e., the part that exceeds spontaneous activity) without any change of the *undriven response* (i.e., spontaneous activity).

## 6.3 Consequences of Multiplicative Scaling: A Simple Model

Most previous neurophysiological studies did not directly test the hypothesis that attention scales responses multiplicatively. Nevertheless, almost all of the available data are consistent with that type of effect, and a few studies even provide direct support for multiplicative scaling by attention. For example, Treue and Martinez-Trujillo (1999) have recently examined the effects of attention on direction tuning in the middle temporal visual area and the medial superior temporal area (MT and MST). Consistent with the results from area V4 presented above, they report that attention increases the height, but does not systematically alter the width, of tuning curves for direction of motion. A further case in point is that, in area V4, the spatial profiles of receptive fields appear to scale multiplicatively when attention is directed at different locations near the receptive field (Connor et al., 1996, 1997). Finally, when orientation tuning curves are measured in inferotemporal cortex for reward-contingent and non-reward-contingent stimuli, they differ only by a multiplicative factor (Vogels and Orban, 1994). Whereas psychophysical evidence raises the possibility that, in the context of much more demanding visual tasks, attention may change not only the height but also the width of neuronal tuning curves (Lee et al., 1999; Braun et al., chapter 11 in this volume), the available neurophysiological evidence suggests that the most common effect of attention in visual cortex is a multiplicative scaling of responses. If true, this would greatly simplify our understanding of the actions and consequences of visual attention.

Figure 6.4 schematizes our current understanding of how attention affects sensory processing. The framework illustrated there is similar to a computational model for attention (Cohen et al., 1992). The framework considers individual neurons or groups of neurons (small boxes) that represent either sensory information (left panel) or information about the attentional state (right panel). The sensory representation further distinguishes between the left and right visual fields (horizontal axis) and two levels of processing (vertical axis). At level 1, units have smaller receptive fields (narrow boxes) than at level 2 (wide boxes), which receives converging inputs from level 1. The units of the attentional representation are neither sensory nor motor, but encode specific information about the current behavioral state, namely, the locus of attention within the visual field. These units become active as soon as the subject learns which visual hemifield will be relevant to the task, and remain active as long as the subject continues to pay attention to this hemifield. Attentional units are connected selectively with sensory units that cover the same part of the visual field.

The mechanisms that initiate and maintain the activity of attentional units are not considered here. However, neural signals of the type postulated here have been observed in the parietal cortex of human subjects while they perform a spatial attention task (Corbetta and Shulman, chapter 1 in this volume).

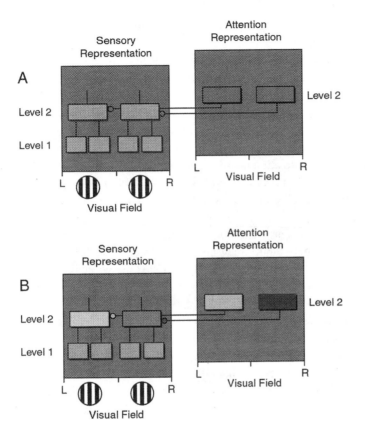

**Figure 6.4**

A model for spatial attention. Each small box represents a unit (i.e., a neuron or group of neurons) responding to a particular location in visual space. Receptive field size increases with each level of processing (levels 1 and 2). Only units responding to vertical stimuli are shown. Unit activity is indicated by shading and reflects either the stimuli in the receptive field (sensory representation) or the amount of attention directed at the receptive field (attention representation). Attentional units are selectively connected to sensory units with similar receptive fields. (*A*) Responses without attentional modulation. None of the attentional units is differentially activated, so that sensory activation remains uniform. (*B*) Responses with attentional modulation. Attention is directed toward one stimulus (lighter shade) and away from the other stimulus (darker shade). The modulatory input from attentional units multiplicatively scales the response of sensory units. As a result, responses increase (lighter shade) in the attended part and decrease (darker shade) in the ignored part of the visual field.

The sensory units in figure 6.4 are assumed to prefer vertical stimulus orientation. (Units preferring other orientations are not relevant to the argument and are omitted.) Units at level 2 inherit this preference from units at level 1. In figure 6.4A, optimally oriented stimuli are presented in both visual hemifields, and elicit moderate responses from the sensory units on each side, as indicated by their intermediate shading. Attentional units are not activated, and thus do not influence the sensory response in any way. In figure 6.4B, the same stimuli are presented, but now attention units are activated differentially, resulting in more attention being allocated to the left visual hemifield (lighter shading) and less attention to the right visual hemifield (darker shading). As a result of the differential input from attention units, sensory units at level 2 respond more strongly to (attended) stimuli on the left and less strongly to (ignored) stimuli on the right. We propose that the effect of this corresponds to a multiplicative scaling. Sensory units at level 1 are not modulated by attention, so responses at this level remain unchanged.

The simple framework of figure 6.4 accounts for most of the attentional effects that have been described in visual cortex. It produces stronger responses when attention is directed at stimuli in or near the receptive field and weaker responses when it is directed at stimuli far from the receptive field. Because the effect of the attention units is strictly multiplicative, the stimulus selectivity of cortical neurons remains unchanged.

## 6.4  Consequences of Multiplicative Scaling: An Expanded Model

Furthermore, the framework presented here may also account for the more complex effects of attention observed with more than one stimulus present in the receptive field (Moran and Desimone, 1995; Luck et al., 1997; Reynolds and Desimone, chapter 7 in this volume). When two stimuli are placed inside the receptive field of a neuron (in area V2, area V4, or inferotemporal cortex), the response is generally dominated by the attended stimulus. For example, if one stimulus drives the cell well and the other does not, shifting attention from one to the other can dramatically reduce the response, as if the ignored stimulus had been partially filtered out of the receptive field. Similar effects have been observed in areas MT and MST when two moving stimuli are placed within the receptive field (Treue and Maunsell, 1996).

Figure 6.5 shows how our framework can be extended to accommodate these effects. In this version, a third level of sensory representation has been added, at which receptive fields are large enough to contain both visual hemifields. We assume that activity at level 3 simply reflects the average of all inputs from level 2. Neurophysiological studies of how neurons respond to two stimuli in their receptive field suggest that the response to

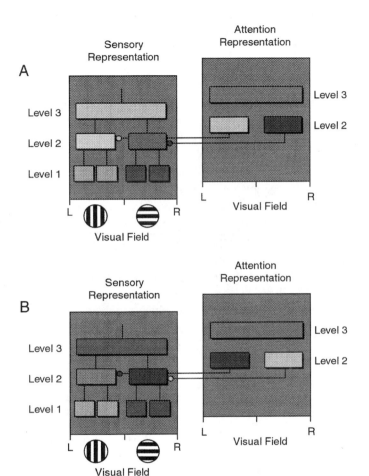

**Figure 6.5**
An extended model for spatial attention. An additional level of processing has been added, in which units have even larger receptive fields. Once again, only units responding to vertical stimuli are shown. However, the visual field contains both vertical and horizontal stimuli, so that some units receive excitatory input (lighter shading) and others units receive inhibitory input (darker shading). (A) Attention directed to the left visual field (preferred stimulus). In this case, attention enhances the excitatory stimulus and attenuates the inhibitory stimulus. At the next level (level 3), the combined effect is a response increase. (B) Attention directed to the right visual field (nonpreferred stimulus). Here attention enhances the inhibitory and attenuates the excitatory stimulus, so that the combined effect is a response *decrease* at level 3. In both cases, the activity at level 3 is determined primarily by the attended stimulus, as if the ignored stimulus had been filtered out of the visual scene. This model accounts for most effects of attention in primate visual cortex.

a stimulus pair typically approximates the average of the responses to each stimulus alone (Britten, 1995; van Wezel et al., 1996; Recanzone et al., 1997).

The most interesting case is when the two hemifields are stimulated differently. For example, assume that the (preferred) stimulus in the left hemifield *excites* the depicted sensory units, whereas the (nonpreferred) stimulus in the right hemifield *inhibits* these units. In figure 6.5A, attention units are more active in the left hemifield than in the right hemifield, corresponding to attention shifted toward the left hemifield (which contains the preferred stimulus). If level 2 responses are scaled multiplicatively by attention, then the excitatory response on the left is amplified and the inhibitory response on the right is attenuated. Thus, the net effect will be increased activity at level 3, because stronger excitation from the left is combined with weaker inhibition from the right. In figure 6.5B, attention is shifted to the right side (which contains the nonpreferred stimulus). In this case, multiplicative scaling amplifies inhibition on the right and attenuates excitation on the left side of level 2. The net effect will be reduced activity at level 3, because stronger inhibition is combined with weaker excitation. Thus, the effect of attention at level 3 is qualitatively consistent with neurophysiological results observed when two stimuli are in the receptive field of a neuron and attention is shifted from one to the other (Moran and Desimone, 1985; Treue and Maunsell, 1996; Luck et al., 1997).

The simple model outlined in figure 6.5 also explains the otherwise puzzling observation that the effect of attention can be far larger when there are two stimuli rather than one stimulus in the receptive field (Moran and Desimone, 1985; Treue and Maunsell, 1996). Between figure 6.5A and 6.5B, the change in activity at level 3 is larger than any change at level 2. The reason is that excitatory and inhibitory responses at level 2 are summed at level 3, so that modest changes at level 2 can combine to produce a far larger change at level 3. The model can also explain what has been described as shrinking receptive fields. If one were to map the receptive field of the level 3 unit, one would obtain different results with attention shifted to the left or the right. In figure 6.5A, the left half of the receptive field would appear more responsive, whereas in figure 6.5B the right half would appear this way. In effect, the receptive field would appear to have shifted toward or shrunk around the attended stimulus in either condition. This is how the effect of shifting attention between two stimuli in the receptive field has been described (Moran and Desimone, 1985), and experiments measuring the spatial profile of receptive fields as attention shifts to different locations have also found this sort of effect on spatial selectivity (Connor et al., 1996, 1997).

Although the results presented earlier show only multiplicative scaling by attention, the theoretical framework outlined here clearly predicts effects that are not multiplicative. In particular, multiplicative scaling at a lower level produces nonmultiplicative effects at the next higher level, such as the shifting or shrinking of the receptive field described for units at level 3. Unless countered or compensated for by special mechanisms, such non-multiplicative effects are a necessary consequence of attention acting selectively at lower processing levels with smaller receptive fields.

However, it seems possible that nonmultiplicative effects are limited to the spatial profile of receptive fields. Whereas spatial profiles grow systematically larger at successive levels of visual processing (Maunsell and Newsome, 1987), the same cannot be said for other receptive field properties. For example, tuning curves for stimulus orientation do not become systematically broader or narrower at successive levels of processing. For this reason, the effect of attention on tuning curves (other than spatial profiles) may simply be multiplicative at all levels of processing (Maunsell and McAdams, 1999).

One implication of the framework in figure 6.5 is that attention should be able to act directly on lower levels of sensory representation, rather than introduce a modulation at the highest level that then passes to lower levels *via* feedback connections. The ability to act directly on lower levels would readily explain how attention can operate at a smaller scale than the receptive field. Selective effects on different parts of the receptive field would be more difficult to explain if attentional modulations originate at higher levels with large receptive fields and reach lower levels with small receptive fields only indirectly, via feedback connections (but see Tsotsos et al., chapter 14 in this volume).

Just like the sensory representation, the attentional representation also contains multiple levels of units (figure 6.5), and units at higher levels are responsible for larger regions of the visual field. At every level, attentional units make connections with the corresponding sensory level. Thus, there would also be a connection at level 3 of the attentional and sensory representations (not shown). The existence of multiple scales of attentional representation accounts for the fact that attention can focus narrowly or disperse widely across the visual field, as required by a given situation (the ''zoom lens'' property of attention; Egly and Homa, 1984; Eriksen and St. James, 1986). However, the attentional representation may not extend to the very smallest scales of sensory representation, because the spatial resolution of attention is far poorer than the spatial resolution of the sensory representation (He et al., 1996). As a result, attentional modulations may be largely limited to later stages of visual cortex where receptive fields are larger. Consistent with this, the effect of attention tends to be stronger in later stages of visual cortex (Maunsell, 1995) and is often rather modest in area V1 (Haenny and Schiller, 1988; Motter, 1993; Luck et al., 1997; McAdams and Maunsell, 1999; but see Ito et al., chapter 5 in this volume; Heeger et al., chapter 2 in this volume).

Although the horizontal axis in figure 6.5 represents visual field location, other axes could be added to accommodate the effect of attending to values along other stimulus dimensions, such as orientation (Moran and Desimone, 1985; Haenny et al., 1988;

Maunsell et al., 1991), direction of motion (Ferrera et al., 1994), and color (Moran and Desimone, 1985; Motter, 1994a, 1994b).

In summary, most effects of attention in primate visual cortex are accommodated by the framework outline here. It accounts for the increase in neuronal responses when previously ignored stimuli become the focus of attention and, more specifically, for the multiplicative scaling of responses to the entire range of stimuli from preferred to nonpreferred. Our framework also explains how attention can act at a smaller scale than the receptive field, and why the modulation by attention may be stronger when there are two stimuli, rather than one stimulus, inside the receptive field.

Two aspects of this framework may appear daunting or unreasonable. First, it postulates a neuronal representation of the behavioral significance of a location or feature, that is, of information which is neither sensory nor motor. There is limited evidence that can bear on the existence of such a representation, on how it might be created from the sensory or nonsensory cues that determine behavioral significance, or how it can persist long after such cues cease to be available. Nevertheless, the fact that attention improves performance only at a selected location demonstrates that this location must be represented somewhere within the brain. In fact, several studies have described neuronal activity that may subserve an attentional representation. For example, the activity of neurons in parietal cortex encodes the position of behaviorally significant locations in the visual field, and this activity persists even in the absence of any sensory stimulus (Andersen, 1988; Colby, 1998). The sustained activity that is commonly observed at higher levels of visual cortex may encode the behavioral significance of stimulus attributes other than location (Fuster and Jervey, 1982; Miyashita and Chang, 1988; Koch and Fuster, 1989; Assad and Maunsell, 1995; Eskandar and Assad, 1999). Because many such neurons represent sensory information as well as behavioral significance, the division between attentional and sensory representations may not be sharp. In short, although the form in which behaviorally relevant locations and attributes are represented remains an important question, the existence of such a representation is not in doubt.

The second challenging aspect of the model in figure 6.5 is that it requires highly specific connections between attentional and sensory representations. Although the necessary degree of specificity is certainly a challenge, similar specificity is needed to create and maintain topographic maps in sensory representations (Kaas et al., 1990; Gilbert and Wiesel, 1992; Swindale, 1996). Presumably, many of these connections are established in development, so that the tasks used in typical attention experiments can build on abilities that are more or less innate. For example, primates are likely to be highly practiced at attending selectively to a particular spatial location (Posner, 1980). In sum, although the framework outlined here poses serious challenges, they are challenges that the nervous system must be able to address.

## 6.5   Conclusions

The evidence presented here suggests that attention directly alters sensory responses, and that its quantitative effect corresponds to a multiplicative scaling of responses. If this general description of the effect of attention is correct, it will have several important implications.

One implication would be that the attentional modulation of sensory cortex involves no special circuits or dedicated mechanisms. Attention-related signals about behavioral significance would use some of the same neuronal circuits that are used by sensory signals. A multiplicative scaling of responses, without any change in the sharpness of tuning, is often the result of sensory–sensory interactions (Britten and Newsome, 1998; McAdams and Maunsell, 1999). For example, the neuronal interactions that determine orientation tuning in area V1 have been described as a multiplicative scaling (Carandini and Heeger, 1994; Carandini et al., 1997).

If sensory and attention signals use the same neuronal mechanisms, there is no reason to expect special circuits or neurotransmitter systems that are specifically related to attention. The only distinction between axons carrying purely sensory signals and those carrying attention signals may in fact be the nature of the information being conveyed. This possibility applies not only to attention signals but also to other feedback signals, such as the motor signals (efference copy) that may multiplicatively scale certain sensory responses in parietal cortex (gain change; Andersen et al., 1985).

The observation of substantially increased response strength with no change in response selectivity offers a simple explanation for the behavioral effects of selective visual attention. Namely, focusing attention on a stimulus is similar or equivalent to increasing the intensity of that stimulus. Like attention, increased intensity typically results in stronger responses but does not change sharpness of tuning (Dean, 1981; Holub and Morton-Gibson, 1981; Albrecht and Hamilton, 1982; Sclar and Freeman, 1982; Skottun et al., 1987; Geisler and Albrecht, 1997). It may therefore prove useful to think of attention as equivalent to higher intensity or salience. It seems possible that the behavioral advantages associated with selective attention, such as reduced thresholds and faster reaction times, can be explained by changes in sensory cerebral cortex that make attended stimuli appear more intense or more salient.

### Acknowledgement

The experiment described here were supported by NIH R01 EY0591 and an award from the Human Frontier Science Program. JHRM is an Investigator with the Howard Hughes Medical Institute.

# References

Albrecht, D. G., and Hamilton, D. B. (1982). Striate cortex of monkey and cat: Contrast response function. *J. Neurophysiol.* 48: 217–237.

Andersen, R. A. (1988). Visual and visual-motor functions of the posterior parietal cortex. In P. Rakic and W. Singer (eds.), *Neurobiology of neocortex* (pp. 285–295). Chichester: John Wiley.

Andersen, R. A., Essick, G. K., and Siegel, R. (1985). The encoding of spatial location by posterior parietal neurons. *Science* 230: 456–458.

Assad, J. A., and Maunsell, J. H. R. (1995). Neural correlates of inferred motion in primate posterior parietal cortex. *Nature* 373: 518–521.

Brefczynski, J. A., and DeYoe, E. A. (1999). A physiological correlate of the "spotlight" of visual attention. *Nature Neurosci.* 2: 370–374.

Britten, K. H. (1995). Spatial interactions within monkey middle temporal (MT) receptive fields. *Soc. Neurosci. Abst.* 21: 663.

Britten, K. H., and Newsome, W. T. (1998). Tuning bandwidths for near-threshold stimuli in area MT. *J. Neurophysiol.* 80: 762–770.

Carandini, M., and Heeger, D. J. (1994). Summation and division by neurons in primate visual cortex. *Science* 264: 1333–1336.

Carandini, M., Heeger, D. J., and Movshon, J. A. (1997). Linearity and normalization in simple cells of the macaque primary visual cortex. *J. Neurosci.* 17: 8621–8644.

Cohen, J. D., Servan-Schreiber, D., and McClelland, J. L. (1992). A parallel distributed processing approach to automaticity. *Am. J. Psychol.* 105: 239–269.

Colby, C. L. (1998). Action-oriented spatial reference frames in cortex. *Neuron* 20: 15–24.

Connor, C. E., Gallant, J. L., Preddie, D. C., and Van Essen, D. C. (1996). Responses in area V4 depend on the spatial relationship between stimulus and attention. *J. Neurophysiol.* 75: 1306–1308.

Connor, C. E., Preddie, D. C., Gallant, J. L., and Van Essen, D. C. (1997). Spatial attention effects in macaque area V4. *J of Neurosci* 17: 3201–3214.

Corbetta, M., Akbudak, E., Conturo, T. E., Snyder, A. Z., Ollinger, J. M., Drury, H. A., Linenweber, M. R., Petersen, S. E., Raichle, M. E., Van Essen, D. C., and Shulman, G. L. (1998). A common network of functional areas for attention and eye movements. *Neuron* 21: 761–773.

Dean, A. F. (1981). The variability of discharge of simple cells in the cat striate cortex. *Exp. Brain Res.* 44: 437–440.

Desimone, R., and Duncan, J. (1995). Neural mechanisms of selective visual attention. *Ann. Rev. Neurosci.* 18: 193–222.

Egly, R., and Homa, D. (1984). Sensitization of the visual field. *J. Exp. Psychol. Hum. Percep. Perf.* 10: 778–793.

Eriksen, C. W., and St. James, J. D. (1986). Visual attention within and around the field of focal attention: A zoom lens model. *Percep. Psychophys.* 40, 225–240.

Eskandar, E. N., and Assad, J. A. (1999). Dissociation of visual motor and predictive signals in parietal cortex during visual guidance. *Nature Neurosci.* 2: 88–93.

Ferrera, V. P., Rudolph, K. K., and Maunsell, J. H. R. (1994). Responses of neurons in the parietal and temporal visual pathways during a motion task. *J. Neurosci.* 14: 6171–6186.

Fuster, J. M., and Jervey, J. P. (1982). Neuronal firing in the inferotemporal cortex of the monkey in a visual memory task. *J. Neurosci.* 2: 361–375.

Geisler, W. S., and Albrecht, D. G. (1997). Visual cortex neurons in monkeys and cats: Detection, discrimination and identification. *Vis. Neurosci.* 14: 897–919.

Gilbert, C. D., and Wiesel, T. N. (1992). Receptive field dynamics in adult primary visual cortex. *Nature* 356: 150–152.

Goldberg, M. E., Musil, S. Y., Colby, C. L., Duhamel, J. R., and Olson, C. R. (1994). Cortical mechanisms for voluntary and involuntary attention: Posterior cingulate and lateral intraparietal areas in the monkey. In B. Albowitz, K. Albus, U. Kuhnt, H. C. Nothdurft, and P. Wahle (eds.), *Structural and functional organization of the neocortex* (pp. 267–278). Berlin: Springer-Verlag.

Haenny, P. E., Maunsell, J. H. R., and Schiller, P. H. (1988). State dependent activity in monkey visual cortex. II. Extraretinal factors in V4. *Exp. Brain Res.* 69: 245–259.

Haenny, P. E., and Schiller, P. H. (1988). State dependent activity in monkey visual cortex. I. Single cell activity in V1 and V4 on visual tasks. *Exp. Brain Res.* 69: 225–244.

He, S., Cavanagh, P., and Intriligator, J. (1996). Attentional resolution and the locus of visual awareness. *Nature* 283: 334– 337.

Heinze, H. J., Mangun, G. R., Burchert, W., Hinrichs, H., Scholz, M., Munte, T. F., Gos, A., Scherg, M., Johannes, S., Hundeshagen, H., et al. (1994). Combined spatial and temporal imaging of brain activity during visual selective attention in humans. *Nature* 372: 543–546.

Henry, G. H., Bishop, P. O., Tupper, R. M., and Dreher, B. (1973). Orientation specificity and response variability of cells in the striate cortex. *Vis. Res.* 13: 1771–1779.

Holub, R. A., and Morton-Gibson, M. (1981). Response of visual cortical neurons of the cat to moving sinusoidal gratings: Response-contrast functions and spatiotemporal interactions. *J. of Neurophysiol.* 46: 1244–1259.

Kaas, J. H., Krubitzer, L. A., Chino, Y. M., Langston, A. L., Polley, E. H., and Blair, N. (1990). Reorganization of retinotopic cortical maps in adult mammals after lesions of the retina. *Science* 248: 229–231.

Kastner, S., De Weerd, P., Desimone, R., and Ungerleider, L. G. (1998). Mechanisms of directed attention in the human extrastriate cortex as revealed by functional MRI. *Science* 282: 108–111.

Koch, K. W., and Fuster, J. M. (1989). Unit activity in monkey parietal cortex related to haptic perception and temporal memory. *Exp. Brain Res.* 76: 292–306.

Lee, D. K., Itti, L., Koch, C., and Braun, J. (1999). Attention activates winner-take-all competition among visual filters. *Nature Neurosci.* 2: 375–381.

Lu, Z.-L., and Dosher, B. A. (1998). External noise distinguishes attention mechanism. *Vis. Res.* 38: 1183–1198.

Luck, S. J., Chelazzi, L., Hillyard, S. A., and Desimone, R. (1997). Neural mechanisms of spatial selective attention in areas V1, V2, and V4 of macaque visual cortex. *J. Neurophysiol.* 77: 24–42.

Mack, A., and Rock, I. (1998). *Inattentional blindness.* Cambridge, MA.: MIT Press.

Mangun, G. R., Buonocore, M. H., Girelli, M., and Jha, A. P. (1998). ERP and fMRI measures of visual spatial selective attention. *Hum. Brain Mapping* 6: 383–389.

Martinez, A., Anllo-Vento, L., Sereno, M. I., Frank, L. R., Buxton, R. B., Dubowitz, D. J., Wong, E. C., Hinrichs, H., Heinze, H. J., and Hillyard, S. A. (1999). Involvement of striate and extrastriate visual cortical areas in spatial attention. *Nature Neurosci.* 2: 364–369.

Maunsell, J. H. R. (1995). The brain's visual world: Representations of visual targets in cerebral cortex. *Science* 270: 764–769.

Maunsell, J. H. R., and McAdams, C. J. (1999). Effects of attention on neuronal response properties in visual cerebral cortex. In M. Gazzaniga (ed.), *The cognitive neurosciences,* 2nd ed. (pp. 315–324). Cambridge, MA: MIT Press.

Maunsell, J. H. R., and Newsome, W. T. (1987). Visual processing in monkey extrastriate cortex. *Ann. Rev. Neurosci.* 10: 363–401.

Maunsell, J. H. R., Sclar, G., Nealey, T. A., and DePriest, D. D. (1991). Extraretinal representations in area V4 in the macaque monkey. *Vis. Neurosci.* 7: 561–573.

McAdams, C. J., and Maunsell, J. H. R. (1999). Effects of attention on orientation-tuning functions of single neurons in macaque cortical area V4. *J. of Neurosci.* 19: 431–441.

Miyashita, Y., and Chang, H. S. (1988). Neuronal correlate of pictorial short-term memory in the primate temporal cortex. *Nature* 331: 68–70.

Moran, J., and Desimone, R. (1985). Selective attention gates visual processing in the extrastriate cortex. *Science* 229: 782– 784.

Motter, B. C. (1993). Focal attention produces spatially selective processing in visual cortical areas V1, V2, and V4 in the presence of competing stimuli. *J. Neurophysiol.* 70: 909–919.

Motter, B. C. (1994a). Neural correlates of attentive selection for color or luminance in extrastriate area V4. *J. of Neurosci.* 14: 2178–2189.

Motter, B. C. (1994b). Neural correlates of feature selective memory and pop-out in extrastriate area V4. *J. Neurosci.* 14: 2190–2199.

Mountcastle, V. B., Motter, B. C., Steinmetz, M. A., and Sestokas, A. K. (1987). Common and differential effects of attentive fixation on the excitability of parietal and prestriate (V4) cortical visual neurons in the macaque monkey. *J. Neurosci.* 7: 2239–2255.

O'Craven, K. M., and Savoy, R. L. (1995). Attentional modulations of activation in human MT shown with functional magnetic resonance imaging (fMRI). *Invest. Ophthalmol. Vis. Sci.,* 36: S856.

O'Regan, J. K., Rensink, R. A., and Clark, J. J. (1999). Change-blindness as a result of "mudsplashes." *Nature* 398: 34.

Posner, M. I. (1980). Orienting of attention. *Q. J. Exp. Psychol.* 32: 3–25.

Recanzone, G. H., Wurtz, R. H., and Schwarz, U. (1997). Responses of MT and MST neurons to one and two moving objects in the receptive field. *J Neurophysiol.* 78: 2904–2915.

Rensink, R. A., O'Regan, J. K., and Clark, J. J. (1997). To see or not to see: The need for attention to perceive changes in scenes. *Psychol. Sci.* 8: 368–373.

Sclar, G., and Freeman, R. D. (1982). Orientation selectivity in the cat's striate cortex is invariant with stimulus contrast. *Exp. Brain Res.* 46: 457–461.

Simons, D. J., & Levin, D. T. (1997). Change blindness. *Trends Cog. Sci.* 1: 261–268.

Skottun, B. C., Bradley, A., Sclar, G., Ohzawa, I., and Freeman, R. D. (1987). The effects of contrast on visual orientation and spatial frequency discrimination: A comparison of single cells and behavior. *J. Neurophysiol.* 57: 773–786.

Spitzer, H., Desimone, R., and Moran, J. (1988). Increased attention enhances both behavioral and neuronal performance. *Science* 240: 338–340.

Swindale, N. V. (1996). The development of topography in the visual cortex: A review of models. Network: Comput. Neural Syst. 7: 161–247.

Tootell, R. B. H., Hadjikhani, N., Hall, E. K., Marrett, S., Vanduffel, W., Vaughan, J., and Dale, A. M. (1998). The retinotopy of visual spatial attention. *Neuron* 21: 1409–1422.

Treue, S., and Martinez-Trujillo, J. C. (1999). Feature-based attention influences motion processing gain in macaque visual cortex. *Nature* 399: 575–579.

Treue, S., and Maunsell, J. H. R. (1996). Attentional modulation of visual motion processing in cortical areas MT and MST. *Nature* 382: 539–541.

van Wezel, R. J. A., Lankheet, M. J. M., Verstraten, F. A. J., Maree, A. F. M., and van de Grind, W. A. (1996). Responses of complex cells in area 17 of the cat to bi-vectorial transparent motion. *Vis. Res.* 36: 2805–2813.

Vogels, R., and Orban, G. A. (1994). Activity of inferior temporal neurons during orientation discrimination with successively presented gratings. *J. Neurophysiol.* 71: 1428–1451.

Watanabe, T., Sasaki, Y., Miyauchi, S., Putz, B., Fujimaki, N., Nielsen, M., Takino, R., and Miyakawa, S. (1998). Attention-regulated activity in human primary visual cortex. *J. Neurophysiol.* 79: 2218–2221.

# 7 Neural Mechanisms of Attentional Selection

**John H. Reynolds and Robert Desimone**

## 7.1  Introduction

The visual system is limited in its capacity to process information. One of the ways the brain overcomes this capacity limitation is to break complex scenes into manageable parts and to process these one at a time. For example, when we know in advance where an important object will appear, we can attend to its location. When we do, we can identify the object quickly and accurately, regardless of how many other objects may be present in the scene. Experiments with monkeys trained to perform visual tasks reveal direct neural correlates of attentional selection. When multiple stimuli appear within a neuron's receptive field, the firing rate of the cell is determined primarily by the attended stimulus. Unattended stimuli have very little control over neuronal responses, and are thus effectively filtered out of the neuronal signal.

These results can be understood within the context of a simple model cortical circuit. The responses of the model neurons of this circuit accurately reproduce the changes in firing rate observed when attention is directed to one of two stimuli inside the receptive field. The model also makes several predictions. First, it predicts that when attention is directed to a location within the receptive field, this will increase the neuron's sensitivity to stimuli appearing at that location. Thus, the model offers an explanation for the finding that people are more sensitive to attended than to unattended stimuli. The model also predicts that when two stimuli appear within the receptive field, the more salient stimulus will exert greater control over neuronal responses than the less salient stimulus, except when the less salient stimulus is attended. In the latter case, attention to the less salient stimulus will cause it to gain control over neuronal responses. Thus, the model offers an explanation for how attention might enable the visual system to process weak, but behaviorally relevant, stimuli even when they appear among highly salient distractor stimuli.

## 7.2  Limited Capacity

Our visual system is very adept at compensating for its limited information-processing capacity. We are therefore often fooled into thinking that when we look at a scene, we see everything, all at once. However, under some conditions, this capacity limitation is revealed. For example, we may feel momentarily overwhelmed when we search for an object in a cluttered room. Accordingly, psychophysical studies have shown that the amount of time required to find an object increases with the number of other objects in a visual scene and with the heterogeneity of the scene (e.g., Treisman and Gelade, 1980; Duncan and Humphreys, 1989; Wolfe, 1989). If the visual system were unlimited in capacity, we could find any object immediately, by simultaneously analyzing everything before us.

This capacity limitation is related to the physiological properties of the neurons that make up the visual system. As visual information traverses the successive cortical areas of the ventral visual stream that underlie object recognition (Ungerleider and Mishkin, 1982), the sizes of receptive fields increase from less than a degree of visual angle in primary visual cortex (area V1) to approximately 20 degrees of visual angle in area TE (Desimone and Schein, 1987; Desimone et al., 1984; Gattass et al., 1988). The number of objects in a scene that will fall within a single receptive field naturally tends to increase with receptive field size, reaching a peak in higher order visual areas with large receptive fields.

Thus, a likely explanation for why we are unable to fully process a complex visual array in a single moment is that that the neurons which make up the visual system are limited-capacity channels. Neurons in higher order areas with large receptive fields are overwhelmed when many visual stimuli appear simultaneously within their receptive fields. Consistent with this idea, studies that have examined how attention modulates the responses of neurons in the macaque visual system have found that the strongest modulations occur when multiple stimuli appear within the neuron's receptive field. Understanding the nature of these modulations offers insight into the neural mechanisms that subserve selective visual attention.

## 7.3   Attentional Modulation of Neuronal Responses in the Ventral Stream

Moran and Desimone (1985) found a direct neural correlate of attentional selection in area V4. They presented pairs of stimuli within the receptive field of ventral stream neurons, and measured the response that was elicited when the monkey attended to one of the two elements of the pair. One of the stimuli was chosen to be of a shape and color that would elicit a strong response when it appeared alone in the receptive field of the cell (*preferred* stimulus). The other stimulus was of a shape and color that would, when presented alone, elicit a weaker response (*poor* stimulus). They found that when the monkey attended to the preferred stimulus, the response to the pair was much stronger than it was when the monkey attended to the poor stimulus. These large changes in firing rate depended on the presence of multiple stimuli within the receptive field. When the poor stimulus was moved to a position outside the receptive field, the firing rate no longer depended on which of the two stimuli was attended.

### 7.3.1   The Biased Competition Model

Desimone and Duncan (1995) have proposed that this attentional modulation requires the presence of multiple stimuli in the receptive field because attention operates by biasing competition between the populations that respond to each of the stimuli. According to this *biased competition* hypothesis, multiple stimuli in the visual field activate populations of neurons that automatically engage in competitive interactions, which are assumed to be mediated through local, intracortical connections. When attention is directed to a stimulus, this is thought to be accompanied by feedback signals generated within areas outside the classical visual system. These signals feed into extrastriate visual cortex and bias the competition in favor of neurons that respond to the attended stimulus. As a result, neurons that respond to the attended stimulus remain active while suppressing neurons that respond to the ignored stimuli.

### 7.3.2   Sensory Interactions and Attentional Modulation

Recently, two studies have been conducted to test this model. According to the model, when two stimuli appear together simultaneously, they activate populations of neurons that engage in competition with one another. The strength of these competitive interactions is predicted to diminish if the stimuli appear asynchronously, because the two populations will not be active at the same time. To test this, Luck and colleagues (1997) presented two stimuli within the receptive field of neurons in areas V2 and V4 and varied their relative timing. Like Moran and Desimone, Luck and colleagues found that the response to a pair of stimuli was strongly suppressed when attention was directed to the poor stimulus. However, consistent with the prediction of the biased competition model, this attention effect was greatly diminished when the two stimuli appeared asynchronously.

Reynolds et al. (1999) tested two additional predictions of the biased competition model. First, according to the model, competition occurs automatically. Therefore, these competitive interactions should be observed even when attention is directed away, to a location outside the receptive field. For example, imagine that we record from a neuron and elicit a response by presenting its preferred stimulus. If we then present an additional stimulus that is a poor stimulus for the recorded neuron but an effective stimulus for a competing population of neurons, this should suppress the response of the recorded neuron. Similarly, if we begin with a poor stimulus, and add an additional stimulus of the preferred shape and color for the recorded neuron, this should generate excitatory input to the recorded neuron and increase the response.

To test this, we have directed monkeys to attend away from the neuronal receptive field, and presented two stimuli inside the receptive field, individually or as a pair. We found that the effect of adding the second stimulus depends on the neuron's selectivity for the two individual stimuli. If the added stimulus is a relatively poor stimulus, it typically suppresses the response elicited by the preferred stimulus. If the added stimulus is relatively more preferred, it typically increases the neuron's response. If the two stimuli individually elicit identical responses, then the response to the pair is typically indistinguishable from the response elicited by either stimulus alone.

This is illustrated in figure 7.1, which shows the responses of a typical cell to a vertical green bar (*reference* stimulus), three different *probe* stimuli, and the three resulting stimulus pairs. For probes eliciting a lower response than the reference (figure 7.1A), the effect of adding the probe was suppressive. For probes eliciting roughly the same response as the reference (figure 7.1B), the pair response was similar to responses to the probe stimulus and reference stimulus presented alone. For probes eliciting a stronger response than the reference stimulus (figure 7.1C), the addition of the probe caused an increase in the cell's mean response.

This relationship held across probes, as illustrated in figure 7.1D, which shows the relationship between selectivity for reference and probe (horizontal axis) versus the change in response that resulted from adding the probe (vertical axis), across all sixteen stimuli. Points labeled A, B, and C correspond to the examples shown in the panels of figures 7.1A, B, and C. The effect of adding the probe was roughly proportional to the neuron's selectivity for reference stimulus and probes, with poorer probes being more suppressive.

**Figure 7.1**
Responses of a single neuron in area V4 with attention directed away from the receptive field. (*A*) Firing rate, in spikes per second, as a function of time (black bar at bottom indicates stimulus duration). A vertical green bar (reference stimulus) elicited a moderately strong response, which peaked at 25 spikes per second (solid line). A vertical yellow bar (probe stimulus) elicited little or no response (dashed line). Both stimuli together (pair stimulus) elicited an intermediate response substantially less than the reference stimulus (dotted line). (*B*) An alternative probe stimulus (oblique blue bar) elicited a response comparable to the reference stimulus when presented alone (dashed line). In this case, the response to the pair stimulus was indistinguishable from the response to the reference stimulus (dotted line). (*C*) Yet another probe stimulus (oblique green bar) elicited a stronger response than the reference stimulus when presented alone (dashed line). Here, the response to the pair was larger than the response to the reference (dotted line). (*D*) Across sixteen different probe stimuli (including the three appearing in panels *A, B,* and *C*), the addition of the probe tended to cause the neuron's response to move toward the response that was elicited by the probe when it was presented alone. This is illustrated here in terms of a positive correlation between selectivity and sensory interaction. Average responses were computed during a 250 ms interval beginning 70 ms after stimulus onset. *Selectivity* was defined as the probe response minus the reference response, normalized by the highest response to any stimulus. Positive selectivity indicates that the probe elicits a stronger response than the reference. *Sensory interaction* was defined as the pair response minus the reference response, again normalized by the highest response to any stimulus. Positive sensory interaction indicates that the pair elicits a stronger response than the reference alone.

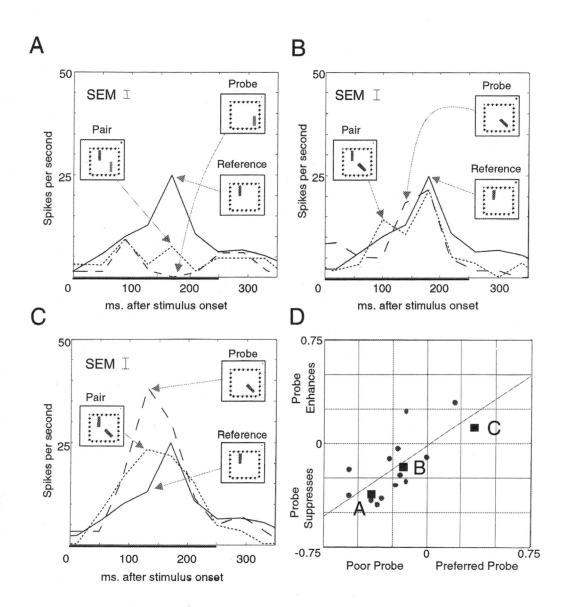

Across a large population of neurons in areas V2 and V4, the pair response was roughly the average of the responses elicited by the individual elements of the pair presented one at a time.

These data are incompatible with some possible models of sensory processing in areas V2 and V4, such as models in which the response to a pair of stimuli is greater than the response to the preferred stimulus appearing alone or less than the response to the poor stimulus alone. They are also incompatible with models in which the pair is treated as a third, independent stimulus with its own, arbitrary response. However, the finding that the addition of a second stimulus drives the neuronal response toward the response elicited when that stimulus appears alone is predicted by the biased competition model.

The model also predicts that when attention is directed to one of two stimuli, the response to the pair should be driven toward the response that would be elicited by the attended stimulus appearing alone. According to the model, when attention is directed to one of the stimuli, this biases the competition in favor of the population of cells that respond to the attended stimulus. When attention is directed to the preferred stimulus, this should reduce or eliminate the suppression caused by the presence of the poor stimulus. To test this, we directed the monkey to attend to the preferred stimulus. As predicted by the biased competition model, this eliminated most of the suppressive effect of the poor stimulus. This is illustrated in figure 7.2A. The upper line (thin, solid) shows the response of a single neuron in area V2 to a stimulus that was very effective in driving the neuron. The lower line (thin, dashed) shows the response to a stimulus that was of a poor orientation and color for the cell. The dotted line in the middle shows the response to the pair of stimuli presented together. For this neuron, adding the poor stimulus suppressed the response that was elicited by the preferred stimulus, but this suppression was almost completely eliminated when attention was directed toward the preferred stimulus (thick solid line).

Likewise, attending to a poor stimulus eliminated the response increase caused by adding a preferred stimulus within the receptive field. This is illustrated in figure 7.2B, which shows the response of a neuron in area V2 that responded very weakly to a vertical bar (lower thin, solid line). A horizontal bar elicited a strong response when it was presented alone (upper thin dashed line), and adding the horizontal bar strongly increased the neuronal response (middle dotted line). However, when the monkey attended to the poor stimulus (vertical bar), the increase in response caused by the addition of the horizontal bar was largely eliminated (thick solid line). Across the population of neurons that were modulated by attention, attending to one of the two stimuli eliminated 80% of the effect (increase or decrease) of the unattended stimulus.

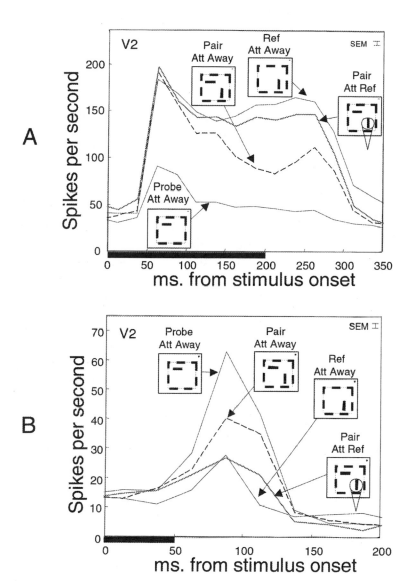

**Figure 7.2**

Attention filters out unattended stimuli. (*A*) Responses of a single neuron in area V2. A (vertical) reference stimulus elicited a strong response (thin solid line), and a (horizontal) probe stimulus a weak response (dashed line), when presented alone. When presented together, the pair elicited an intermediate response (dotted line). However, the suppression caused by the addition of the probe was almost completely eliminated when attention was directed at the reference (thick solid line). Attention effectively filtered the unattended probe out of the neuronal signal. (*B*) Another neuron responded weakly to a vertical reference stimulus (thin solid line) and strongly to a horizontal probe stimulus (dashed line). Adding the preferred probe stimulus to the reference stimulus increased the response (dotted line). When attention was directed to the reference stimulus, this eliminated most of the increase caused by the addition of the probe (thick solid line). In effect, the neuron responded as though the ignored probe stimulus were not present.

### 7.3.3   An Implementation of the Biased Competition Model

There are a number of ways in which biased competition could be implemented by the cortex. The model circuit appearing in figure 7.3 is a simple feedforward competitive neural network that implements the biased competition model. It was developed to provide an existence proof that the biased competition model can satisfy the constraints provided by the above-described experiments.

The model is composed of two sets of neurons. The circle in the upper part of figure 7.3 represents the neuron whose response we are recording (the output neuron). The two circles below represent populations of afferent neurons that respond independently to the two individual stimuli, and send excitatory and inhibitory input to the output neuron. When one of the two stimuli appears, its afferent population is active and the other afferent population is silent. The response of the neuron to either individual stimulus is assumed to depend on the relative amount of excitatory and inhibitory input feeding into the output neuron from this afferent population. Thus, when the stimulus on the left appears alone, it activates the population on the left, which sends a strong excitatory input and a weaker inhibitory input to the output neuron. As a result, the output neuron is strongly activated. In contrast, the stimulus on the right activates an input population that sends a weaker excitatory input and a stronger inhibitory input to the output neuron. Thus, when it is activated, it elicits a weak response from the output neuron. That is, the stimulus on the right is, by definition, a poor stimulus for the output neuron.

When the two stimuli appear together, their excitatory inputs are assumed to be additive, as are their inhibitory inputs. Hence, the effect of adding the poor stimulus is to reduce the relative amount of excitatory input, causing a reduction in the response of the output neuron, as we observed experimentally. Simulations of this model have shown that it can reproduce the relationships between individual stimulus responses and paired stimulus responses observed in the recording data (Reynolds et al., 1999).

Attention is assumed to modulate the efficacy of synapses projecting from the population of neurons that is activated by the attended stimulus. Because the inputs from the two channels are assumed to be additive, the ratio of total excitatory to total inhibitory inputs is driven toward the ratio that obtained when the attended stimulus appeared alone. The model thus predicts that the firing rate will move toward the rate observed when the attended stimulus was presented alone, as we found to be the case for neurons in macaque areas V2 and V4. The model provides a possible explanation for how the attended stimulus might come to have greater control over the response of the neuron, thereby filtering the unattended stimulus out of the visual stream.

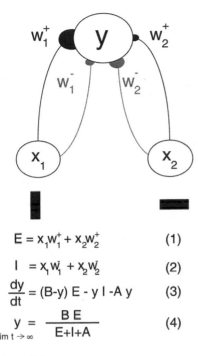

$$E = x_1 w_1^+ + x_2 w_2^+ \qquad (1)$$

$$I = x_1 w_1^- + x_2 w_2^- \qquad (2)$$

$$\frac{dy}{dt} = (B-y)\,E - y\,I - A\,y \qquad (3)$$

$$\lim_{t \to \infty} y = \frac{B\,E}{E+I+A} \qquad (4)$$

**Figure 7.3**
A simple implementation of the biased competition model. The top circle represents the recorded neuron, whose firing rate is designated $y$. The two circles below represent populations of input neurons that respond independently to the reference and probe stimuli, and project to the recorded neuron. The average responses of the input populations are designated $x_1$ and $x_2$. Black lines indicate excitatory projections from each input population to the recorded neuron. Gray lines indicate the inhibitory projections, which are assumed to depend on inhibitory interneurons (not shown). The variables $w_1^+$ and $w_2^+$ represent the magnitudes, or weights, of the excitatory projections from the two input populations, and $w_1^-$ and $w_2^-$ represent the weights of the inhibitory projections. Equations 1 and 2 state, respectively, that the total excitatory and inhibitory inputs to the cell are the responses of the input populations, weighted, respectively, by their excitatory and inhibitory weights. Equation 3 describes the change in the response of the output neuron over time. Equation 4 describes the equilibrium response of the recorded neuron, which depends on the total mix of excitatory and inhibitory input. The parameters $A$ (response decay rate) and $B$ (maximal response) are constants. Therefore, the equilibrium response depends on the relative contributions of excitatory and inhibitory inputs (equation 4). Adding probe to reference will drive the response from its reference-alone toward its probe-alone level. Attention is assumed to increase the signal from attended stimuli by increasing the efficacy of the relevant synapses. This drives the response toward the level that would be observed for the attended stimulus alone. The model is described further in Reynolds et al. (1999).

### 7.4  Further Predictions of Biased Competition

#### 7.4.1  Baseline Shift

The model also offers an explanation for several other previously reported results, such as the observation that the spontaneous firing rate of ventral stream neurons increases when attention is directed to a location within the receptive field (Luck et al., 1997). According to the model, attention increases the efficacy of synapses projecting from afferent neurons whose receptive fields are at the attended location. Therefore, spontaneous activity among these afferents is predicted to activate the measured neuron more strongly, in turn increasing its spontaneous firing rate. This increase in spontaneous activity is predicted to depend on the magnitude of inputs from the afferent neurons. Consistent with this, Luck and colleagues found that the increase in spontaneous activity is larger when attention is directed to the center of the receptive field (stronger afferent projections), versus a position near the edge of the receptive field (weaker afferent projections). Likewise, in human brain imaging studies using fMRI, Kastner and colleagues found an increase in activity in several cortical visual areas when subjects attended to a location in space prior to the presentation of an expected target stimulus (Kastner et al., 1999). This increase was retinotopically specific, in that it occurred only at the retinotopical location of the focus of attention.

#### 7.4.2  Attention to a Single Receptive Field Stimulus

The model is also consistent with spatial attention effects that have been observed using single stimuli within the receptive fields of ventral stream neurons (Moran and Desimone, 1985; Haenny et al., 1988; Spitzer et al., 1988; Maunsell et al., 1991). These studies have found no change or small increases in firing rate when attention was directed to the receptive field stimulus. According to the model, attention increases the efficacy of synapses feeding from afferents that are activated by the attended stimulus. Therefore, the model predicts increased responses when attention is directed to a single stimulus, provided that the stimulus does not already saturate the neuronal response. We have simulated the model with a single receptive field stimulus, using the same parameters derived to fit the responses to pairs measured by Reynolds and colleagues (1999). The model predicted a mean increase of 17.5% in neuronal response to a single stimulus with attention, which falls within the range of effects previously reported with a single stimulus inside the receptive field.

#### 7.4.3  Bottom-Up Salience Biasing Competition

In addition, the model predicts that when attention is directed away from the receptive field, variations in the relative salience of stimuli appearing within the receptive field should bias the neuron's response in favor of the more salient stimulus. For example, consider the case when the response to a preferred stimulus is suppressed by the addition of a poor stimulus. According to the model, increasing the intensity or salience of the poor stimulus (e.g., by increasing luminance contrast) should increase the average firing rate of the input population responding to the poor stimulus. This will increase the strength of inputs from that stimulus, resulting in greater suppression of the response to the pair. Thus, the poor stimulus is predicted to become increasingly suppressive with increased intensity or salience (contrast), even if it elicits a significant excitatory response on its own. Finally, the model predicts that attending to a less salient stimulus can counteract the influence of a more salient stimulus in the same receptive field, if attention is assumed to increase synaptic efficiency enough so that input from the less salient, but attended, stimulus is stronger than input from the more salient, but unattended, stimulus. Thus, the model offers a way to explain how attention could filter out highly salient distractor stimuli so as to enable less salient, but behaviorally relevant, stimuli to allow higher order cortical areas to influence behavior appropriately.

## 7.5   Biased Competition: From Sensory Input to Motor Output?

Recent experiments suggest that similar mechanisms may be at work in a variety of cortical areas, supporting other functions in addition to spatial attention, including searching for an object stored in memory and selecting a target for saccadic eye movements. Several studies have found that the responses of neurons in inferior temporal cortex to a preferred stimulus are suppressed when a second, nonpreferred stimulus is added inside the receptive field (Miller et al., 1993; Rolls and Tovee, 1995), suggesting that competitive interactions may also occur in this area. Chelazzi and colleagues (1993) have found that competitive interactions can be biased in favor of objects held in working memory. In their experiment, a monkey saw and held in memory a visual stimulus (cue item). After the stimulus disappeared, the computer screen went blank for a brief a delay period, which was succeeded by an array of stimuli. The monkey's task was to make a saccade to the stimulus that matched the cue item that had appeared earlier (figure 7.4A). The locations of the stimuli varied from trial to trial, so during this blank period, the monkey knew what stimulus it was to search for, but it could not know where this stimulus would appear. During this delay, neurons maintained an elevated firing rate (figure 7.4B). However, unlike the spatially selective elevation in spontaneous activity that is observed when a monkey attends to a given location, this elevated firing rate encoded the identity of the stimulus that had been stored in memory. It was highest when the stimulus stored in memory had elicited a strong neuronal response when it was present.

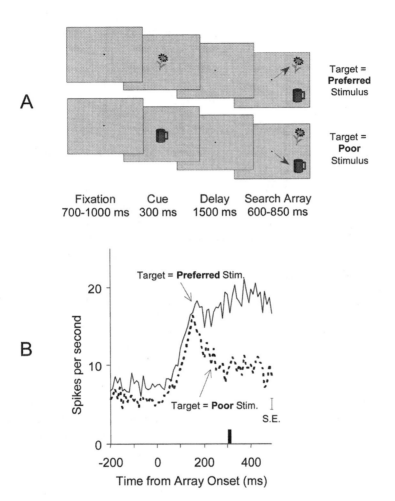

**Figure 7.4**
Responses of neurons in inferior temporal cortex during memory-guided search. (*A*) Task. Monkeys fixated a spot on a computer screen. A central cue appeared (here, either the flower or the cup). After a delay, two or more stimuli appeared within the receptive field, and the monkey had to saccade to the stimulus that had appeared earlier as the cue. Sometimes (upper four panels), the cue was a preferred stimulus for the cell (here, the flower). On separate trials (lower four panels) the cue was a poor stimulus (the cup). (*B*) Neuronal responses. During the delay, inferotemporal neurons showed an elevated baseline activity that reflected the cue stored in memory. The spontaneous firing rate was higher on trials in which the cue was a preferred stimulus for the cell, relative to trials when the cue was a poor stimulus. After the search array appeared, the response separated, either increasing or decreasing, depending on whether the cue was, respectively, a preferred or poor stimulus for the cell. This separation occurred before the onset of the saccade, which is indicated by the vertical bar on the horizontal axis. After Chelazzi et al. (1993).

After the delay period, an array of randomly positioned stimuli appeared inside the receptive field, and the monkey was rewarded if it made a saccade to the stimulus that matched the stimulus held in memory. When the array first appeared, it elicited a response that was typically intermediate between the responses to the individual stimuli presented one at a time. However, about 100 ms before the onset of the saccade, the competition was suddenly resolved in favor of the stimulus that had earlier been stored in memory. Thus, memory-guided search for a stimulus at an unknown location appears to depend on the same competitive mechanisms that are involved in spatial attention.

Several recent experiments also suggest the operation of biased competitive mechanisms in the dorsal stream of processing, which is involved in processing information about stimulus motion. Treue and Maunsell (1996) found that attention modulates the responses of directionally selective neurons in areas MT and MST in a manner very similar to what we have observed for color- and shape-selective neurons in the ventral stream. They have reported that the response to a single stimulus is increased in magnitude when the stimulus is attended. However, much larger attention effects were found when attention was directed to one of two stimuli simultaneously moving in opposite directions in the receptive field. When the monkey attended to a stimulus moving in the neuron's preferred direction of motion, the response was greater than when attention was directed to a stimulus moving in the opposite direction.

Recanzone et al. (1997) have also recorded responses of neurons in areas MT and MST, and have found a pattern of data that is consistent with competitive interactions between stimuli. The response to a stimulus moving in a nonpreferred direction was increased by the addition of a second stimulus moving in the preferred direction. Likewise, the response to a stimulus moving in nonnull direction for the cell was suppressed by the addition of a stimulus moving in the null direction. Britten and Heuer (1999) have also recently recorded the responses of neurons in area MT when two stimuli appeared either alone or together inside the receptive field. They found that the response to the pair was significantly less than the sum of the two individual responses, and suggested that this may be evidence for inhibitory interactions among neurons in area MT.

It appears that related mechanisms may also be at work at the transition from visual processing to eye movement control. Schall and Hanes (1993) have shown that neuronal responses in the frontal eye field are strongest when a pop-out target stimulus appears inside the receptive field. These responses are suppressed when the target appears just outside the receptive field, near its border. Schall and Hanes have suggested that this results from mutual inhibition, and may reduce the responses of neurons that encode eye movements to locations near the target. This could reduce the probability of erroneously making a saccade to a nearby nontarget.

Basso and Wurtz (1997) have provided evidence that can be interpreted as supporting a similar biased competitive circuit within the superior colliculus (SC). They have recorded the responses of buildup neurons in the intermediate layers of the superior colliculus, which receive input from the frontal eye fields, and participate in the control of eye movements. In one condition, the monkey did not know in advance which of several potential targets would be selected for an eye movement. SC responses were lower when there were more possible targets in the search array. Such a reduced response would be expected to arise from mutual inhibition between populations of neurons coding the different possible target locations. When the monkey knew in advance which of the stimuli was to be the target of the eye movement, the response was no longer suppressed by the presence of additional distractors. This is exactly what would be expected if the competition were resolved in favor of the known target, possibly as a result of signals generated in the frontal eye fields, which specify which of the stimuli would be selected for an eye movement.

## 7.6   Conclusions

Findings from single-unit recording studies of visual attention, memory-guided search, and the selection of targets for a saccadic eye movement all seem to have a similar "signature of mechanism." When multiple stimuli appear together, they seem to activate mutually suppressive interactions between neurons with contrasting response properties. In each area where these interactions have been observed, it has proven possible to bias neuronal responses in favor of a desired stimulus, providing a mechanism by which the nervous system can select a desired stimulus out of a cluttered visual world. Taken together, these results appear to suggest that biased competition may be a basic computational strategy which has been adopted throughout the visual system, the oculomotor system, and possibly in other modalities as well.

## References

Basso, M. A., and Wurtz, R. H. (1997). Modulation of neuronal activity by target uncertainty. *Nature* 389: 66–69.

Britten, K. H., and Heuer, H. W. (1999). Spatial summation in the receptive fields of MT neurons. *J. Neurosci.* 19: 5074–5084.

Chelazzi, L., Miller, E. K., Duncan, J., and Desimone, R. (1993). A neural basis for visual search in inferior temporal cortex. *Nature* 363: 345–347.

Desimone, R., Albright, T. D., Gross, C. G., and Bruce, C. (1984). Stimulus-selective properties of inferior temporal neurons in the macaque. *J. Neurosci.* 4: 2051–2062.

Desimone, R., and Duncan, J. (1995). Neural mechanisms of selective visual attention. *Ann. Rev. Neurosci.* 18: 193–222.

Desimone, R., and Schein, S. (1987). Visual properties of neurons in area V4 of the macaque: Sensitivity to stimulus form. *J. Neurophysiol.* 57: 835–868.

Duncan, J., and Humphreys, G. W. (1989). Visual search and stimulus similarity. *Psychol. Rev.* 96: 433–458.

Gattass, R., Sousa, A. P., and Gross, C. G. (1988). Visuotopic organization and extent of V3 and V4 of the macaque. *J. Neurosci.* 8: 1831–1845.

Haenny, P. D., Maunsell, J. H. R., and Schiller, P. H. (1988). State dependent activity in monkey visual cortex. II. Retinal and extraretinal factors in V4. *Exp. Brain Res.* 69: 245–259.

Kastner, S., Pinsk, M. A., De Weerd, P., Desimone, R., and Ungerleider, L. G. (1999). Increased activity in human visual cortex during directed attention in the absence of visual stimulation. *Neuron* 22: 751–761.

Luck, S. J., Chelazzi, L., Hillyard, S. A., and Desimone, R (1997). Neural mechanisms of spatial selective attention in areas V1, V2, and V4 of macaque visual cortex. *J. Neurophysiol.* 77: 24–42.

Maunsell, J. H. R., Sclar, G., Nealey, T. A., and DePriest, D. D. (1991). Extraretinal representations in area V4 in the macaque monkey. *Vis. Neurosci.* 7: 561–573.

Miller, E. K., Gochin, P. M., and Gross, C. G. (1993). Suppression of visual responses of neurons in inferior temporal cortex of the awake macaque by addition of a second stimulus. *Brain Res.* 616: 25–29.

Moran, A. J., and Desimone, R. (1985). Selective attention gates visual processing in the extrastriate cortex. *Science* 229: 782–784.

Recanzone, G. H., Wurtz, R. H., and Schwarz, U. (1997). Responses of MT and MST neurons to one and two moving objects in the receptive field. *J. Neurophysiol.* 78: 2904–2915.

Reynolds, J. H., Chelazzi, L., and Desimone, R. (1999). Competitive mechanisms subserve attention in macaque areas V2 and V4. *J. Neurosci.* 19: 1736–1753.

Rolls, E. T., and Tovee, M. J. (1995). The responses of single neurons in the temporal visual cortical areas of the macaque when more than one stimulus is present in the receptive field. *Exp. Brain Res.* 103: 409–420.

Schall, J. D., and Hanes, D. P. (1993). Neural basis of saccade target selection in frontal eye field during visual search. *Nature* 366: 467–469.

Spitzer, H., Desimone, R., and Moran, J. (1988). Increased attention enhances both behavioral and neuronal performance. *Science* 240: 338–340.

Treisman, A., and Gelade, G. (1980). A feature-integration theory of attention. *Cog. Psychol.* 12: 97–136.

Treue, S., and Maunsell, J. H. R. (1996). Attentional modulation of visual motion processing in cortical areas MT and MST. *Nature* 382: 539–541.

Ungerleider, L. G., and Mishkin, M. (1982). Two cortical visual systems. In J. Ingle, M. A. Goodale, and R. J. W. Mansfield (eds.), *Analysis of visual behavior* (pp. 549–586).

Wolfe, J. M. (1989). Guided search: An alternative to the feature integration model for visual search. *J. Exp. Psychol. Hum. Percep. Perf.* 15: 419–433.

# 8 From Attention to Action in Frontal Cortex

Kirk G. Thompson, Narcisse P. Bichot, and Jeffrey D. Schall

## 8.1 Introduction

The purpose of the visual system is to transform light into action. For example, consider the visual search illustrated in figure 8.1, in which the observer must locate a T among many Ls. The observer makes a series of gaze shifts to inspect the elements in the array. Before each gaze shift, two selection processes have to take place (e.g., Allport 1987; Pashler 1991; Coles et al., 1995). The first process selects a stimulus to guide action, and the second selects the action. In this chapter, we will review our investigations into the processes by which visual stimuli are selected as targets for gaze shifts.

Recognition is growing that overt eye movements and covert shifts of visual attention are guided by a common mechanism. Several experiments have shown a cost in perceptual reliability or saccade latency if attention is directed away from the target for a saccade (e.g., Hoffman and Subramaniam, 1995; Kowler et al., 1995; Deubel and Schneider, 1996). In addition, directing attention seems to influence the production of saccades (Sheliga et al., 1995; Kustov and Robinson, 1996). Further evidence is the common manner in which bottom-up factors influence visual selection for attention and saccades. Visual conspicuousness drives covert (e.g., Theeuwes, 1991) and overt (Theeuwes et al., 1998) selection. In fact, nontarget elements that resemble the target can be inadvertently selected covertly (e.g., Kim and Cave, 1995) or overtly (Findlay, 1997; Zelinsky and Sheinberg, 1997; Motter and Belky, 1998; Bichot and Schall, 1999b).

Top-down factors also influence visual selection. Cognitive strategies can override both covert (e.g., Bacon and Egeth, 1994) and overt (e.g., Bichot et al., 1996; Nodine et al., 1996) selection of conspicuous target stimuli. In addition, target selection is influenced by implicit memory representations arising through short-term priming of location or stimulus features for covert (e.g., Maljkovic and Nakayama, 1994, 1996) and overt orienting (Bichot and Schall, 1999a; McPeek et al., 1999). Target selection is also influenced by long-term priming of target properties across sessions (Bichot and Schall, 1999b). Finally, an explicit memory representation is needed to identify the unique target during conjunction search (e.g., Treisman and Sato 1990; Bacon and Egeth, 1997).

To explain all of these observations, most models of covert attention (e.g., Koch and Ullman, 1985; Treisman, 1988; Cave and Wolfe, 1990; Olshausen et al., 1993; Wolfe, 1994) and overt saccade generation (e.g., Findlay and Walker, 1999) postulate the existence of a map of salience derived from converging bottom-up and top-down influences. Peaks on the salience map that develop through winner-take-all competitive interactions represent locations that have been selected for further processing and can, but need not necessarily, lead to orienting saccadic eye movements.

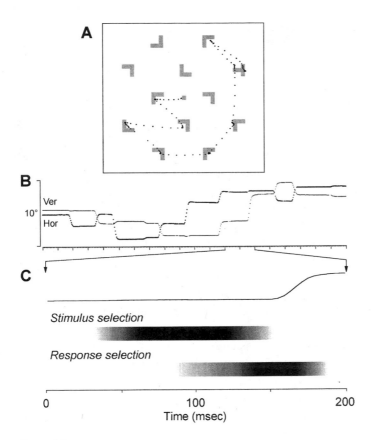

**Figure 8.1**
(A) Pattern of gaze shifts made by a monkey searching for a randomly oriented T among Ls. The T among L array appeared after the monkey fixated the central spot. On this trial the monkey's first saccade was to the left, followed by a sequence of eye movements around the perimeter of the array. (B) The same sequence of saccades plotted as horizontal (thick) and vertical (thin) eye position as a function of time. (C) A segment of the scan path, including the first saccade to the target, is expanded to illustrate the stimulus selection and response selection processes in (B). These processes precede each saccade. Modified from Schall and Thompson (1999).

## 8.2  Frontal Eye Field

This chapter focuses on our investigations of the frontal eye field (FEF), an area in prefrontal cortex that contributes to transforming visual signals into saccade commands (reviewed by Schall, 1997). FEF has two facets, one motor and the other sensory.

The evidence for the motor function of FEF is compelling. Low intensity microstimulation of FEF elicits saccades (e.g., Bruce et al., 1985). This direct influence is mediated by a population of neurons that discharge specifically before and during saccades (Bruce and Goldberg, 1985; Hanes and Schall, 1996; Hanes et al., 1998). The neurons in FEF that generate movement-related activity are located in layer 5 and innervate the superior colliculus (Segraves and Goldberg, 1987) and parts of the neural circuit in the brain stem that generate saccades (Segraves, 1992). These neurons provide the motor plan for voluntary eye movements. In other words, their activity reflects the outcome of the motor response selection process, which is what movement to make. Electrophysiological data indicate the sufficiency of FEF activity to produce gaze shifts. Recent reversible inactivation studies provide evidence for the necessity of FEF to produce saccades. Recent work has demonstrated that reversible inactivation of FEF impairs monkeys' ability to make saccades (Dias et al., 1995; Sommer and Tehovnik, 1997). These findings complement earlier observations that ablation of FEF causes an initially severe impairment in saccade production that recovers in some respects over time (e.g., Schiller et al., 1987; Schiller and Chou, 1998; see also Rivaud et al., 1994).

The evidence for the visual function of FEF is equally compelling. FEF is connected with extrastriate visual areas in both the dorsal stream and the ventral stream (e.g., Baizer et al., 1991), and the projections between extrastriate visual cortex and FEF are topographically organized (Schall, Morel, et al., 1995; Stanton et al., 1995). The central field representation of retinotopically organized areas such as V4, TEO, and MT, as well as areas that overrepresent the *central* field (e.g., caudal TE), project to the ventrolateral portion of FEF. This part of FEF produces short amplitude saccades (Bruce et al., 1985). The peripheral field representation of retinotopically organized areas, as well as areas that overrepresent the *peripheral* visual field (e.g., PO and MSTd), project to the dorsomedial part of FEF. This part of FEF produces larger amplitude saccades. The anatomical evidence also reveals a large degree of convergence of afferents from multiple extrastriate visual areas in FEF. Specifically, the data suggest that individual neurons in FEF may receive signals representing the color, form, depth, and direction of motion of objects in the image. Such convergence seems desirable for a system to select targets for gaze shifts, regardless of the visual properties of the target. In addition to the connections with visual cortex, FEF is connected with prefrontal cortex areas 12, 46, and 9 (e.g., Stanton et al., 1993). In fact, quantitative analyses of the connectivity between cortical visual areas indicate that FEF is a uniquely well-connected node in the network (Jouve et al., 1998).

As a result of the extensive innervation from extrastriate visual cortical areas, physiological recordings in the FEF of monkeys trained to shift gaze to visual targets have found that roughly half of the neurons have visual responses (Mohler et al., 1973; Bruce and Goldberg, 1985; Schall, 1991). Consistent with the extensive convergence of visual signals in FEF, the neurons do not typically exhibit any selectivity for stimulus features like orientation, color, or direction of motion. The time at which FEF visual neurons respond to flashed stimuli coincides with the latencies of visual responses in dorsal stream areas such as MT (Nowak and Bullier, 1997; Schmolesky et al., 1998). In fact, many neurons in FEF respond to visual stimuli before some neurons in area V1 do. Although FEF visual neurons do not respond selectively for stimulus features such as color or orientation, around half of the visually responsive neurons generate an enhanced response to stimuli that will be the target for a saccade (Goldberg and Bushnell, 1981). The research reviewed below demonstrates how these visually responsive neurons in FEF participate in the selection of visual targets for saccades (see also Schall and Bichot, 1998; Schall and Thompson, 1999). What does this selection process in FEF represent? In this chapter, we will develop the claim that the activation of FEF visual neurons represents a salience map in which stimulus locations are selected on the basis of visual conspicuousness, prior knowledge, and internal random variability (Thompson and Bichot, 1999).

## 8.3   The Role of Visual Conspicuousness in Selection

We will first review our work that addresses bottom-up influences on attention and eye movements. The term "bottom-up" refers to the usually automatic allocation of attention based exclusively on the properties of the image. A stimulus that is conspicuously different in one or more visual attributes from neighboring stimuli is most likely to be attended and fixated. The visual search paradigm has been used extensively to investigate visual selection and attention (Treisman, 1988; Wolfe, 1998). In a visual search task, multiple stimuli are presented, and from among them a target is discriminated. Search is efficient if stimuli differ along basic visual feature dimensions, for example, color, form, or direction of motion. This kind of search is referred to as "pop-out." In contrast, if targets and distractors resemble each other, or no single feature clearly distinguishes the two types of stimuli, then search becomes less efficient (e.g., Duncan and Humphreys, 1989).

We have investigated how the brain selects targets for visually guided saccades by recording the activity of neurons in the FEF of monkeys trained to shift gaze to the pop-out target in either of two complementary visual search arrays (Schall and Hanes, 1993; Schall, Hanes, et al., 1995; Thompson et al., 1996). As shown in figure 8.2, we found that visually responsive neurons in FEF initially responded indiscriminately to the target or the distractor of the search array in their receptive field. The absence of feature-selective responses in FEF during visual search is consistent with earlier work (Mohler et al., 1973). However, before saccades were generated, a discrimination process proceeded by which most visually responsive cells in FEF ultimately signaled the location of the pop-out target stimulus. Thus, the activity of FEF visual neurons participates in the visual selection process. The movement-related activity in FEF was the same immediately before saccades to the target presented alone or with distractors (Hanes et al., 1995; Schall, Hanes, et al., 1995). But this should not be surprising, because the same saccade was generated in both conditions. Complementary observations in FEF have been made in monkeys scanning

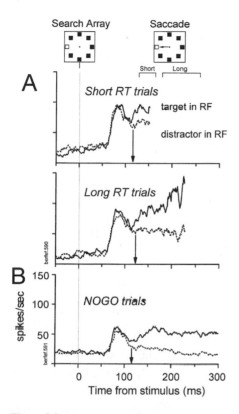

**Figure 8.2**
Visual selection of a conspicuous target. The neural activity of a single FEF visual neuron is shown following presentation of a pop-out search array during (A) GO search and (B) NOGO search. Each plot shows the activation when the oddball stimulus appeared in the receptive field (RF) (*solid line*) and when distractors appeared in the receptive field (*dotted line*). The trials are aligned on the time of search array (*top*) presentation. (A) The time course of activation during a block of GO search trials. The monkey was instructed to make saccades to the oddball of the search array. The activation during subsets of trials in which reaction times (RT) were short and long are shown separately. The plots of neural activity end at the mean reaction time for each group. The ranges of reaction times for the short and long trials are indicated across the top. (B) The time course of activity during a block of NOGO trials. The monkey was instructed to withhold eye movements. The times of target discrimination (arrows) were approximately the same in all three subsets of trials, showing a dissociation between the visual selection of a stimulus and the production of saccades. Modified from Thompson et al. (1996) and Thompson et al. (1997).

complex images (Burman and Segraves, 1994) and selecting a target based on a motion cue (Kim and Shadlen, 1999).

An obvious and important question about this selection process is, When does it occur? A corollary question is How does the time of target selection in FEF relate to when the saccade is made? These are particular instances of questions that have a long tradition in psychology because reaction time is one of the original and basic quantitative measures of behavior. A working hypothesis of experimental psychology is that behavioral response times are composed if more or less distinct stages of processing (Donders, 1868; Sternberg, 1969). For example, the time taken to identify and select a stimulus corresponds to the perceptual stage of processing, and the time taken to prepare and execute a movement corresponds to the motor stage of processing. We analyzed the time course of saccade target discrimination in FEF to evaluate the hypothesis that the random variability of saccade latency is due to variability in the time taken to select the target for the saccade. We found that the large majority of FEF visually responsive neurons discriminate the target from a distractor in a pop-out search at a fairly constant interval after search array presentation (figure 8.2A) (Thompson et al., 1996). This finding indicates that at least under the conditions of pop-out search, the visual system requires a relatively constant period of time to locate potential targets, and additional timing variability is introduced in the time to prepare and execute the eye movement. Other work has described how postperceptual response preparation processes (Hanes and Schall, 1996) and states of readiness (Everling et al., 1998; Pare and Munoz, 1996; Dorris and Munoz, 1998) contribute to reaction time variability.

To examine further the dissociation of visual selection in FEF from saccade production, we tested the hypothesis that the selection observed in FEF requires saccade planning and execution. FEF activity was recorded while monkeys were instructed to maintain fixation during presentation of a pop-out search array (Thompson et al., 1997). Although no saccade was made to the pop-out stimulus, FEF neurons still discriminated the oddball stimulus from distractors at the same time and to the same degree as when a gaze shift was produced (figure 8.2B). Thus, the visual selection observed in FEF does not require saccade planning. Coupled with the evidence that attention is allocated automatically to the pop-out target in a search array (reviewed by Egeth and Yantis, 1997), this finding suggests that FEF may play a role in covert orienting of visual attention. This conclusion is supported by recent brain imaging studies showing that a region in human frontal cortex including FEF is activated in association with both attention and saccade tasks (Nobre et al., 1997; Corbetta et al., 1998).

To summarize, current data indicate that the evolution of visually evoked activity in FEF represents the process of selecting conspicuous targets. This selection process seems to represent not only the target for an overt gaze shift but also the location of a covert attention shift. The stimulus properties that distinguish a target from distractors are represented in appropriate areas of visual cortex in which a concomitant selection process occurs (e.g., Luck et al., 1997; Chelazzi et al., 1998; Treue and Maunsell, 1999; McAdams and Maunsell, 1999; Reynolds and Desimone, chapter 7 in this volume). Most likely, the selection observed in FEF is conveyed by the afferents from the various visual areas. However, FEF also provides feedback connections to extrastriate visual cortex (Baizer et al., 1991; Schall, Morel, et al., 1995), so we should not overlook the possibility that the state of neural activity in FEF can influence neural processing in visual cortex.

## 8.4  The Influence of Knowledge on the Selection Process

The influence of top-down factors on gaze behavior has been shown elegantly by Yarbus (1967), among other researchers (reviewed by Viviani, 1990). The term ''top-down'' is used to refer to internal influences, such as the memory and expectations of the observer. Although conspicuous objects attract gaze, knowledge of what to look for also strongly influences the guidance of gaze. The same type of selective visual behavior is observed in both humans and other primates, such as macaque monkeys (Keating and Keating, 1993; Burman and Segraves, 1994).

Numerous studies have demonstrated the influence of top-down factors on visual selection. Cognitive strategies can override both covert (e.g., Bacon and Egeth, 1994) and overt (e.g., Bichot et al., 1996; Nodine et al., 1996) selection of pop-out targets. Expectations can affect visual selection even when the stimuli of interest are conspicuous. Subjects are faster at finding a pop-out target when the feature distinguishing target from distractors remains constant than when it varies from trial to trial (Bravo and Nakayama, 1992; Maljkovic and Nakayama, 1994). Similar effects have been observed on eye movements (Bichot and Schall, 1999b; McPeek et al., 1999). Repetition of target position on successive trials also improves performance (Maljkovic and Nakayama, 1996). Recent work has shown that viewers detect targets faster if they are embedded in previously experienced visual display configurations even though observers do not recognize the repetition (Chun and Jiang, 1998).

In some cases, knowledge can override conspicuousness. For example, experts are more likely than novices to ignore conspicuous but irrelevant parts of a visual image from their field of expertise (e.g., Nodine et al., 1996; Chapman and Underwood, 1998; Nodine and Krupinski, 1998). Other work using simpler visual search displays also shows that, under some circumstances, cognitive strategies can prevent conspicuous stimuli from capturing attention (Bacon and Egeth, 1994). Such observations stress the extent to which visual selection is under voluntary control, and we have investigated how such control is expressed in the brain.

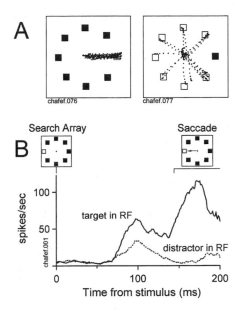

**Figure 8.3**
Visual selection of a learned target during pop-out search. (*A*) Saccades made by a monkey trained in only one instance of the visual search array, a red target among green distractors. When presented with an array in which the target and distractor colors were switched, instead of looking at the conspicuous green stimulus, this monkey looked only at one of the red distractors. (*B*) The time course of activation of a single FEF visual neuron in this monkey when the red target (solid line) was in the receptive field and when a green distractor (dotted line) was in the receptive field. Activity is plotted beginning at the time of search array presentation. The range of saccadic reaction times is shown. Unlike neurons recorded in monkeys that learned to perform generalized oddball search tasks (see figure 8.2), the initial visual response of this neuron discriminated the target from distractors. Modified from Bichot et al. (1996).

To study the effects of training experience on gaze behavior and associated neural activity, we trained monkeys exclusively with search arrays that contained a target of a constant color among distractor items of another constant color (Bichot et al., 1996). Control monkeys were trained to make a saccade to a target distinguished by the uniqueness of its color relative to all other items in the display (i.e., the display sometimes contained a red target among green distractors, and sometimes a green target among red distractors). Control monkeys shifted gaze according to visual salience, but the experimental monkeys persistently directed gaze to stimuli possessing the known target color (figure 8.3A). In other words, when experimental monkeys were presented with the search array complementary to that on which they had been trained, they shifted gaze to the distractors and not to the target, even though the target was of unique color. As described above, FEF neurons in monkeys trained to perform a general visual search do not exhibit color selectivity, but their activity evolves to signal the location of the unique stimulus. In monkeys trained exclusively on targets of one color, however, about half of FEF neurons show selectivity for stimuli of that color, which takes the form of a suppression of the initial visual responses to stimuli of the distractor color (figure 8.3B). How might this initial selective response arise in FEF? One possibility is that appropriate bias signals are delivered to FEF from other prefrontal areas responsible for executive control and strategy. Recent studies have demonstrated that the selective properties of prefrontal neurons can change according to rules or strategies (e.g., Asaad et al., 1998; Rainer et al., 1998, Rainer et al., 1999; White and Wise, 1999).

In many situations, objects of interest cannot be located solely on the basis of their visual features. In such cases, which are exemplified by a visual search for a conjunction of features such as color and shape, an explicit memory representation is needed to identify the target (e.g., Treisman and Sato, 1990; Bacon and Egeth, 1997). We investigated how the brain combines knowledge with visual processing to locate targets for eye movements by training monkeys to perform a visual search for a target defined by a unique combination of color and shape (feature conjunction) (figure 8.4). The color–shape combination defining the target was changed randomly between sessions. We observed two separate top-down influences on gaze behavior and the neural selection process: visual similarity to the target and the history of target properties (Bichot and Schall, 1999a, 1999b). The evidence for the influence of visual similarity was that monkeys made occasional errant saccades during this conjunction search that tended to direct gaze to distractors which resembled the current target. Similar observations have been made with human observers during covert (Kim and Cave, 1995) and overt orienting (Findlay, 1997; Motter and Belky, 1998; but see Zelinsky, 1996). Physiological recordings in FEF revealed that when monkeys successfully shifted gaze to the target, FEF neurons not only discriminated the target from distractors but also discriminated among the nonselected distractors exhibiting more activation for distractors that shared a target feature and a distractor that shared none.

Thus, the pattern of neural discrimination among nonselected distractors corresponded to the pattern of errors that reveal the allocation of attention. These behavioral and neurophysiological findings support the hypothesis that the target in at least some conjunction visual searches can be detected efficiently on the basis of visual similarity (Duncan and Humphreys, 1989), most likely through parallel processing of the individual features that define the stimuli (Wolfe et al., 1989; Cave and Wolfe, 1990; Treisman and Sato, 1990). The correspondence between the pattern of neural selection observed in FEF and the results of studies and predictions of models of visual attention (e.g., Cave et al., 1999) is further evidence that the selection in FEF predicts the allocation of visual attention.

The history of stimulus presentation across sessions also affected the selection process during conjunction search. If an error was made, monkeys showed a significant tendency

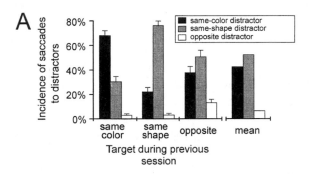

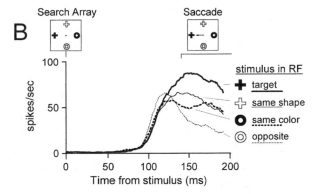

**Figure 8.4**
Visual selection during conjunction search. (*A*) Gaze pattern in conjunction search during neural record-ings. Incidence of saccades to distractors having the same color (*black*) or the same shape (*gray*) as the target, or having features opposite to the target (*unfilled*) is shown as a function of the target properties in the pre-vious session. Error bars show the standard error. If they made an error, monkeys tended to shift gaze to a distractor that resembled the target, especially if the distractor had been the target in the previous experi-mental session. (*B*) Time course of activity of an FEF neuron during conjunction search when the target stim-ulus (thick solid line), same-color distractor (thin solid line), same-shape distractor (thick dotted line), and opposite distractor (thin dotted line) fell in its receptive field. The plots begin at the time of search array presentation. The range of latencies of saccades to the target are indicated. When this neuron was recorded, the target was the same shape as the target of the previous session. Modified from Bichot and Schall (1999a).

(in addition to the visual similarity tendency just described) to shift gaze to the distractor that had been the target in the previous session. Recordings from FEF neurons during trials with correct saccades to the conjunction target revealed a corresponding difference in activation among distractors, resulting in more activation for distractors that had been the search target during the previous session. This effect, which may be a form of long-term priming, revealed itself across sessions that were at least a day apart and persisted throughout each experimental session. The longer duration of this influence distinguishes this learning effect from the short-term priming during pop-out searches that lasts for about 10 trials or 30 seconds in humans (Maljkovic and Nakayama, 1994) as well as monkeys (Bichot and Schall, 1999b).

## 8.5 Selection of Ambiguous Targets

In the visual search studies just described and in other studies that have examined the neural processes involved in visual choices, the choice of behavioral response was dictated explicitly by differences in the visual stimuli (e.g., Glimcher and Sparks, 1992; di Pelligrino and Wise, 1993; Schlag-Rey et al., 1997; Gottlieb et al., 1998; Asaad et al., 1998). In other words, the external stimuli completely dictated the correct response. The real world is rarely as clear as the laboratory. Often behavioral choices must be made on the basis of incomplete or unclear information. We have investigated the sensory and motor activity in FEF of monkeys responding to an ambiguous stimulus that could result in either of two mutually exclusive perceptual reports (Thompson and Schall, 1999; Thompson and Schall, 2000). The phenomenon of backward masking was used to create a condition in which the same physical stimulus might or might not be detected and localized. The experiment was designed to discourage guessing by requiring monkeys to report either the perceived presence or the absence of a target.

Figure 8.5 shows the activity of a visually responsive FEF neuron during *hit trials,* on which the target appeared and was correctly detected; *miss trials,* on which the target

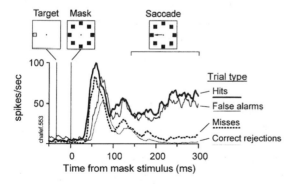

**Figure 8.5**
Visual selection of an ambiguous target during visual masking. The time course of activity of a single FEF visual neuron during the backward masking task is plotted separately for hits (thick solid lines), misses (thick dotted lines), false alarms (thin solid lines), and correct rejections (thin dotted lines). The activity is aligned on the time of mask presentation at 0 ms. The target appeared 33 ms before the mask on hits and misses. The range of saccade latencies during hits and false alarms is indicated at the top. Modified from Thompson and Schall (1999) and Thompson and Schall (2000).

appeared but was not detected; *false alarm trials,* on which no target appeared but the monkey reported one present; and *correct rejection trials,* on which no target appeared and the monkey correctly reported that no target was present. The monkey's behavior on hits and false alarms was the same; it made a saccade indicating perception of a target. Likewise, the monkey's behavior on misses and correct rejections was the same; it maintained fixation on the central spot, indicating a perceived absence of a target.

It is generally thought that visual responses in prefrontal cortex register sensory activity that reaches awareness to guide voluntary behavior (e.g., Crick and Koch, 1995). We were surprised to find that virtually all visually responsive neurons in FEF responded at short latencies to the target stimulus whether or not the monkey reported its presence (on hits and misses). Monkeys shifted gaze to the masked stimulus when the initial visual response to the target stimulus was only slightly stronger. Monkeys also made frequent errors of indicating target presence when there was none (false alarms), and we found that false alarms were made when visual neurons responded slightly more strongly to the mask stimulus. Thus, for nearly every visually responsive FEF neuron, when the early sensory responses were slightly greater, the target was reported as being present. This difference was small, often only one or two spikes in the period before the response to the mask. We believe it is unlikely that this difference in the initial visual activation arises de novo in FEF. Most likely, the difference observed reflects variations in visual activation in earlier stages of the visual pathway, perhaps even originating in the retina and propagating throughout the visual system.

Regardless of how the differences in activation came to be, the initial visual activation occurring immediately before the mask response predicts reasonably well whether monkeys will generate a "yes" or a "no" report (Thompson and Schall, 1999). We postulate that the initial visual responses in FEF represent the evidence upon which the detection decision is based. In terms of signal detection theory the early visual response is the dependent variable along a decision axis (Green and Swets, 1966). When this visual response is slightly greater than otherwise, it crosses a threshold on this axis such that the monkey responds that the target was there. Further studies are required to identify where in the visual system the differences in the initial visual responses arise, as well as the nature of the neural decision threshold.

In addition to the early visual response differences, many of the visually responsive FEF neurons exhibited a prolonged phase of elevated activity that occurred specifically during trials on which the target was reported as being present (hits and false alarms) but not during trials on which the target was reported as being absent (misses and correct rejections). For the neuron shown in figure 8.5, this second phase of differential activity began around 100 ms following mask presentation and continued until the saccade.

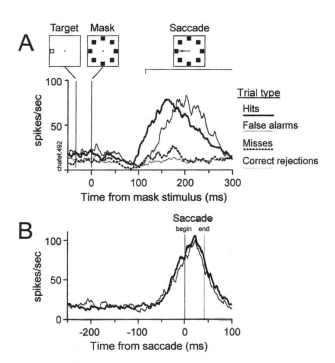

**Figure 8.6**
Response selection of an ambiguous target during visual masking. (*A*) The time course of activity of a single FEF movement neuron during the backward masking task is plotted separately for hits, misses, false alarms, and correct rejections. Conventions are the same as in figure 8.5. (*B*) The activity of the same FEF movement neuron associated with hits and false alarms aligned on the time of saccade initiation.

What does this late, enhanced activation on hits and false alarms represent? As reviewed above, FEF is commonly regarded as a motor area. Thus, one must ask whether the late activation after the mask response is related to visual processing or to motor programming. To address this question, we compared the selective activity of movement neurons against that of visual neurons.

Figure 8.6 shows the activity of a movement neuron during the visual masking task. Movement neurons in FEF are distinguishable from the visual neurons in several ways. First, movement neurons exhibited little or no modulation of activity on misses or on correct rejections, but exhibited strong activation associated with the saccade on hits and false alarms. Further, the magnitude and pattern of movement-related activity was the same for hits as it was for false alarms (figure 8.6B). And finally, the time of the late selective response in visual neurons was synchronized with the time of target presentation, but onset of movement cell activity began progressively later on trials with progressively longer saccade latencies (Thompson and Schall, 2000).

These results indicate further that visual neurons and movement neurons in FEF are functionally distinct. FEF movement neurons provide a motor command appropriate to produce the overt behavioral report through a gaze shift. In contrast, the relationship of visual neurons to saccade execution appears to be more distal than that of the movement neurons. However, the later period of activity of the visual neurons was clearly related more to the behavioral response than to the physical stimulus. Therefore, we think that the selective signal observed in the visual neurons represents a signal that is not just visual but not quite motor, that is, the signal is not dictated solely by the retinal image but it is not an explicit motor command.

## 8.6 Conclusions

The findings we have reviewed suggest the following general conclusions. The data reveal neurophysiological correlates of two selection processes that have been theorized to be necessary for the execution of a voluntary movement: the selection of the *stimulus* that guides the action and the selection of the *action* itself. It seems clear that the activity of movement neurons in FEF corresponds to the selection and preparation of the action. We believe it is equally clear that the selection process observed in visual neurons in FEF corresponds to the selection of stimuli. This neural selection occurs during visual search for a conspicuous target as well as during visual search that requires a memory representation. The neural selection also occurs when an ambiguous sensory signal is selected for further processing. We hypothesize that this visual selection process corresponds to the allocation of covert attention that precedes purposive gaze shifts.

The data also indicate how the selection process observed in frontal cortex may be related to the selection processes observed in visual cortical areas. Whereas the role of visual cortex is to analyze what is where in the image, we suggest that one role of FEF is to represent locations that could receive orienting responses. Figure 8.7 (plate 5) diagrams the hypothesis that FEF contains a map of visual salience. To illustrate this, consider performance of a conjunction visual search. Each element in the array is distinct, but none is conspicuously different from the others. The properties of the elements in the image are processed by populations of neurons discriminating shape, color, and direction of motion, among other features. For the color–shape conjunction, the motion map does not contribute to the selection process, but the units responding to the particular color and shape at each location are activated. These feature maps correspond conceptually to the processing that occurs in striate and extrastriate visual cortex. In models of visual search,

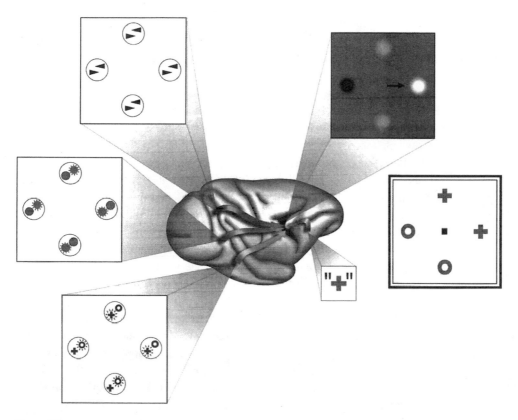

**Figure 8.7**
Frontal-eye fields as a salience map. Consider the task of finding the target in the conjunction visual search display shown at the right in the double border. To locate the target, the elementary features of color and shape must be determined. Visual shape (*lower left*), color (*center left*), and motion (*upper left*) are portrayed as being analyzed across the visual field by topographic maps in different parts of extrastriate visual cortex. Each circle enclosing a pair of features represents a hypercolumn in the cortex; the actual organization is more complicated. The starburst design around one feature indicates activation at different locations in the color and shape maps resulting from the stimuli in the visual search display; the motion map is not activated because the search display is static. The convergence of the activation from the feature maps into FEF is portrayed on a rendering of a macaque brain. This search for a conjunction of color and shape cannot be accomplished with visual processing alone because the properties of the stimuli do not completely specify which is the target. To locate the target correctly, a memory representation must influence the activation in the salience map. The square enclosing the red ✚ symbolizes a memory representation of the correct target that is portrayed as influencing FEF through a projection from ventral prefrontal cortex. The panel issuing from FEF (*upper right*) indicates the state of activation in a salience map that guides orienting in the search array. The location in the salience map corresponding to the red ✚ has the highest activation (white), the locations with stimuli that are the same shape or color as the target have intermediate activation (gray), and the location with the stimulus that is neither the same shape nor the same color as the target has minimal activation. Compare with figure 8.4B. The arrow in the salience map (*upper right*) indicates the cover or overt orienting resulting from the pattern of activation. See text for discussion. (See plate 5 for color version.)

the feature maps converge onto another map of the visual field that represents the locations of targets for orienting.

Consistent with this architecture as reviewed above, FEF receives convergence from many extrastriate visual areas. When the desired target is distinctly different from other stimuli in the image, then these bottom-up projections are sufficient to guide action. In many situations, though, such as conjunction search, a memory representation must be combined with the outcome of visual processing to guide the search for the target. To perform this function, models of visual search include a top-down influence on the salience map. Similarly, FEF is also innervated by areas in prefrontal cortex that can represent the properties of the desired target as well as the influence of strategy and context. The level of activation in the salience map represents the likelihood that the represented stimulus will receive additional processing through covert or overt orienting. In figure 8.7 the correct target receives the highest activation and distractors that are the same shape or same color as the target receive some activation. Overall, the data we have reviewed suggest that the visually evoked activation in FEF represents the selection of stimuli for further action, whether the selection is guided by external stimulus properties, knowledge, or self-generated decision criteria.

We are not suggesting that FEF is the only map of visual salience in the brain. Several lines of evidence suggest a similar function for the superior colliculus (e.g., Basso and Wurtz, 1998; reviewed by Findlay and Walker, 1999) and posterior parietal cortex (e.g., Robinson et al., 1995; Steinmetz and Constantinides, 1995; Gottlieb et al., 1998). It seems clear, then, that the functional salience map is distributed among distinct, but interconnected, concurrently active visuomotor structures. Moreover, the representation of salience to select locations for further processing seems to be a useful theoretical construct that can organize current data and guide further empirical and theoretical efforts.

## Acknowledgement

Our research has been supported by the National Eye Institute, the McDonnell-Pew Program in Cognitive Neuroscience, and the McKnight Endowment Fund for Neuroscience.

## References

Allport, A. (1987). Selection for action: Some behavioral and neurophysiological considerations of attention and action. In H. Heuer & A. F. Sanders (eds.), *Perspectives on perception and action* (pp. 395–419). Hillsdale, NJ: Laurence Erlbaum.

Asaad, W. F., Rainer, G., and Miller, E. K. (1998). Neural activity in the primate prefrontal cortex during associative learning. *Neuron* 21: 1399–1407.

Bacon, W. F., and Egeth, H. E. (1994). Overriding stimulus-driven attentional capture. *Percep. Psychophys.* 55: 485–496.

Bacon, W. F., and Egeth H. E. (1997). Goal-directed guidance of attention: Evidence from conjunctive visual search. *J. Exp. Psych. Hum. Percep. Perf.* 23: 948–961.

Baizer, J. S., Ungerleider, L. G., and Desimone, R. (1991). Organization of visual inputs to the inferior temporal and posterior parietal cortex in macaques. *J. Neurosci.* 11: 168–190.

Basso, M. A., and Wurtz, R. H. (1998). Modulation of neuronal activity in superior colliculus by changes in target probability. *J. Neurosci.* 18: 7519–7534.

Bichot, N. P., and Schall, J. D. (1999a). Effects of similarity and history on neural mechanisms of visual selection. *Nature Neurosci.* 2: 549–554.

Bichot, N. P., and Schall, J. D. (1999b). Saccade target selection in macaque during feature and conjunction visual search. *Vis. Neurosci.* 16: 81–89.

Bichot, N. P., Schall, J. D., and Thompson, K. G. (1996). Visual feature selectivity in frontal eye fields induced by experience in mature macaques. *Nature* 381: 697–699.

Bravo, M. J., and Nakayama, K. (1992). The role of attention in different visual search tasks. *Percep. Psychophys.* 51: 465–472.

Bruce, C. J., and Goldberg, M. E. (1985). Primate frontal eye fields. I. Single neurons discharging before saccades. *J. Neurophysiol.* 53: 603–635.

Bruce, C. J., Goldberg, M. E., Bushnell, M. C., and Stanton, G. B. (1985). Primate frontal eye fields. II: Physiological and anatomical correlates of electrically evoked eye movements. *J. Neurophysiol.* 54: 714–734.

Burman, D. D., and Segraves, M. A. (1994). Primate frontal eye field activity during natural scanning eye movements. *J. Neurophysiol.* 71: 1266–1271.

Cave, K. R., Kim, M.-S., Bichot, N. P., and Sobel, K. V. (2000). Visual selection within a hierarchical network: The FeatureGate model. *Cog. Psychol.*

Cave, K. R., and Wolfe, J. M. (1990). Modeling the role of parallel processing in visual search. *Cog. Psychol.* 22: 225–271.

Chapman, P., and Underwood, G. (1998). Visual search of driving situations: Danger and experience. *Perception* 27: 951–964.

Chelazzi, L., Duncan, J., Miller, E. K., and Desimone, R. (1998). Responses of neurons in inferior temporal cortex during memory-guided visual search. *J. Neurophysiol.* 80: 2918–2940.

Chun, M. M., and Jiang, Y. (1998). Contextual cueing: Implicit learning and memory of visual context guides spatial attention. *Cog. Psychol.* 36: 28–71.

Coles, M. G. H., Smid, H. G. O. M., Scheffers, M. K., and Otten, L. J. (1995). Mental chronometry and the study of human information processing. In M.D. Rugg and M. G. H. Coles (eds.), *Electrophysiology of mind: Event-related brain potentials and cognition* (pp. 86–131). Oxford: Oxford University Press.

Corbetta, M., Akbudak, E., Conturo, T. E., Snyder, A. Z., Ollinger, J. M., Drury, H. A., Linenweber, M. R., Petersen, S. E., Raichle, M. E., Van Essen, D. C., and Shulman, G. L. (1998). A common network of functional areas for attention and eye movements. *Neuron* 21: 761–773.

Crick, F., and Koch, C. (1995). Are we aware of neural activity in primary visual cortex? *Nature* 375: 121–123.

Deubel, H., and Schneider, W. X. (1996). Saccade target selection and object recognition: Evidence for a common attentional mechanism. *Vis. Res.* 36: 1827–1837.

Dias, E. C., Kiesau, M., and Segraves, M. A. (1995). Acute activation and inactivation of macaque frontal eye field with GABA-related drugs. *J. Neurophysiol.* 74: 2744–2748.

di Pellegrino, G., and Wise, S. P. (1993). Visuospatial versus visuomotor activity in the premotor and prefrontal cortex of a primate. *J. Neurosci.* 13: 1227–1243.

Donders, F. C. (1868). On the speed of mental processes. Trans. W. G. Koster. In *Attention and performance II* (pp. 412–431). Amsterdam: North-Holland, 1969.

Dorris, M. C., and Munoz, D. P. (1998). Saccadic probability influences motor preparation signals and time to saccadic initiation. *J. Neurosci.* 18: 7015–7026.

Duncan, J., and Humphreys, G. W. (1989). Visual search and stimulus similarity. *Psychol. Rev.* 96: 433–458.

Egeth, H. E., and Yantis, S. (1997). Visual attention: Control, representation, and time course. *Ann. Rev. Psychol.* 48: 269–297.

Everling, S., Dorris, M.C., and Munoz, D.P. (1998). Reflex suppression in the anti-saccade task is dependent on prestimulus neural processes. *J. Neurophysiol.* 80: 1584–1589.

Findlay, J. M. (1997). Saccade target selection during visual search. *Vis. Res.* 37: 617–631.

Findlay, J. M., and Walker, R. (1999). A model of saccade generation based on parallel processing and competitive inhibition. *Behav. Brain Sci.* 22: 661–674.

Glimcher, P. W., and Sparks, D. L. (1992). Movement selection in advance of action in superior colliculus. *Nature* 355: 542–545.

Goldberg, M.E., and Bushnell, M.C. (1981). Behavioral enhancement of visual responses in monkey cerebral cortex. II. Modulation in frontal eye fields specifically related to saccades. *J. Neurophysiol.* 46: 773–787.

Gottlieb, J. P., Kusunoki, M., and Goldberg, M. E. (1998). The representation of visual salience in monkey parietal cortex. *Nature* 391: 481–484.

Green, D. M., and Swets, J. A. (1966). *Signal detection theory and psychophysics.* New York: Wiley.

Hanes, D. P., Patterson, W. F., and Schall, J. D. (1998). The role of frontal eye field in countermanding saccades: Visual, movement and fixation activity. *J. Neurophysiol.* 79: 817–834.

Hanes, D. P., and Schall, J. D. (1996). Neural control of voluntary movement initiation. *Science* 274: 427–430.

Hanes, D. P., Thompson, K. G., and Schall, J. D. (1995). Relationship of presaccadic activity in frontal and supplementary eye field to saccade initiation in macaque: Poisson spike train analysis. *Exp. Brain Res.* 103: 85–96.

Hoffman, J. E., and Subramaniam, B. (1995). The role of visual attention in saccadic eye movements. *Percep. Psychophys.* 57: 787–795.

Jouve, B., Rosenstiehl, P., and Imbert, M. (1998). A mathematical approach to the connectivity between the cortical visual areas of the macaque monkey. *Cereb. Cortex* 8: 28–39.

Keating, C. F., and Keating, E. G. (1993). Monkeys and mug shots: Cues used by rhesus monkeys (Macaca mulatta) to recognize a human face. *J. Comp. Psychol.* 107: 131–139.

Kim, J. N., and Shadlen, M. N. (1999). Neural correlates of a decision in the dorsolateral prefrontal cortex of the macaque. *Nature Neurosci.* 2: 176–185.

Kim, M.-S., and Cave, K. R. (1995). Spatial attention in search for features and feature conjunctions. *Psychonom. Sci.* 6: 376–380.

Koch, C., and Ullman, S. (1985). Shifts in selective visual attention: Towards the underlying neural circuitry. *Hum. Neurobiol.* 4: 219–227.

Kowler, E., Anderson, E., Dosher, B., and Blaser, E. (1995). The role of attention in the programming of saccades. *Vis. Res.* 35: 1897–1916.

Kustov, A. A., and Robinson, D. L. (1996). Shared neural control of attentional shifts and eye movements. *Nature* 384: 74–77.

Luck, S. J., Chelazzi, L., Hillyard, S. A., and Desimone, R. (1997). Neural mechanisms of spatial selective attention in areas V1, V2, and V4 of macaque visual cortex. *J. Neurophysiol.* 77: 24–42 .

Maljkovic, V., and Nakayama, K. (1994). Priming of pop-out: I. Role of features. *Mem. Cog.* 22: 657–672.

Maljkovic, V., and Nakayama, K. (1996). Priming of pop-out: II. The role of position. Percep. Psychophys. 58: 977–991.

McAdams, C.J., and Maunsell, J.H.R. (1999). Effects of attention on orientation-tuning functions of single neurons in macaque cortical area V4. *J. Neurosci.* 19: 431–441.

McPeek, R. M., Maljkovic, V., and Nakayama, D. (1999). Saccades require focal attention and are facilitated by a short-term memory system. *Vis. Res.* 39: 1555–1566.

Mohler, C. W., Goldberg, M. E., and Wurtz, R. H. (1973). Visual receptive fields of frontal eye field neurons. *Brain Res.* 61: 385–389.

Motter, B. C., and Belky, E. J. (1998). The guidance of eye movements during active visual search. *Vis. Res.* 38: 1805–1815.

Nobre, A. C., Sebestyen, G. N., Gitelman, D. R., Mesulam, M. M., Frackowiack, R. S. J., and Frith, C. D. (1997). Functional localization of the system for visuospatial attention using positron emission tomography. *Brain* 120: 515–533.

Nodine, C. F., and Krupinski, E. A. (1998). Perceptual skill, radiology expertise, and visual test performance with NINA and WALDO. *Acad. Radiol.* 5: 603–612.

Nodine, C. F., Kundel, H. L., Lauver, S. C., and Toto, L. C. (1996). Nature of expertise in searching mammograms for breast masses. *Acad. Radiol.* 3: 1000–1006.

Nowak, L. G., and Bullier, J. (1997). The timing of information transfer in the visual system in extrastriate cortex of primates, In K. Rockland, A. Peters, and J. Kaas (eds.), *Cerebral cortex,* vol. 12 (pp. 205–241). New York: Plenum Press.

Olshausen, B. A., Anderson, C. H., and Van Essen, D. C. (1993). A neurobiological model of visual attention and invariant pattern recognition based on dynamic routing of information. *J. Neurosci.* 13: 4700–4719.

Pare, M., and Munoz, D.P. (1996). Saccadic reaction time in the monkey: Advanced preparation of oculomotor programs is primarily responsible for express saccade occurrence. *J. Neurophysiol.* 76: 3666–3681.

Pashler, H. (1991). Shifting visual attention and selecting motor responses: Distinct attentional mechanisms. *J. Exp. Psychol. Hum. Percep. Perf.* 17: 1023–1040.

Rainer, G., Asaad, W. F., and Miller, E. K. (1998). Selective representation of relevant information by neurons in the primate prefrontal cortex. *Nature* 393: 577–579.

Rainer, G., Rao, S. C., and Miller, E. K. (1999). Prospective coding for objects in primate prefrontal cortex. *J. Neurosci.* 19: 5493–5505.

Rivaud, S., Müri, R. M., Gaymard, B., Vermersch, A. I., and Pierrot-Deseilligny, C. (1994). Eye movement disorders after frontal eye field lesions in humans. *Exp. Brain Res.* 102: 110–120.

Robinson, D. L., Bowman, E. M., and Kertzman, C. (1995). Covert orienting of attention in macaques. II. Contributions of parietal cortex. *J. Neurophysiol.* 74: 698–712.

Schall, J. D. (1991). Neuronal activity related to visually guided saccades in the frontal eye fields of rhesus monkeys: Comparison with supplementary eye fields. *J. Neurophysiol.* 66: 559–579.

Schall, J. D. (1997). Visuomotor areas of the frontal lobe. In K. Rockland, A. Peters, and J. H. Kaas (eds.), *Extrastriate cortex of primates,* vol. 12 of *Cerebral Cortex* (pp. 527–638). New York: Plenum Press.

Schall, J. D., and Bichot, N. P. (1998). Neural correlates of visual and motor decision processes. *Curr. Opin. Neurobiol.* 8: 211–217.

Schall, J. D., and Hanes, D. P. (1993). Neural basis of saccade target selection in frontal eye field during visual search. *Nature* 366: 467–469.

Schall, J. D., Hanes, D. P., Thompson, K. G., and King, D. J. (1995). Saccade target selection in frontal eye field of macaque. I. Visual and premovement activation. *J. Neurosci.* 15: 6905–6918.

Schall, J. D., Morel, A., King, D. J., and Bullier, J. (1995). Topography of visual cortical afferents to frontal eye field in macaque: Functional convergence and segregation of processing streams. *J. Neurosci.* 15: 4464–4487.

Schall, J. D., and Thompson, K. G. (1999). Neural selection and control of visually guided eye movements. *Ann. Rev. Neurosci.* 22: 241–259.

Schiller, P. H., and Chou, I. H. (1998). The effects of frontal eye field and dorsomedial frontal cortex lesions on visually guided eye movements. *Nature Neurosci.* 1: 248–253.

Schiller, P. H., Sandell, J. H., and Maunsell, J. H. R. (1987). The effect of frontal eye field and superior colliculus lesions on saccadic latencies in the rhesus monkey. *J. Neurophysiol.* 57: 1033–1049.

Schlag-Rey, M., Amador, N., Sanchez, H., and Schlag, J. (1997). Antisaccade performance predicted by neuronal activity in the supplementary eye field. *Nature* 390: 398–401.

Schmolesky, M. T., Wang, Y., Hanes, D. P., Thompson, K. G., Leutgeb, S., Schall, J. D., and Leventhal, A. G. (1998). Signal timing across the macaque visual system. *J. Neurophysiol.* 79: 3272–3278.

Segraves, M. A. (1992). Activity of monkey frontal eye field neurons projecting to oculomotor regions of the pons. *J. Neurophysiol.* 68: 1967–1985.

Segraves, M. A., and Goldberg, M. E. (1987). Functional properties of corticotectal neurons in the monkey's frontal eye fields. *J. Neurophysiol.* 58: 1387–1419.

Sheliga, B. M., Riggio, L., and Rizzolatti, G. (1995). Spatial attention and eye movements. *Exp. Brain Res.* 105: 261–275.

Sommer, M. A., and Tehovnik, E. J. (1997). Reversible inactivation of macaque frontal eye field. *Exp. Brain Res.* 116: 229–249.

Stanton, G. B., Bruce, C. J., and Goldberg, M. E. (1993). Topography of projections to the frontal lobe from the macaque frontal eye fields. *J. Comp. Neurol.* 330: 286–301.

Stanton, G. B., Bruce, C. J., and Goldberg, M. E. (1995). Topography of projections to posterior cortical areas from the macaque frontal eye fields. *J. Comp. Neurol.* 353: 291–305.

Steinmetz, M. A., and Constantinidis, C. (1995). Neurophysiological evidence for a role of posterior parietal cortex in redirecting visual attention. *Cereb. Cortex* 5: 448–456.

Sternberg, S. (1969). The discovery of processing stages: Extensions of Donders' method. *Acta Psychol.* 30: 276–315.

Theeuwes, J. (1991). Cross-dimensional perceptual selectivity. *Percep. Psychophys.* 50: 184–193.

Theeuwes, J., Kramer, A. F., Hahn, S., and Irwin, D. E. (1998). Our eyes do not always go where we want them to go: Capture of the eyes by new objects. *Psychol. Sci.* 9: 379–385.

Thompson, K. G., and Bichot, N. P. (1999). Frontal eye field: A cortical salience map. *Behav. Brain Sci.* 22: 699–700.

Thompson, K. G., Bichot, N. P., and Schall, J. D. (1997). Dissociation of target selection from saccade planning in macaque frontal eye field. *J. Neurophysiol.* 77: 1046–1050.

Thompson, K. G., Hanes, D. P., Bichot, N. P., and Schall, J. D. (1996). Perceptual and motor processing stages identified in the activity of macaque frontal eye field neurons during visual search. *J. Neurophysiol.* 76: 4040–4055.

Thompson, K. G., and Schall, J. D. (1999). The detection of visual signals by macaque frontal eye field during masking. *Nature Neurosci.* 2: 283–288.

Thompson, K. G., and Schall, J. D. (2000). Antecedents and correlates of visual detection and awareness in macaque prefrontal cortex. *Vis. Res.* 40: 1523–1538.

Treisman, A. (1988). Features and objects: The fourteenth Bartlett memorial lecture. *Q. J. Exp. Psychol.* 40A: 201–237.

Treisman, A., and Sato, S. (1990). Conjunction search revisited. *J. Exp. Psychol. Hum. Percep. Perf.* 16: 459–478.

Treue S., and Maunsell, J.H. (1999). Effects of attention on the processing of motion in macaque middle temporal and medial superior temporal visual cortical areas. *J. Neurosci.* 19: 7591–7602.

Viviani, P. (1990). Eye movements in visual search: Cognitive, perceptual and motor control aspects. In E. Kowler (ed.), *Eye movements and their role in visual and cognitive processes* (pp. 353–393). New York: Elsevier.

White, I. M., and Wise, S. P. (1999). Rule-dependent neuronal activity in the prefrontal cortex. *Exp. Brain Res.* 126: 315–335.

Wolfe, J. M. (1994). Guided search 2.0: A revised model of visual search. *Psychol. Bull. Rev.* 1: 202–238.

Wolfe, J. M. (1998). Visual search. In H. Pashler (ed.), *Attention* (pp. 13–74). Hove, UK: Psychology Press.

Wolfe, J. M., Cave, K. R., and Franzel, S. L. (1989). Guided search: An alternative to the feature integration model for visual search. *J. Exp. Psychol. Hum. Percep. Perf.* 15: 419–433.

Yarbus, A. L. (1967). *Eye movements and vision.* New York: Plenum Press.

Zelinsky, G. J. (1996). Using eye saccades to assess the selectivity of search movements. *Vis. Res.* 36: 2177–2187.

Zelinsky, G. J., and Sheinberg, D. L. (1997). Eye movements during parallel-serial search. *J. Exp. Psychol. Hum. Percep. Perf.* 23: 244–262.

# 9 Separating Attention from Chance in Active Visual Search

Brad C. Motter and James W. Holsapple

## 9.1 Introduction

Finding an object in a cluttered scene is a typical problem in everyday vision. Despite the evident difficulty of processing the large amount of information in such a scene, we have a remarkable ability to locate one particular object in the midst of numerous distracting objects. In some situations, a distinguishing feature, such as color, can lead us more or less directly to the desired object in a heterogeneous scene. However, even in the absence of distinguishing features, the search is typically far more efficient than an object-by-object sequence of visual fixations. Actual search rates are significantly faster, and can be attained only by processing more than one object during each fixation. The superiority of actual search over an object-by-object strategy implies, therefore, that target objects can be detected at some distance from the point of fixation.

A major emphasis of previous work on visual search has been to discover the constraints that govern search performance while fixation is maintained. One focus of this research has been the conditions under which target objects are found quickly in a spatially parallel manner, as opposed to a slower serial scan of the objects in the display. Following Neisser (1967), it was recognized that certain features are processed in parallel and thus may serve as a basis for guiding attention. Objects may be localized, even counted, when they possess distinguishing features (Sagi and Julesz, 1985). On the other hand, when a target object is distinguished only by a particular combination of features, its discovery requires some form of focal attentive scrutiny. The mechanism of this focal attentive scrutiny is thought to be a covert scanning process, in which a focus of attention is directed serially to different objects within the scene (Treisman, 1988). This view is based on the well-known fact that attention can be willfully shifted away from the point of fixation during maintained fixation (Eriksen and Hoffman, 1972; Posner, 1980). Such covert shifts of attention are presumed to be the basis for detecting target objects while maintaining the direction of gaze.

Unlike saccadic eye movements, covert shifts of attention away from the point of fixation are not accompanied by a realignment of the retinal receptor gradient with the newly attended object. Although spatial resolution falls off with increasing retinal eccentricity, acuity is usually not a limiting factor in visual search because object size typically far exceeds acuity thresholds. However, acuity is not the only measure that decreases with retinal eccentricity. The retinal receptor gradient also provides the basic structural framework for lateral interactions that strongly constrain object visibility. Whereas acuity depends directly on receptor density, the spatial range of lateral interactions is more pliable, and may vary widely between observers (Toet and Levi, 1991). Unfortunately, relatively little is known about the spatial range of the attentional processes underlying visual search, especially during *active visual search,* which combines shifts of attention with eye movements.

Here we formally examine the spatial range of attentional processing during active visual search by modeling the probability of target discovery as a function of retinal eccentricity. We conclude that the attentional mechanism can be conceptualized as the spatial distribution of the conditional probability of target detection, corrected for chance contributions. For displays with discrete objects, as typically used in visual search studies, the combination of this spatial probability distribution with a random walk through the set of relevant objects fully accounts for all aspects of search performance.

## 9.2   Methods

In a previous study, we investigated visual search among elements of different orientation and color (Motter and Belky, 1998b). Measuring the probability of target detection as a function of target eccentricity, we found that target detection was likely only within a fairly limited region around the point of fixation. Here we use the same methods to study visual search among randomly rotated Ts and Ls, all of the same color. Specifically, the task is to locate either a single T among numerous Ls, or a single L among numerous Ts (figure 9.1). Two rhesus monkeys served as subjects, and eye position was measured with an implanted scleral coil. The measurement of eye position was calibrated at the beginning of each daily session. We chose a monochrome display of Ts and Ls in order to minimize

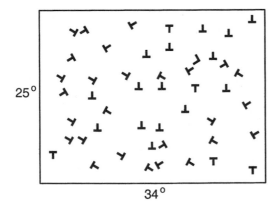

**Figure 9.1**
Search display containing forty-eight stimuli. Search starts from an initial fixation at center of display. Target for each trial was randomly selected and positioned (an L in this display). Subjects had to find and fixate target for 600 ms. Border frame was not present in actual display.

feature selective guidance and to concentrate on attentional processes. All stimulus items were randomly oriented in steps of 60°. The Ts and Ls were formed by combining two red bars measuring $1.25° \times 0.25°$ of visual angle. Stimulus items were placed randomly in a rectangular display area of $34° \times 25°$ in arrays of 6, 12, 24, 48, or 96 items. The number of items varied from trial to trial. The target item (T or L) was randomly selected for each trial and the animal was cued by presenting it at the center of the display for 1–1.5 s immediately before the array presentation (Motter and Belky, 1998b). The animal was trained to locate the target and to fixate on it for 600 ms. A target was always present, and the initial fixation was always at the center of the display. The experimental protocol and all procedures were approved by the VA Medical Center's Animal Care and Use Committee.

## 9.3    Contribution of Attention and Chance to Target Detection

Although one might suppose that fixations are directed at pairs or clusters of items, an examination of eye movement records shows that most saccades accurately land near one item, bringing it into the fovea (Motter and Belky, 1998a). This was also true in the present case of visual search among Ts and Ls (figure 9.1). The distances between fixation and the nearest item is shown in figure 9.2. More than 90% of saccades land within 1.5° of the item center, and more than 70% within 1° (the junction of the two bars composing the T or L was taken to be the center). Thus, visual search proceeds largely by a sequence of object fixations.

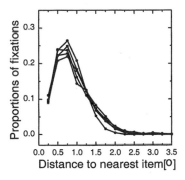

**Figure 9.2**
Fixations target individual stimuli. Curves depict distributions of the distances between fixation center and the center of the nearest stimulus. The five superimposed curves are the results for visual search experiments conducted with each search array size (6, 12, 24, 48, or 96 items). The decrease in the proportion of fixations as zero separation distance is approached (left side) reflects the smaller radius within which fixations could occur, resulting in fewer total fixations.

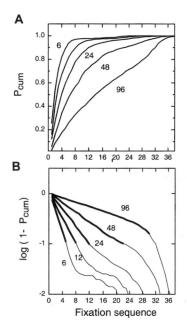

**Figure 9.3**
Determination of the probability of target discovery, $P$, from the cumulative probability. (*A*) Cumulative probability ($P_{cum}$) of capturing the target as a function of the number of required fixations for each of the five array sizes. (*B*) Replot of the ordinate of (*A*) in terms of $\log(1 - P_{cum})$. The linear form of the curves indicates that the fixation-by-fixation probability of target discovery did not change during the trial. This implies a sampling with replacement and little, if any, memory of previously sampled sites. The bold portions of the curves were used to estimate the slopes and calculate $P$. Data shown are for one subject.

If search is a strict random walk through the $N$ items in a display, then for each fixation the probability of target discovery is simply $1/N$. Following previous models of search behavior (Engel, 1977; Krendel and Wodinsky, 1960; Williams, 1966), the rate at which a search progresses can be summarized in terms of survivor functions. Figure 9.3A shows the cumulative probability ($P_{cum}$) of target detection as a function of the number of fixations since the start of the trial, for search arrays of different sizes. The number of fixations required to find the target is typically far less than the total number of items ($N$). The detection of the target on a given fixation was defined by whether or not the next saccade captured the target. Starting with the cumulative probability ($P_{cum}$), we would like to derive the probability of detecting the target during an individual fixation ($P_{ind}$). Assuming for the moment that $P_{ind}$ is constant over time, the cumulative probability of *not* finding the target after $f$ fixations is simply the product of *not* detecting the target during $f$ sequential fixations:

$$1 - p_{cum}(f) = (1 - P_{ind})^f \tag{1}$$

or

$$\log(1 - P_{cum}(f)) = f \times \log(1 - P_{ind}).$$

Clearly the above relationship is a linear function of fixations if $P_{ind}$ is a constant. $P_{ind}$ can be found by determining the slope, $m$, of the plot of $\log(1 - P_{cum})$ against fixation number and then solving the relationship:

$$P_{ind} = 1 - 10^{m}. \tag{2}$$

As shown in Fig. 9.3B, the slopes of the resulting plots are in fact mostly linear, indicating that $P_{ind}$ was constant during most fixations. Departures from linearity occur as the cumulative probability curves approach their asymptotic value. For cumulative probabilities in the range of 0.0 to 0.90, the curves are well fit by linear functions. Thus, the overall search rate (i.e., the number of fixations to target detection) can be summarized by a single parameter $P_{ind}$. Note that for a strictly random walk, $P_{ind}$ is expected to be $1/N$. The actual values observed for two animals are substantially larger and are listed in table 9.1.

The significance of a constant $P_{ind}$ is that search proceeds as if the probability of detecting the target is the same for every fixation and every trial. If there was a memory of non-target locations, and it would accumulate with each fixation, then $P_{ind}$ would gradually increase and the slope of the curves in figure 9.2B would increase. If present at all, any such effect in our data is evidently very small. However, we cannot entirely rule out a slight cumulative change in slope over the first few fixations. A memory for $m$ non-target locations would reduce the set of possible target locations to $N$-$m$. A memory holding just a few non-target locations (say, 1 to 3) would matter only when the array size is so small that the difference between $N$ and $N$-$m$ is significant. We conclude that memory for non-target locations does not play a major role in visual search, consistent with the findings of Horowitz and Wolfe (1998).

**Table 9.1**
Estimates of the Probability, $P$, of Target Discovery on Each Fixation for Two Subjects

| Array size | Pind estimate | | |
| --- | --- | --- | --- |
| | 1/N | C | L |
| 6 | .167 | .377 | .320 |
| 12 | .083 | .253 | .207 |
| 24 | .042 | .179 | .139 |
| 48 | .021 | .101 | .087 |
| 96 | .010 | .055 | .038 |

The fact that $P_{ind}$ is larger than $1/N$ for all size arrays (table 9.1) shows that information about more than one item is processed during each fixation. To estimate how much more, we have to remove the chance contribution to $P_{ind}$. The approach outlined here will be used again in another context. In general, there are two reasons why a given fixation may be followed by a saccade to the target. The first reason is that attentional processing of items at some distance from the point of fixation happens to reveal the target, and triggers a saccade to the corresponding location. The second reason is that attentional processing does not reveal the target, but that the next saccade is made to a random item that *by chance* turns out to be the target. Therefore, the total probability of target detection ($P_{tot}$) includes a non-chance component due to attentional processing ($P_a$) as well as a chance component ($P_c$). Taking into account also the possibility that the target is discovered both by attentional processing and by chance,

$$P_{tot} = P_a \times (1 - P_c) + P_c \times (1 - P_a) + P_a \times P_c$$

or

$$P_{tot} = P_c + P_a \times (1 - P_c). \tag{3}$$

Solving for the attentional component yields

$$P_a = (P_{tot} - P_c)/(1 - P_c). \tag{4}$$

With the help of equation (4) we can compute the attentional component of the probability of target detection from our measured total probability ($P_{tot}$) and the chance probability ($P_c = 1/N$). The results of this calculation are shown in figure 9.4. Clearly, chance plays

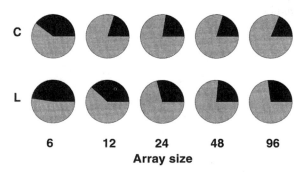

**Figure 9.4**
Probability of target discovery attributable to the separate chance and attentive components as a function of array set size. Pie charts show relative contributions of attentive ($P_a$, light shade) and chance ($P_c$, dark shade) components for two subjects, C and L. During active visual search, chance plays a major role in the discovery of targets, especially for small arrays of relevant stimuli.

a significant role in target detection, and for small arrays (6 items) the contributions of attentional processing and of chance are almost the same. As array size increases, the attentional contribution increases to about three times that of chance. The changing importance of chance, depending on array size, has not been recognized in previous studies of active visual search.

## 9.4   Spatial Distribution of the Probability of Target Detection

We have seen that active visual search involves a series of saccades to objects in the visual scene. The record of eye movements contains useful information in the target saccades that land on the target, as well as in the non-target saccades that land on items at some distance from the target. In particular, non-target saccades contain information about the radial distribution of target detection, that is, the probability of target detection as a function of target eccentricity relative to the current point of fixation. To compute this function, which we will term $p_{tot}(r)$, one has to measure for every non-target saccade the distance between the fixation point and the target location, and note whether the ensuing saccade was a target or a non-target saccade (Motter and Belky, 1998b). The calculation is based on all saccades during a search trial, except the initial saccade to the display center and the final target saccade (for details, see Motter and Belky, 1998b). The functions $p_{tot}(r)$ that are obtained for visual search among arrays of Ts and Ls are shown in figure 9.5. Different array sizes yield distinct probability distributions that form a series of monotonically decreasing functions. Just as in the previous section, the total probability of target detection combines contributions of attention and of chance. Our next task will be to distinguish these.

To arrive at the detection probability due to attention, we need to remove the probability due to chance from the total probability of target detection. Although the probability due to chance is simply $1/N$, the radial distribution of this probability is not uniform because saccades are not equally likely between all items in the display. In particular, saccades are more likely to target nearby items than items farther away (Motter and Belky, 1998a). To determine the relationship between eccentricity and chance detection of the target, we reasoned that the probability of saccading to the target when it is at eccentricity $r$ from fixation, $p_c(r)$, is the probability of making a saccade to an item at that eccentricity, $p_{SAD}(r)$, times the probability of selecting the target at random from the set of items at that eccentricity, $1/(p_{ISD}(r) \times N)$:

$$p_c(r) = \frac{p_{SAD}(r)}{p_{ISD}(r) \times N}. \tag{5}$$

We used the saccadic amplitude distribution (SAD) of non-target saccades, which presumably are guided purely by chance, to estimate the chance probability of making a

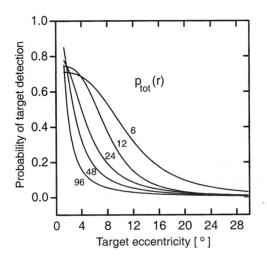

**Figure 9.5**
Spatial sensitivity curves. Curves are obtained by measuring target eccentricity from each fixation during search and noting whether the ensuing saccade captured the target or not. The sensitivity curves are logistic function fits to the data, shown separately for the five array set size conditions. The measured total sensitivity curves contain probabilities incorporating both chance and attentive components.

saccade to an item at a particular eccentricity, $p_{SAD}(r)$. The distribution of interstimulus distances (ISD) was measured for the display used. The saccade distributions $p_{SAD}(r)$ observed for different size arrays, as well as the interstimulus distribution $p_{ISD}(r)$, are shown in figure 9.6. Note that all array sizes exhibit the same interstimulus distribution because items are placed randomly within the display. Because the displays were bounded, the probability of encountering an item at a particular eccentricity, $p_{ISD}(r)$, increased to a maximum—for our display size this was near 12°—and then declined. The fact that the saccade distributions depart substantially from the interstimulus distribution implies that the probability of target detection by chance is not spatially uniform but varies with eccentricity.

The distributions of the radial functions $p_{SAD}(r)$ and $p_{ISD}(r)$ shown in figure 9.6 are averages taken over the entire display. Although these functions actually are locally determined, we have found that the local evaluations of equation 5 in fact result in the same function as the global average $p_c(r)$ (Motter and Holsapple, unpublished observations). Figure 9.7 shows the probability of chance detection, $p_c(r)$, as obtained from the measured distributions $p_{SAD}(r)$ and $p_{ISD}(r)$ with the help of equation 5. For comparison, the total probability of target detection, $p_{tot}(r)$, is shown as well. Chance plays a significant role in target detection; for the display size used, this was especially evident at intermediate

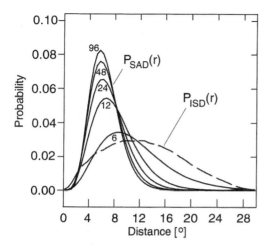

**Figure 9.6**
Saccadic amplitude and interstimulus distance distributions. The five solid curves depict the distribution of saccadic amplitudes (SAD) during active search for each of the array sizes. An orderly shift in the peaks of the SAD curves parallels the increasing density of items (and thus the decreasing average nearest neighbor distance between stimuli). SAD curves are exponential fits to data. The dashed curve depicts the distribution of interstimulus distances (ISD) for the display items. Because items are randomly placed on the display, this distribution is independent of array size.

eccentricities of 4° to 8°. It is important to recognize that the non-uniform distribution of chance detection is a direct result of the differences between $p_{SAD}(r)$ and $p_{ISD}(r)$. Although these distributions differ locally, the integral of $p_c(r)$ over the display is always $1/N$.

Having calculated the probability of chance detection, $p_c(r)$, we can now apply equation 4 and remove its contribution from the total probability of target detection, $p_{tot}(r)$, in order to obtain the desired probability of target detection by attention, $p_a(r)$. The result of this calculation is shown in figure 9.8, for different array sizes (compare figure 9.7). The attentional detection probability $p_a(r)$ retains the same general shape as the total detection probability $p_{tot}(r)$, and the differences due to array size remain as well. However, the main implication of these functions is that any reasonable probability of target detection by attention is limited to a fairly narrow zone around the center of gaze. The size of this zone depends on the density of array items, as shown by the fact that the different distributions collapse if eccentricity is measured in units normalized to array density (Motter and Belky, 1998b). Note that the radial profile of the "detection zone" is independent of any assumptions regarding the nature of the mechanisms that underlie the detection—whether they are limited by the constraints of eccentric vision or an active spatially parallel attentive scan, or whether they involve a serial process of covert scans.

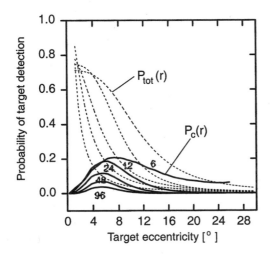

**Figure 9.7**
Spatial distribution of the chance component. Solid curves depict the chance probability of saccading to the target as a function of target eccentricity from fixation. The curves illustrate that when saccades are biased toward targeting items near the current fixation point, there is an accompanying higher probability of discovering the target by chance when it is located nearby. The total sensitivity curves (dashed lines) are shown for comparison.

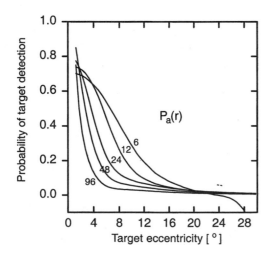

**Figure 9.8**
Spatial distribution of the attentive component. Sensitivity curves depict the attentive probability of detecting and capturing the target as a function of target eccentricity from fixation. These curves were derived by subtracting the chance curves of figure 9.7 from the total sensitivity curves shown in figure 9.5 (see text for details). The attentive component of target detection can be regarded as a focal attentive filter whose strength and areal extent are given by a radially symmetric function based on the curves in this figure.

## 9.5   Overall Probability of Target Detection Deduced from the Spatial Distribution

The preceding sections described two independent analyses of active visual search. The first analysis was based on counting the fixations before target detection, and yielded the total probability of detecting the target on a given fixation. The second analysis was based on the distance between target and fixation, and yielded the total probability of detecting the target at a given distance from fixation. Both analyses distinguished the respective contributions of attention and chance. In this section we demonstrate that the two analyses yield consistent results, as they must. The exercise of attempting this verification proves to be useful because it reveals several constraints on the mechanism underlying target detection by attention.

As we have seen, attention searches only a small zone around the center of gaze effectively. If the effectiveness in this small zone were 100%, that is, if targets in this zone were invariably detected, then the probability of target detection would be the area of the zone divided by the area of the display. However, because the detection probability decreases monotonically with eccentricity (figure 9.8), the overall probability of target detection must be obtained by integrating the spatial distribution of target detection over the area of the display, $A$. To accomplish this, we construct a *spatial* sensitivity function $f_a(r,\phi)$ by rotating $p_a(r)$ around the origin, thus sweeping out an area around the point of fixation. Of course, this assumes that the sensitivity function $f_a(r,\phi)$ is radially symmetric. In a more general analysis, we have found that radial symmetry is indeed a reasonable assumption for the sensitivity function $f_a(r,\phi)$ (Motter and Holsapple, unpublished observations).

When the effective area covered by the sensitivity function $f_a(r,\phi)$ is small relative to the total area of the display, boundaries can be ignored and the desired overall probability of target detection can be obtained by a straightforward integration followed by division by the display area. Unfortunately, the effective search area covers an appreciable fraction of the display, and when gaze rests on an item near the border, much of the effective search area falls outside the bounds of the display. One might expect that in such a case, the sensitivity function $f_a(r,\phi)$ is modified such that attentional resources are redistributed to locations inside the display, rather than wasted on locations outside the display. However, our investigation of this issue finds that the sensitivity distribution remains locally invariant for all locations within the display (Motter and Holsapple, unpublished observations). In light of this result, the integration of the sensitivity function $f_a(r,\phi)$ must take the position of display borders into account.

To properly estimate the overall probability of target detection by attention, we must therefore integrate the sensitivity function $f_a(r,\phi)$ inside the display boundaries and, in addition, average over a representative selection of fixation locations. Because items are placed randomly in the display area, one might think that a random sampling of the display area would be sufficient to generate such a selection. However, the distribution of eye positions is not uniform over the display area, but favors locations between the center and the boundaries of the display. To overcome this difficulty, we used a random sample of actual eye positions as starting points for integrating the sensitivity function $f_a(r,\phi)$. The logic here is that the actual fixations made by the animal enter into the calculation of both the overall probability of target detection by attention and the radial sensitivity function $p_a(r)$.

The integration procedure is illustrated in figure 9.9. The probability of finding a target in an area element $dA = r\ dr\ d\phi$ is given by the ratio $dA/A$, where $A$ is the total area of

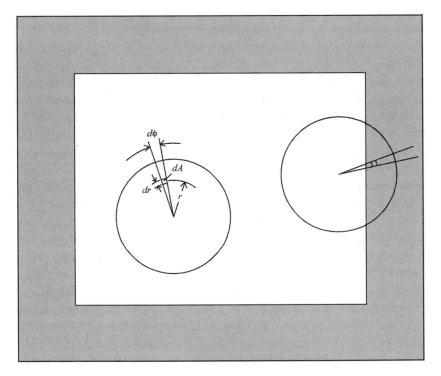

**Figure 9.9**
Cartoon of the integration procedure, showing two fixation positions, A and B, within the display surface boundaries—the white area within the surrounding hatched area. The probabilities associated with each differential element $dA$ falling within the display boundaries were summed for each fixation position. In B, a large portion of the function $f_a(r)$ falls outside the display surface and must be excluded from the integration. Because of this dependence on fixation location within the display, the integration procedure averaged across a large random sample of actual fixation positions.

the display. The probability $dp$ of detecting a target in $dA$ is then simply the product of $f_a(r,\phi)$ and $dA/A$:

$$dp = f_a(r) \frac{r\, dr\, d\phi}{A}. \tag{6}$$

The spatial sensitivity function $f_a(r,\phi)$ was generated by fitting a logistic function to the radial sensitivity function $p_a(r)$. For each eye position, we integrated the probabilities $dp$ contributed by each area element $dA$ falling within the boundaries of the display surface $S$. The overall probability of target detection by attention, $P'_a$, was then calculated by averaging across the $M$ positions in our sample of actual eye positions:

$$P'_a = \frac{1}{M} \sum_i^M \left[ \iint_S f_a(r)(r\, dr\, d\phi/A) \right]_i. \tag{7}$$

We have now arrived at our second estimate for the probability of target detection by attention, $P'_a$, which was calculated from the spatial sensitivity function, $f_a(r,\phi)$, with the help of equation 7. The first estimate, $P_a$, was calculated from the cumulative probability of target detection, $P_{cum}$, with the help of equations 2 and 4. As anticipated, the two values are in close agreement, as shown in figure 9.10.

Given that the two estimates are based on very different assumptions, this result is far from trivial. The first estimate was derived from the cumulative probability of target detection without making any assumptions about the spatial characteristics of attentional processing. In contrast, the integration method that yielded the second estimate obviously relied on a major assumption, namely, that target detection by attention is restricted to a rigid neighborhood around the line of sight. In spite of this restrictive assumption, the integration method nevertheless produced the correct result. The significance of the agreement between the two estimates becomes clear when one realizes that the distribution of display items relative to the point of fixation changes as gaze moves toward the border of the display. If the attentional mechanism underlying the sensitivity function $f_a(r,\phi)$ was some freely allocable resource, one would expect that the sensitivity function $f_a(r,\phi)$ would change near the border of the display. However, such changes did not seem to take place, and a procedure that discarded all sensitivity outside the display border retained just the right amount of sensitivity to predict the correct probability of target detection by attention.

Following equation 3, the total probability of target detection during an individual fixation, $P_{tot}$, is given by

$$P_{tot} = \frac{1}{N} + P_a \times \left(1 - \frac{1}{N}\right). \tag{8}$$

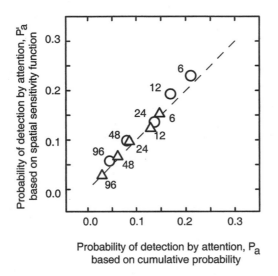

**Figure 9.10**
Probability of target discovery attributable to the attentive search filter. Comparison of the probability estimates from integration of the chance-corrected sensitivity curves with the estimates derived from cumulative probability measures $(P - 1/N)$ verifies that the form of the attentive search filter depicted in figure 9.8 accurately accounts for all search performance beyond chance. Circles are for the same subject as in previous figures; triangles are for second subject; numbers indicate array set size.

Despite all the complications mentioned above, it is important to recognize that the overall probability of detecting the target *by chance* is simply $1/N$. Given that both estimates for the overall probability of detecting the target *by attention* have the same value, it is clear from equation 8 that the total probability of target detection, $P_{tot}$, will also be the same. These results suggest two important conclusions: (1) A simple model of search that sums chance detection and the action of an ''attention filter,'' namely, a radially symmetric sensitivity function, accounts for essentially all aspects of active visual search. (2) To fully account for search performance, it is sufficient to assume an ''attention filter,'' of fixed size and strength, that remains centered on the point of fixation. Thus, the effects of a hypothetical covert scanning process are accurately summarized by the spatial profile of the ''attention filter.''

## 9.6   Discussion

During active visual search, most eye movements shift fixation directly to another item of the search array. Given enough time, the search could therefore be accomplished by accidental target discovery during a purely random walk. Actual search performance, how-

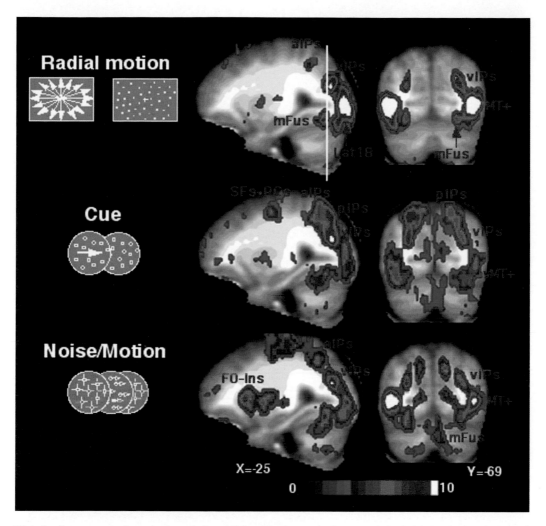

**Plate 1** Group z-maps for activations during radial motion (*top row*), the cue period of trials involving a directional cue (*middle row*), and the noise/motion period of trials involving a directional cue (*bottom row*). A sagittal slice of the left hemisphere is shown in the left column, a coronal slice in the right column. The white line through the sagittal slice in the top left panel shows the location of the coronal slice. The color scale represents the z-score of the activation and all displayed pixels have passed a multiple comparison procedure that includes a Bonferroni correction for the number of hemodynamic response functions used to generate the z-map. aIPs, anterior intraparietal sulcus; pIPs, posterior intraparietal sulcus; vIPs, ventral intraparietal sulcus; SFs-PCs, superior frontal-precentral sulcus; Lo, lateral occipital; FO-Ins, frontal operculum-insula; mFus, mid-fusiform gyrus. See chapter 1.

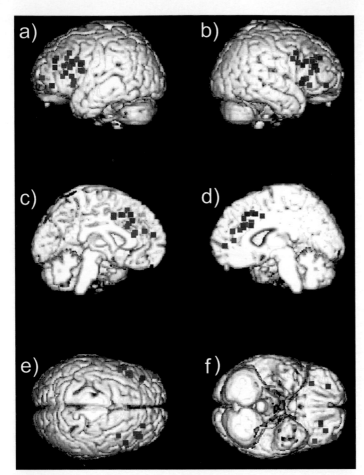

**Plate 2** Frontal activations associated with five different manipulations of cognitive demand, rendered together onto a standard brain using modified SPM software (Wellcome Department of Cognitive Neurology, London): lateral (*a* and *b*) and medial (*c* and *d*) views of each hemisphere, and views of whole brain from above (*e*) and below (*f*). Cognitive demands: green, response conflict; purple, novelty; orange, number of elements; red, delay; blue, perceptual difficulty. See chapter 4.

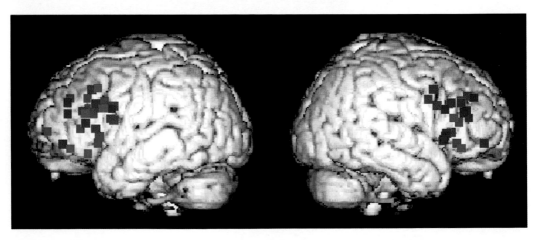

**Plate 3** Lateral views from plate 2, with additional foci (yellow) associated with selective attention to left field (left hemisphere) and right field (right hemisphere). See chapter 4.

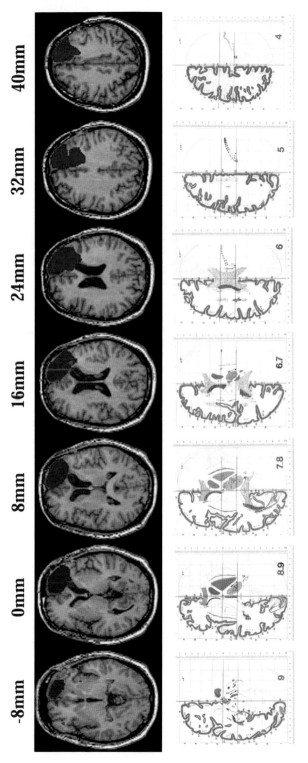

**Plate 4** Horizontal slices (*upper row*) from MRI of a single frontal patient, PP. Using SPM software (Wellcome Department of Cognitive Neurology, London), MRI has been linearly transformed into standard space, and resliced in horizontal sections corresponding to matched sections (*lower row*) from atlas of Talairach and Tournoux (1988; reproduced by permission). Numbers at top indicate z-levels in the space of the atlas; within each section the left of the brain appears to the left. Red region is lesion as traced by the consultant neuroradiologist. Yellow triangles indicate peak activations from Vandenberghe et al. (1997), associated in that experiment with attention to left (left hemisphere) or right (right hemisphere). See chapter 4.

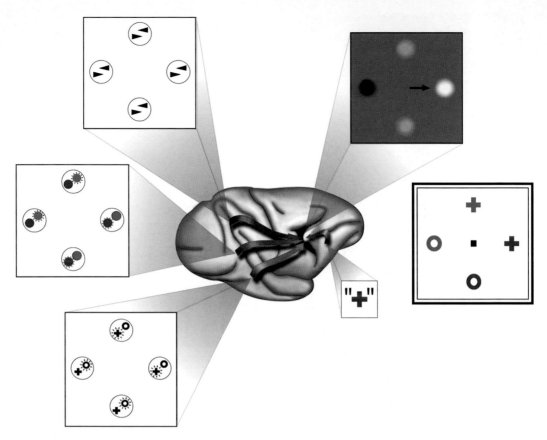

**Plate 5** Frontal eye fields as a salience map. Consider the task of finding the target in the conjunction visual search display shown at the right in the double border. To locate the target, the elementary features of color and shape must be determined. Visual shape (*lower left*), color (*center left*), and motion (*upper left*) are portrayed as being analyzed across the visual field by topographic maps in different parts of extrastriate cortex. Each circle enclosing a pair of features represents a hypercolumn in the cortex; the actual organization is more complicated. The starburst design around one feature indicates the activation at different locations in the color and shape maps representing the stimuli in the visual search display; the motion map is not activated because the search display is static. The convergence of the activation from the feature maps into FEF is portrayed on a rendering of a macaque brain. This search for a conjunction of color and shape cannot be accomplished with visual processing alone because the properties of the stimuli do not specify which is the target. To locate the target correctly, a memory representation must influence the activation in the salience map. The square enclosing the red + symbolizes a memory representation of the target that is portrayed as influencing FEF through a projection from ventral prefrontal cortex. The panel issuing from FEF (*upper right*) indicates the state of activation in a salience map that guides orienting in the search array. The location in the salience map corresponding to the red + has the highest activation (white), the locations with stimuli that are the same shape or color as the target have intermediate activation (gray), and the location with the stimulus that is neither the same shape nor the same color as the target has minimal activation. Compare with figure 8.4b. The arrow in the salience map (*upper right*) indicates the covert or overt orienting resulting from the pattern of activation. See chapter 8.

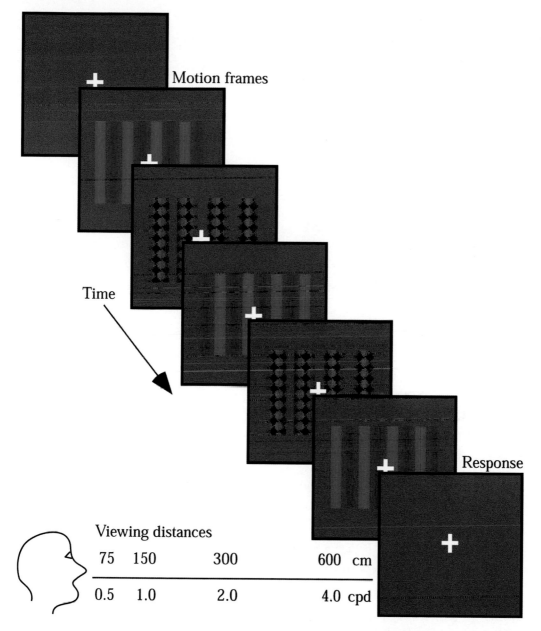

**Plate 6** Procedure using amplification principle in third-order motion to measure the attentional amplification of salience. Even frames are texture-contrast gratings, with unambiguously high salience in the high-contrast texture bands. Odd frames are red–green color gratings, characterized by separate red-saturation and green-saturation values. Motion strength (e.g., as measured by Reichardt and motion energy detectors) is determined by the product of the modulation amplitudes in even and odd frames. When the texture modulation in the even frames is far above threshold, even weak salience modulations in the odd frames can produce apparent motion. Different viewing distances determine the spatial frequency (cycles per degree) of the gratings on the retina. See chapter 10.

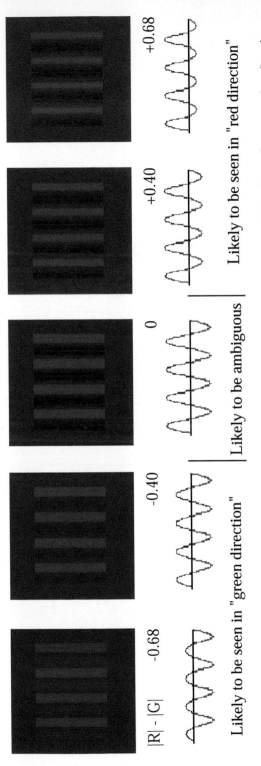

**Plate 7**  Five stimuli with different red advantages. From top to bottom: −0.68, −0.32, 0, +0.32, +0.68. For the displays of plate 6, attending to green (or red) produces apparent motion equivalent to a stimulus approximately one level higher (or lower). See chapter 10.

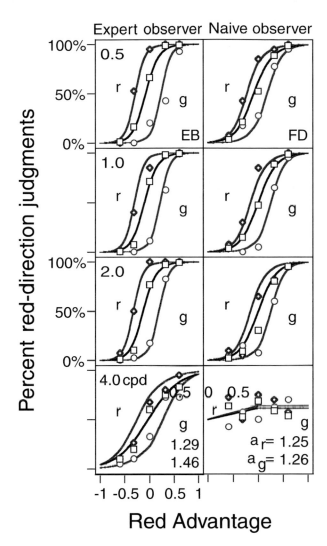

**Plate 8** Results of the attention-amplification experiment. The percent of red-consistent motion judgments versus the red stimulus advantage, $|R| - |G|$, which is the difference $|R|$ of red from background yellow minus the difference $|G|$ of green from background yellow. As red advantage increases, the probability of perceiving motion in the red-consistent direction increases. Five data points are shown for each of four spatial frequencies (rows), three attentional conditions, and two observers (columns). Solid curves are model fits (see figure 10.13a). Middle curves indicate the baseline condition (no attention instructions); curves on right (r) and on left (g) are model fits for the attend-red and attend-green conditions, respectively. The estimated model parameters for the $|R|$ and $|G|$ amplification due to attention, $\alpha_r$ and $\alpha_g$, are indicated in the bottom panel for each observer. See chapter 10.

A

B

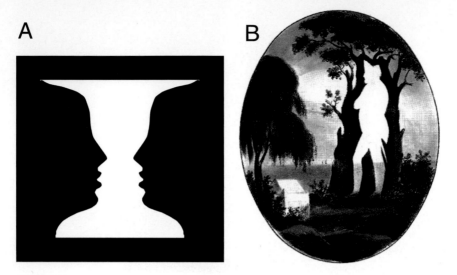

**Plate 9**  Figure-ground ambiguities. (*a*) Ambiguous profiles-vase, after Rubin (1915). (*b*) Forest scene with Napoleon. Normally, trees are seen as figure and the intervening space as ground. However, the intervening space can also be seen as figure when it is attended or has a meaningful shape. (Y&B Associates, after Currier & Ives, ca. 1835.) See chapter 10.

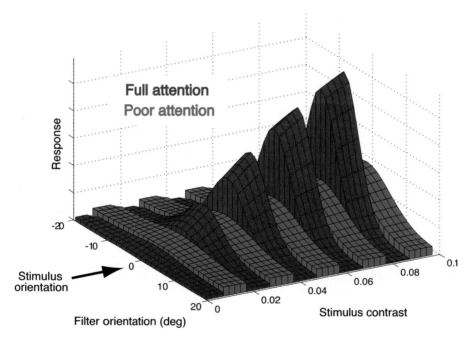

**Plate 10**  Attentional change in the response distribution. Nonlinear responses $R_{\theta\omega}$ of filters tuned to orientations between $-20°$ and $+20°$, to a grating stimulus of orientation $0°$ and contrasts between 0 and 5% (threshold regime). Responses to fully and poorly attended stimuli are represented by the red and blue surfaces, respectively (shown interleaved for clarity). By strengthening a winner-take-all competition among visual filters, attention emphasizes the filters that respond best to the stimulus at hand. This both increases the gain and sharpens the tuning of the filters in question. See chapter 11.

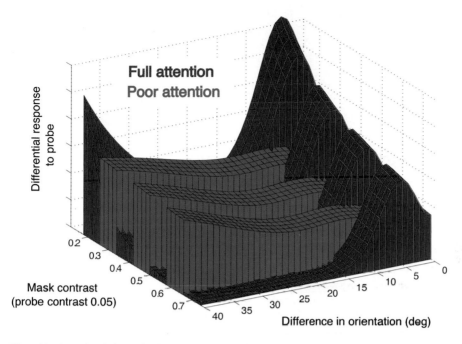

**Plate 11** Attentional change in the response to a weak stimulus component. Incremental response $\Delta R_{\theta\omega}$ of the filter tuned optimally to a weaker stimulus component ("probe," orientation $0°$, contrast 0.05), in the presence of a superimposed, stronger stimulus component ("mask," orientation between $0°$ and $40°$, contrast between 0.1 and 0.75). Response values are given in multiples of the response without mask. For many mask parameters, attention *reduces* the incremental response. This predicts that attention can be counterproductive (i.e., lowers performance of tasks concerning the weaker stimulus component). See chapter 11.

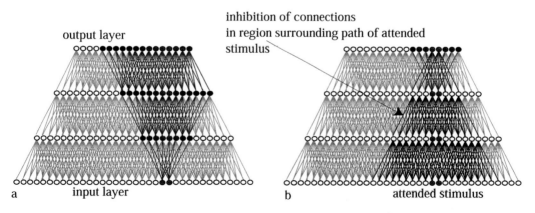

**Plate 12** (*a*) Feedforward activation of the visual processing pyramid and (*b*) its modulation after attentional selection has been applied. Red connections are those affected by the stimulus, gray connections are those which play no role, and black connections are those inhibited by the WTA selection process. The top layer is not inhibited by the top-layer WTA and thus the feedforward divergence of the stimulus to the output layer is seen. If it were inhibited, no other stimulus could reach the output layer, making the system effectively blind to all nonattended stimuli. The model predicts that nonattended stimuli do reach the output layer of the system, but their representation may be incomplete or corrupted by interfering signals (Tsotsos 1997). The shading of the units' colors reflects the assumption that unit weighting profiles are Gaussian in nature. See chapter 14.

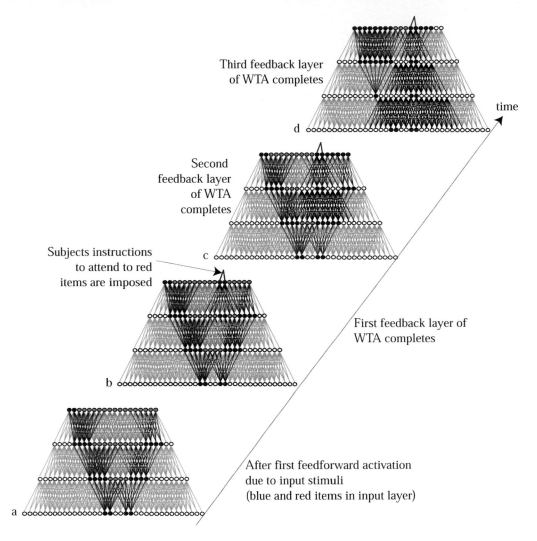

Third feedback layer
of WTA completes

time

d

Second
feedback layer
of WTA
completes

c

Subjects instructions
to attend to red
items are imposed

First feedback layer of
WTA completes

b

After first feedforward activation
due to input stimuli
(blue and red items in input layer)

a

**Plate 13**   A four-step sequence showing attentional modulation when there are two stimuli in the input and the system attends to one. (*a*) The visual processing pyramid at the point where the activation due to two separate stimuli in the input layer has just reached the output layer. No attentional effects are yet in evidence. (*b*) The location selection is applied and two units in the output layer are identified (location cues can be placed anywhere in the visual field prior to a test stimulus). The first WTA stage then takes place, and the largest responses within the next layer of receptive fields of the selected units are found. The connections not corresponding to those largest response units are inhibited. (*c*) The results after the second stage of WTA. (*d*) The results after the third and final stage of WTA. Due to the complexity of the figure, the variations in unit strength due to the Gaussian weighting profile are not shown. See chapter 14.

**Plate 15 [facing page]**   The circuit that implements the hierarchical selection described in the text is shown; this is a conceptual view and is not intended to correspond to specific neurons and their connectivities. A more detailed explanation of this circuit can be found in Tsotsos et al. (1995). See chapter 14.

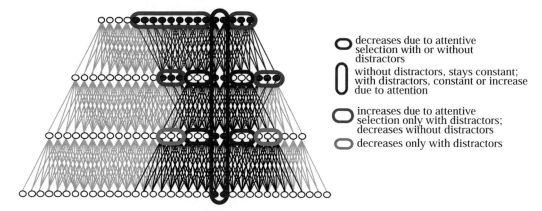

○ decreases due to attentive selection with or without distractors

○ without distractors, stays constant; with distractors, constant or increase due to attention

○ increases due to attentive selection only with distractors; decreases without distractors

○ decreases only with distractors

**Plate 14** Modulation predictions. Following the changes of a particular unit of the pyramid through the four-step sequence of plate 13 leads to the overall changes depicted in this diagram. Specific portions of each layer undergo systematic changes as indicated; the changes depend on whether distractors are present or not (and on which side of the attended stimulus they fall) and their strengths may differ depending on the distance separating the attended stimulus and the distractors. The best way to relate this figure to those of plate 13 is to select a specific unit in the pyramid in plate 13a and track its changes over time, as depicted in the sequence from plate 13a through d. See chapter 14.

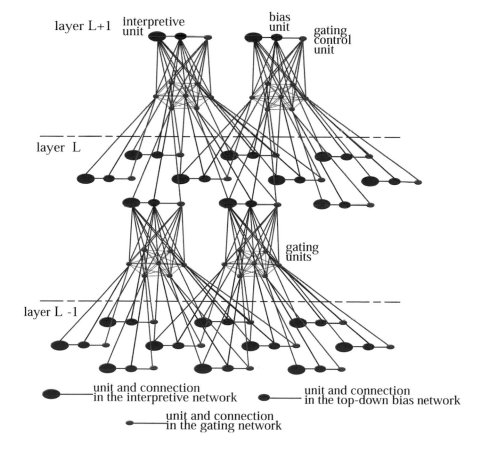

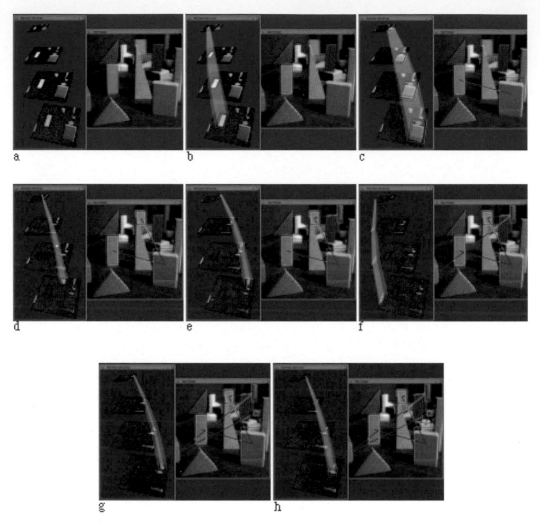

**Plate 16** Example of computer simulation. An image of several colored blocks is the test image. The algorithm is instructed to search for blue regions, and it attempts to do this by searching for the largest, bluest region first. This test image is shown on the right half of each image; the regions selected are outlined in yellow, with blue lines between them showing the system's scan path. The left side of each image shows a four-level visual processing pyramid. The instruction is applied to the pyramid to tune its feature computations, and the result is that the regions within each layer of the pyramid that remain are those which are blue. The left side of (*a*) shows the set of blue of objects found. Then the WTA algorithm selects the largest, bluest one first (*b*), inhibits that region (note it does not appear in *c*), and then repeats the process six more times. The system does not know about objects, only rectangular regions; thus, although it sometimes appears to select whole blocks, this is due solely to fortuitous camera viewpoints. See chapter 14.

ever, is always significantly faster than predicted by chance detection alone, suggesting that more items than the one at the center of gaze are being processed during each fixation. Interestingly, the total probability of target detection, $P$, remains the same during all fixations of a search trial (where $P$ is defined for an ensemble of identical animals viewing the same search array). This implies that the same number of items is processed during every fixation and that there is little or no memory for locations that have already been processed. However, the most important result is that both attention and chance contribute significantly to search performance. This fact follows simply from the observation that the total probability of target detection $P$ always exceeds the probability of detecting a target by chance, $1/N$, but that $1/N$ is always a significant fraction of $P$.

Although it is relatively straightforward to calculate the respective contributions of attention and chance to the total probability of target detection, $P$, it is not so clear how to characterize the spatial process that we associate with active attention and that is presumably is responsible for the analysis of array items at some distance from the center of gaze. We obtain excellent results by postulating a fixed "attention filter," that is, a radial distribution function describing the probability of detecting a target *by attention* at a given distance from the center of gaze. To obtain this function, we first determine the radial distribution of the total probability of target detection, $p(r)$, and then subtract the probability of target detection *by chance*. This is complicated by the fact that the latter quantity varies significantly with eccentricity. Although the probability due to chance is simply $1/N$, the radial distribution of this probability is not uniform because the saccadic amplitude distribution functions are not equal to the interstimulus distance distribution. In particular, saccades are more likely to target nearby items than items farther away (Motter and Belky, 1998a). Thus, the appropriate correction for chance is a radial function $p_c(r)$ that takes into account the spatial biases of saccade lengths and interstimulus distances. When this correction is applied to $p(r)$, the residual distribution function, $p_a(r)$, represents the probability of detecting the target *by attention* as a function of distance from the center of gaze. The function $p_a(r)$ retains the general form of the total probability distribution $p(r)$ and decreases monotonically with eccentricity, but of course is of lower magnitude.

Having determined the respective contributions of attention and chance to the spatial distribution of target detection, $p(r)$, it is natural to ask if one can reconstruct the total probability of target detection, $P$, that is known independently. Accomplishing this increases our confidence that the different contributions have been determined accurately, and the assumptions that enter into the reconstruction tell us something about the nature of the "attention filter." Indeed, when one combines $p_a(r)$ and $p_c(r)$ to obtain, respectively, the overall probabilities of target detection by attention, $P_a$, and by chance, $1/N$, the total probability of target detection, $P$, is almost perfectly matched. This result goes beyond the fact that two different procedures for estimating the total probability of target detection yield the same value. The matching estimates imply, first, that we have correctly identified the functional form of $p_a(r)$ and, second, that attentional resources are "wasted" at the boundary of the display. It is very important to realize that the correct value of $P_a$ is obtained only if $p_a(r)$ is *not* integrated over locations outside the display borders. This leads to two conclusions: (1) Essentially all aspects of search performance can be modeled with the "attention filter" given by the radial function $p_a(r)$. (2) The "attention filter" is locked to the line of sight, and attentional processing resources are lost when the center of gaze approaches the display border.

Although our analysis has isolated the "attention filter" that underlies the total sensitivity function, together with target detection by chance, it does not reveal how this "attention filter" actually works. Broadly speaking, there are two general possibilities. First, information about array items in the vicinity of the center of gaze is gathered through a *serial* process involving covert shifts of attention (e.g., Treisman, 1988; Wolfe, 1996). Second, information about the vicinity is collected by a *parallel* process, that is, simultaneously, without recourse to covert shifts of attention. The second possibility is the simpler one, in that attention operates in a stereotyped manner and at a fixed rate. In addition, the second possibility explains, in an entirely natural fashion, the surprising waste of attentional resources at display borders. In fact, it is quite difficult to reconcile the first possibility with the observed waste of resources, unless one is willing to make several assumptions ad hoc.

Despite the uncertainty about the serial or parallel nature of the "attention filter," our results do allow some general observations. First, due to the spatial characteristics of eye movements (they tend to target items relatively close to the current point of fixation), chance detection contributes significantly to total search performance and must be taken into account before the spatial range and effectiveness of the attentional contribution can be ascertained. Second, and also due to the spatial characteristics of eye movements (they accurately locate items that are too distant to be distinguishable as targets or non-targets), the information that guides eye movements does not appear to be the same as that mediating target detection. In this respect, our observations of accurate saccades to peripheral non-targets are consistent with previous findings that have shown that peripheral stimuli can be selected on the basis of color or luminance even when their shape is not discriminable (Egeth et al., 1984; Motter and Belky, 1998a). It is of interest that these differences may parallel the division of the cortical visual system into parietal and temporal subdivisions that can be described, respectively, as contributing to the guidance of movement and the analysis of visual detail (Mishkin et al., 1983; Goodale and Milner, 1992).

## Acknowledgment

Support was provided by the VA Medical Research Program and the Department of Neuro-surgery, SUNY-Health Science Center at Syracuse, New York.

## References

Egeth, H. E., Virizi, R. A., and Garbart, H. (1984). Searching for conjunctively defined targets. *J. Exp. Psychol. Hum. Percep. Perf.* 10: 32–39.

Engel, F. L. (1977). Visual conspicuity, visual search and fixation tendencies of the eye. *Vis. Res.* 17: 95–108.

Ericksen, C. W., and Hoffman, J. E. (1972). Temporal and spatial characteristics of selective encoding from visual displays. *Percep. Psychophys.* 12: 201–204.

Goodale, M. A., and Milner, A. D. (1992). Separate visual pathways for perception and action. *Trends Neurosci.* 15: 20–25.

Horowitz, T. S., and Wolfe, J. M. (1998). Visual search has no memory. *Nature* 394: 575–577.

Krendel, E. S., and Wodinsky, J. (1960). Search in an unstructured visual field. *J. Optical Soc. America* 50: 562–568.

Krose, B. J. A., and Julesz, B. (1989). The control and speed of shifts of attention. *Vis. Res.* 11: 1607–1619.

Mishkin, M., Ungerleider, L. G., and Macko, K. A. (1983). Object vision and spatial vision: Two central pathways. *Trends Neurosci.* 6: 414–417.

Motter, B. C., and Belky, E. J. (1998a). The guidance of eye movements during active visual search. *Vis. Res.* 38: 1805–1815.

Motter, B. C., and Belky, E. J. (1998b). The zone of focal attention during active visual search. *Vis. Res.* 38: 1007–1022.

Neisser, U. (1967). *Cognitive psychology.* New York: Appleton-Century-Crofts.

Posner, M. I. (1980). Orienting of attention. *Q. J. Exp. Psychol.* 32: 3–25.

Sagi, D., and Julesz, B. (1985). Detection and discrimination of visual orientation. *Perception* 14: 619–628.

Toet, A., and Levi, D. M. (1991). The two-dimensional shape of spatial interaction zones in the parafovea. *Vis. Res.* 32: 1349–1357.

Treisman, A. (1988). Features and objects: The fourteenth Bartlett memorial lecture. *Q. J. Exp. Psychol.* 40A: 201–237.

Williams, L. G. (1966). Target conspicuity and visual search. *Hum. Factors* 8: 80–92.

Wolfe, J. M. (1996). Visual search. In H. Pashler (ed.), *Attention.* London: University College Press.

# 10 Two Computational Models of Attention

**George Sperling, Adam Reeves, Erik Blaser, Zhong-Lin Lu, and
Erich Weichselgartner**

## 10.1 Introduction

### 10.1.1 Attention Models for the Twenty-first Century

Models of attention phenomena should (1) explain or account for significant phenomena and (2) be physiologically plausible. There are other good properties models might have, such as simplicity, parsimony, efficiency, application to naturalistic situations, and so on. Here, we concentrate on two models of visual attention that account for the overall behavior of an observer in psychophysical tasks. Among the many models that have been proposed for attention phenomena, we offer a particular reason for giving especially serious consideration to the ones proposed here. They do not merely predict that an observer should do better in one situation than another, or that an interaction between two variables should be observed under certain circumstances. They account for relatively large amounts of data quite efficiently. "Large amounts" of data means (in 2000) minimally dozens, preferably hundreds, and sometimes more than a thousand data points obtained from each observer in the experiments with, preferably, an average of a hundred or so observations for each of the hundreds of data points. As the number of data points becomes large, the data increasingly constrain possible models. By "account for," we mean that a model accounts for more than 80%, and preferably more than 90%, of the variance in the data.

When a model efficiently accounts for a large amount of data, the concepts embodied in the model, such as an attention window or attention-switching time or attentional amplification, achieve face validity, like the concepts of an electron or of electron spin in physicists' models. The large-scale quantification is essential to make the attention processes analogous to twentieth-century physical concepts. Without such quantification, attention theories are underconstrained, and correspond to speculative theories about the nature of matter that characterized earlier stages of physics.

### 10.1.2 Two Attention Models: Overview

Models will be considered for two phenomena: the time course of attention windows and attention amplification involved in selective attention. Following these two quite well-determined models, a speculative proposal is offered for the overall functional architecture in which these models are embedded.

The first model derives the form of an attention window from psychophysical experiments. Here, we concentrate primarily on the derivation—how a sufficiently detailed data set implies the shape of an attention window and the properties of certain related processes, such as cue interpretation and the storage of attended items in the visual short-term memory. Elsewhere (Sperling and Weichselgartner, 1995), this model has been applied to make accurate, quantitative predictions of the data from the paradigms that have been most widely used to measure shifts of visual attention. In particular, it makes predictions of the pattern of speeded reaction times in response to valid attentional cues (Posner's cost/ benefits paradigm) with traditional go/no-go responses and also with choice reaction-time responses. It predicts the pattern of more accurate responses at locations that have been validly cued, and also has other applications (Sperling and Weichselgartner, 1995). This is the model to consider when there are spatial or temporal attention cues.

The second model describes the processes involved in the attentional amplification of attended features. It shows how the relative importance (salience) of features is determined by bottom-up processes and altered by top-down processes of selective attention, providing a precise description of these processes in terms of the attentional amplification of selected inputs to a salience map. This model provides a general theory, derived from detailed psychophysical data, for how bottom-up and top-down attentional influences combine. It is especially applicable to studies of visual search, in terms of providing a mechanism for so-called guided search. (Note: The ideal attention experiment presents the same stimuli, and records the same responses, in two conditions that differ only in attentional instructions and in the payoff matrices. Typically, search experiments are not formally attention experiments, although they often are considered together with that category. See Sperling and Dosher, 1986 for a detailed review.) The second model also applies to figure–ground segmentation, and to a host of selective-attention paradigms.

The two models use quite different mathematical structures because of the psychophysical phenomena from which they are derived. However, these are merely different aspects of the same underlying control structure, a salience map and associated processes, that is developed in the more speculative overall formulation, and that provides a general framework for combining bottom-up and top-down attentional processes. Together, the two models encompass most of the paradigms that have been used to study attention.

## 10.2   Determining the Time Course and Structure of Attention Windows

### 10.2.1   Measuring Attention Reaction Times

**Indirect Measures of Motor Reaction Time: The Grabbing Response**   The procedure for measuring the reaction time of a shift of visual attention can be best understood by an analogy with an unusual way of measuring a motor reaction time. Imagine an observer, as shown in figure 10.1, seated at a conveyer belt on which balls, about the size of billiard balls, pass by. The speed of the belt has been calibrated so that ten balls pass per second.

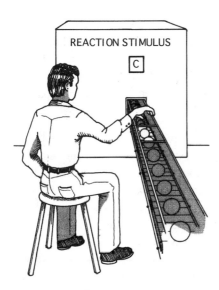

**Figure 10.1**
The grabbing response: an indirect measurement of individual reaction times. Balls are placed on the moving conveyer belt so that a new ball passes the opening every 0.1 s. When a critical "reaction stimulus" appears above the conveyor belt (say, the letter C), the observer reaches into the opening and grabs the first ball possible. A code number inside the ball indicates its place in the sequence, and hence the moment in time at which it passed the opening. This grabbing response is analogous to the procedure in which items from the "next-to-be-attended" stream are admitted to short-term memory because a cue has triggered a shift of attention to that stream.

There is a small opening through which the observer can reach to grab a ball. His task is to monitor a screen until a critical character (a target) appears. In this example, the target is the letter C. As soon as the observer detects a target, his task is to reach into the opening and grab the first ball that he can. Once he has grabbed a ball, he opens it and reads the number painted on the inside.

Suppose the experimenter has arranged the situation so that the number of the ball that is simultaneous with the target is 0, the ball that passes one tenth of a second later is 1, two tenths of a second later is 2, and so on. From the number that is reported by the observer, the experimenter can infer the reaction time of the observer's "grabbing" response on that trial to an accuracy of 1/10 s. From a long series of trials, the experimenter can observe the entire distribution of reaction times for a particular target in a particular environment of nontargets (distractors).

There is a minor problem with this reaction procedure. Suppose that the observer has consistently been grabbing balls numbered 3 and 4. Then, in one trial in which he was not quite prepared, the observer grabs a ball with the number 9. The observer knows he was slow, and might improve his response by calling out a lower number than 9, especially if there were a reward for quick reactions. To eliminate the possibility of cheating, the balls are assigned arbitrary numbers. The experimenter knows the number of the ball that passed the opening at each instant, but the observer does not. The identification number of the ball is of interest only insofar as it indicates the instant at which the ball passed the opening.

**Grabbing Items for Short-term Memory**   The procedure for measuring the grabbing response would be an indirect and unnecessarily complicated procedure for measuring a motor reaction time because direct measures of motor reaction times are easily obtainable. However, there is no direct measurement of an attention reaction time. But the indirect grabbing procedure is easily applied to measuring attention reaction times in a paradigm in which the attention response is to grab one item from a rapidly passing stream of items and enter it into short-term memory. The procedure is as follows.

The observer views two adjacent streams of items, a stream of letters on the left and a stream of numerals on the right. (A stream of items is a spatial location where consecutive frames containing new visual items fall one on top of the other.) Initially, the observer's attention is focused on the stream containing the target, the search stream. When the target is detected, the observer's task is to shift attention to the numeral stream (the measurement stream, the next-to-be-attended stream) and to report the earliest possible numeral. To eliminate eye movements, experience has shown that it is best if the observer maintains fixation on the next-to-be-attended stream throughout the trial. Thereby, when the time to shift attention arrives, there is no urge to move the eyes because they already are fixated on their destination. In the early experiments described here, however, the observer maintained fixation between the two streams, and the streams were centered 1.87° apart (figure 10.2).

The (target-containing) search stream consisted of a sequence of thirty randomly chosen letters of the alphabet. The letters B, I, O, Q, S, and Z were omitted because of their similarity to the numbers 8, 1, 0, 5, and 2. A target letter was embedded at a random position in the middle of the stream. In different blocks of trials, the target was either the letter C or the letter W, or simply an outline square with no letter in the middle. The rate of target stream presentation was 4.6 letters per second (218 ms between consecutive onsets). This rate was chosen to make the target detection task sufficiently difficult that observers had to devote all their attention to it. The rate of the next-to-be-attended stream differed between blocks: 4.6, 6.9, 9.2, or 13.4 numerals per second. (For additional details, see Sperling and Reeves, 1980).

The observers' task was to detect the target letter and then to report the first numeral they could from the numeral stream (i.e., to grab the earliest possible numeral). Addition-

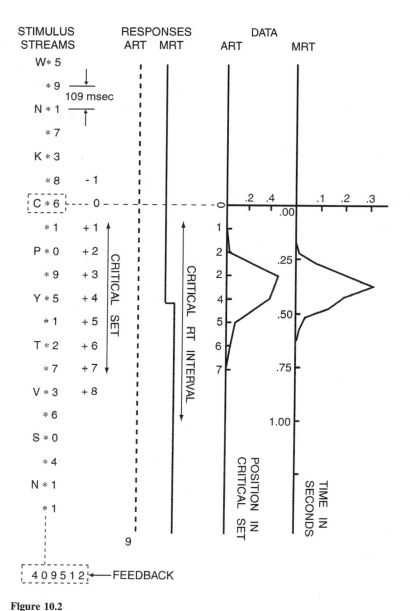

**Figure 10.2**

Attention and motor reaction times (ARTs and MRTs). The subject fixates the central * and attends the letter-containing stream (left) until a target letter (C) is detected, then shifts attention (but not his eyes) to the next-to-be-attended numeral-containing stream, to "grab" and report the first possible numeral. The critical set is a sequence of all-different numerals in the to-be-attended stream, centered on the time when the response is expected. The ART graph shows the histogram of temporal positions from which numerals were reported (middle). In addition to reporting numerals, the subject also made a rapid finger response upon detecting the target letter. The MRT graph shows the histogram of these motor-reaction times (right). Although the abscissa is the same in both ART and MRT graphs, the units of the MRT graph give the actual time in seconds, whereas those of the ART graph indicate the onset times of critical-set items.

ally, the observers were required to make a motor reaction-time response, lifting a finger from a response key. After considerable practice, performance on both these tasks was almost independent (i.e., differed little from control conditions in which either task was performed alone).

**Attention Reaction Times (ARTs)**    Figure 10.2 shows the data for an observer with the target letter C, and the next-to-be-attended stream rate of 9.6 numerals/s. The data show that the observer nearly always reported the numerals occurring 3 or 4 positions after simultaneity, that is, numerals that occurred 327 or 436 ms after target onset. By analogy to the grabbing response, this is a distribution of attention reaction times (ARTs). For comparison, the histogram of motor reaction times (MRTs) shown in figure 10.2 is remarkably similar. Figure 10.2 illustrates that it is possible to obtain as good information about the implicit, unobservable reaction time of an attention-grabbing response as it is about a motor reaction time.

Reeves (1977) obtained 17 pairs of motor and attention reaction times in a variety of conditions. The ART and MRT distributions are not always quite as similar as in figure 10.2, although they are highly correlated. An increase in difficulty of target detection causes a somewhat greater increase in mean ART than in mean MRT. This implies that the target is processed somewhat more fully before an ART (as opposed to an MRT) is initiated.

**Reporting Four Numerals**    To obtain more information about the attention microprocesses that underlie ART performance, it is useful to gather more extensive data than are illustrated in figure 10.2. The ''grabbing'' procedure described above was elaborated to require the observer to report not merely the first numeral that he could from the numeral stream, but the earliest four. In all other respects the procedure was identical. The observer merely had to, after reporting one numeral from the numeral stream as before, now report three more numerals. Control experiments showed that when the observer was reporting four numerals, the first-reported numeral had the same statistical properties as the only reported numeral when the observer was reporting just one. Thus, the three additional numeral reports are obtained at no cost.

**Single-Item Data**    Figure 10.3 shows a complete set of data for one observer and one target. It shows the four reported numerals at each of the four numeral rates. There are eight temporal positions at which numeral reports are recorded, 4 such eight-point curves per figure panel, and four figure panels, for a total of 128 data points.

**Data from Pairs of Items**    Figure 10.4 shows a different aspect of the data from the same experiment and same conditions as in figure 10.3. These data are used to test a strength model of visual short-term memory, and are based on the method of paired

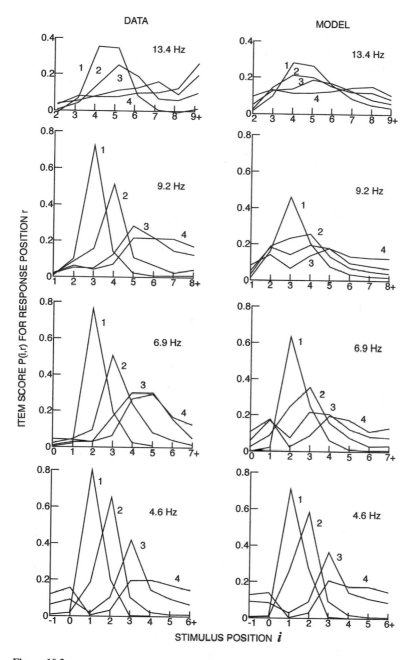

**Figure 10.3**
Data and model predictions for a modified attention-gating experiment ("Report four numerals!"). The abscissa is the position $i$ of the reported items from the to-be-attended stream. The ordinate $P_i(r)$ is the estimated probability of reporting the item from stimulus position $i$ in response position $r$. The curves labeled 1, 2, 3, 4 represent $r$, the first-, second-, third-, and fourth-reported items within a response. In all graphs, there is a progression from left to right of the response items: earlier response items tend to come from earlier stimulus positions. The speed of the to-be-reported stream is indicated in terms of the number of items per second (13.4 to 4.6). The left column shows the data for one subject; the right column shows the model fit to these data. (See text for details.)

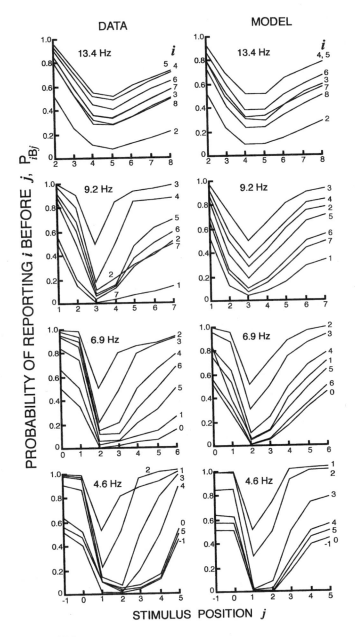

**Figure 10.4**
The probability $P_{iBj}$ of reporting an item from stimulus position $i$ earlier in the response than an item from stimulus position $j$ as a function of $j$. Target and stimulus speeds are as in figure 10.3. The left column shows data for one subject; the right column shows the model fit to these data. Each curve represents a particular stimulus position $i$ (indicated at extreme right, adjacent to the curve). Model curves are perfectly laminar (do not cross); their relative heights therefore precisely represent the relative strengths of the memory representation of the indicated stimulus positions.

comparisons. Suppose two numerals, *i, j* occur in the same response. If numeral *i* is reported *before* numeral *j,* we write *iBj;* otherwise we write *jBi.* We regard being reported first as "winning" or achieving primacy in short-term memory. Each trial is analogous to a sports or chess tournament in which we are given the order of the four best competitors (the four reported positions).

There is an extensive mathematical development that deals with precisely this situation: determining the relative strength of different players, even when they may not have played against each other, by determining how they fare against common opponents. The relevant data are *paired comparisons:* the collection of available *iBj* pairs.[1]

Figure 10.4 shows $P_{iBj}$, the observed probability of reporting position *i* before position *j,* as a function of *j.* Each curve is for a different *i.* In order to display continuous curves, we arbitrarily (but logically) define $P_{iBi} = 0.5$. There are seven critical positions for which data were collected, and this results in twenty-one independent $P_{iBj}$ values in each panel, yielding eighty-four data points in the four panels. The top panel of figure 4 (numeral rate 13.4/s) shows that position 5 is the strongest: 90% of the time it is reported before position 2, 80% of the time before position 3, and never less than 50% of the time before any other position. However, position 5 is in a virtual tie with position 4, which is second strongest. Third strongest is position 6, followed by positions 7, 3, 8, and 2.

**Laminarity and Folding**    The data have two interesting properties: laminarity and folding. Laminarity means that the curves do not cross. A failure of laminarity means a circle: *iBj* and *jBk,* but *kBi* (instead of the expected *iBk*). The data predicted by the model are perfectly laminar (righthand panels, figure 10.4). The real data have 5% crossings, and statistical analysis shows that this number, although very small, is slightly higher than the number (2–3%) that would would be expected by chance. To a very good approximation, however, laminarity holds for the real data. This means that, to a very good approximation, the data can be described by a strength model.[2]

A strength model means that the order of reporting an item from a position, except for random variation, is determined entirely by the memory strength of the position. The strongest position occurs roughly 300–400 ms after the target. Item strength is roughly symmetric around the strongest position. Items from weaker positions before and after the strongest position alternate in the response. This property is *folding.*

### 10.2.2    Model for a Temporal Attention Window: The Engine

The properties of laminarity and folding in the item pairs of the panels of figure 10.4, and the progression of the individual item reports from chaotic to orderly in the panels of figure 10.3, can be nicely encapsulated in an attention-gating model. This is a model of an attention window that gates the flow of information from the input to short-term memory. The engine of the model is illustrated in figure 10.5, which shows the time course of the attention window.

The strength of an item in memory is determined by the height of the window function during the time the item is visually available, which is the time from its initial exposure until it is overwritten by the next item. (A more elaborate model would assume that an item is stored in *sensory memory* and that its availability decays exponentially. For the short time intervals under consideration here, this is an unnecessary complication.) The integral of visual availability over time determines total attention strength. The laminarity property then implies that items are reported in order of their strength, independent of when they might have occurred within the attention window.

The attention window principle is much like the old Compur-Rapid camera shutter that opened a diaphragm embedded within the lens to expose the whole image and then closed it. This type of shutter opens over a period of tens of milliseconds and then closes with a similar time course. If such a shutter had photographed the stimulus array, and the observer then reported items from the photograph simply in order of their clarity in the final image, it would correspond exactly to the presumed process here.

### 10.2.3   Model for a Temporal Attention Window: The Full Model

Just as a car needs more than an engine to make it useful, so an attention model needs more than an attention window. To generate data, a representation of both input streams is needed, as well as an explicit response-generating mechanism. The target-detecting and -interpreting mechanism is represented in the model[3] by a simple delay $\tau$.

**The Temporal Attention Window (Attention-Gating Function)**   The attention window must be represented by a causal function. It cannot be a normal density function, because this begins at $-\infty$ and therefore is not causal. The simplest causal function is an exponential decay function, that is, a one-stage RC circuit (first-order Gamma function). The absolutely instantaneous onset from zero to maximum value makes this function unrealistic. The next simplest function is two successive, identical RC stages (a second-order Gamma), and that is what was chosen to represent the shape of the attention window. The Gamma function controls the gate to short-term memory.

**The Next-to-Be-Attended Pathway**   The next-to-be-attended stream from which the response items will be chosen is represented in the top row of figure 10.5. Items are assumed to be visually available until they are overwritten. Their access to memory is determined by the attention gate, which at each instant of time multiplies the next-to-be-attended-item by the height of the attention window. The integrated product determines strength in memory. Item strength is subject to random variation, represented as added noise. Items are output in order of their net strength.

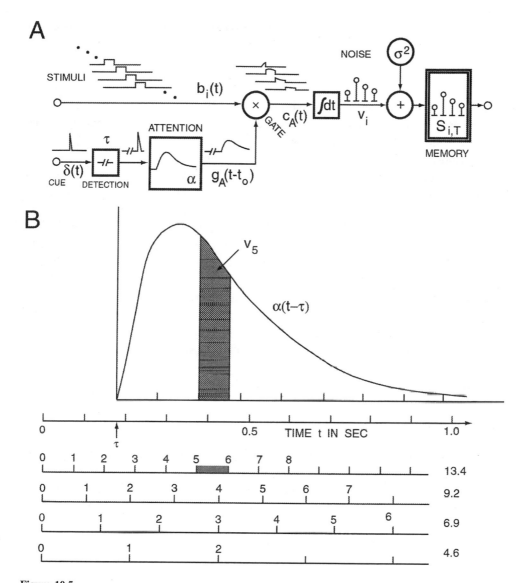

**Figure 10.5**
Model for the attention gating experiment. (*A*) Block diagram of the model. There are two input streams: the upper one receives the stream of to-be-attended items, $l(t)$; the lower one receives the target—the cue to switch attention, $\delta(t)$. Detection of the target occurs after a delay $\tau$, at which time an attention window is generated, as represented by the box $\alpha$. The attention window is produced by two consecutive RC stages, each with time constant $\alpha$. Although items of the to-be-attended stream are presented instantaneously, they are visually available until the arrival of a subsequent item, as indicated by $b_i(t)$. The attention gate, $\times$, multiplies the visual information $b_i(t)$ by the attention window to produce $c_A(t)$, the temporal function that describes the instantaneous availability of the *i*th item. The integral $v_i = \int c_A(t)dt$ gives the strength of item *i*. On a particular trial *T*, strength is perturbed by random Gaussian noise with variance $\sigma^2$ to produce the net strength of item $S_{i,T}$ in short-term memory. Response items are output in order of their net strength. (*B*) Detailed illustration of the attention window. The curve $\alpha(t - \tau)$ describes the time course of an attention window. The strength of a particular item (here, item 5) is given by the area $v_5$ under the window during the time that item 5 is visually available. The example is for a presentation rate of 13.4 items per second. Slower rates would produce bigger areas under the attention window.

**Efficiency**   The model has only three estimated parameters: $\tau$, the time needed to detect and interpret the target, which in this instance is also the cue to shift attention; $\alpha$ (the effective width of the attention window is $\alpha\sqrt{2}$); and $\sigma$, the standard deviation of the memory noise. In effect, $\sigma$ scales the memory strength, because it determines by how much two positions, $i$ and $j$, must differ in strength in order for position $i$ to be reported before position $j$ with a probability $P$. Without noise, the order of report would be completely deterministic.

The parameter $\tau$ has nothing to do with the attention mechanism *per se;* it reflects the processes that detect and interpret the cue. Thus only two attention parameters need to be estimated from the data: the width of the attention window and the power of the memory noise. The model with one detection and two attention parameters generates the 212 predictions shown in figures 10.3 and 10.4. These predictions account for 0.85 to 0.90 of the variance of the data, depending on the observer and the condition. For example, changing to another target generates a new set of 212 points but requires only one new parameter ($\tau$, which characterizes the speed of target detection). Accounting for 0.85 to 0.90 of the variance is not perfect prediction, but it is impressively efficient. Three targets were investigated for each observer so, with five estimated parameters, the model accounts for 636 data points per observer.

### 10.2.4   Extended Attention Models

**One Attentional Episode**   The attention-gating model implies that, for items accumulated within a single attention window, observers have no intrinsic information about the temporal order in which items were entered into memory. In the absence of information provided by lower-level processes such as apparent motion, and in the absence of correlations between successive items (as might occur with meaningful words), the attribute used to order memory items is their memory strength. In this theory, discriminating the temporal order of two successive events requires two successive attention windows.[4]

**Two Consecutive Attentional Episodes**   When two successive attention episodes occur, such as detecting a target (and remembering it) and then switching attention to a next-to-be-attended stream (and remembering items from that stream), observers can discriminate memory items that belong to the target stream from items that belong to the next-to-be-attended stream. They can discriminate these two episodes even when the target is embedded in the next-to-be-attended stream and does not itself differ from other items, as illustrated below.

Figure 10.6 illustrates two successive attention episodes. The task of the observer was to attend a single stream of characters until a target was detected, and then to report that target and the next three characters. The target was one of the characters in the stream

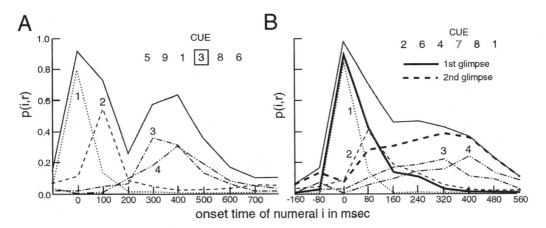

**Figure 10.6**
Attention windows generated by two successive attention episodes. The subject (EW) monitors a stream of items until a cued item occurs. He then attempts to report the cued item and the subsequent three items. (A) The probability of reporting items from a particular stream position when the cue is an outline square around the target item (as shown). The envelope curve indicates the cumulative probability of reporting an item from a particular stream position in any of the four responses. The four curves under the envelope, ordered from left to right, indicate the probability of reporting an item from position $i$ in the first, second, third, and fourth response positions, respectively. (B) Here the target item is more intense than other items. In addition to reporting each item, the subject indicated whether it was in the first glimpse (thick solid curve) associated with the target or in the second glimpse (thick dashed curve) associated with a subsequent voluntary shift of attention. The form of the second glimpse coincides exactly with subject EW's results in the ART experiment (i.e., when reporting items from a next-to-be-attended stream with no requirement to report the cue in the attended stream; see figure 10.2).

that either had greater luminous intensity than the other characters or was surrounded by an outline square. In addition to reporting four characters, the observer reported whether each character was associated with the target (described by the observers as the first glimpse) or with a second group of characters (second glimpse). Observers were able to report the target almost 100% of the time, and frequently the next occurring item. These constituted the first glimpse. The second glimpse had precisely the same distribution of items as the items in an attention shift from one location to another (as described above).

In terms of mechanisms, the two successive glimpses described by the observers correspond to two consecutive memory episodes. The distinction between the two episodes (glimpses) is quite clear. For both episodes, the memory structure maintains successive items simultaneously—unlike visual sensory memory (iconic memory), in which the contents are overwritten by succeeding items. Accessing the contents of such a memory requires a memory access code, usually called a retrieval cue. For the target item, the retrieval cue is simple: it is "all the items that are stored in association with an outline square (or with a sudden intensity increase)." For the second episode, the access code is an internally generated code: "all the items that are associated with the attention window created in such-and-such circumstances and at such-and-such a time." (The observer does not have direct access to the attention window itself, only to its contents and to their context.) It is not surprising that items associated with a brief visual retrieval cue are much more tightly grouped in time and more reliably reported than items associated with an internally generated retrieval cue.

**Multiple Attention Episodes: Discrete Spotlight Model**   Visual attention can be well represented by a spotlight model that is actually used in many theaters. In the model or in the theater, there is a collection of available spotlights. For convenience, they are numbered in the order of their use, so that the same physical spotlight may have many numbers. A spotlight $i$ illuminates some portion of the stage; its spatial distribution of illumination is given by $f_i(x,y)$. Only one spotlight is turned on at a time. The lighting program is a sequence of immediately consecutive events designated as episodes $E_i$, each characterized by a starting time, an ending time, and a spatial distribution of light, as illustrated in figure 10.7A. When, at time $t_i$, power is switched from spotlight $i - 1$ to spotlight $i$, the transfer of power takes a nonnegligible amount of time. Thereby, there is a certain amount of unavoidable overlap in the light from adjacent successive episodes during the transfer period (figure 10.7B). The time course of the transfer of power from one spotlight to another is described by a temporal function $G(t - t_i)$. This function is a cumulative probability distribution function that increases monotonically from zero to unity as $t$ increases (figure 10.7A). For example, in switching from the initial spotlight with light distribution $f_0(x,y,t)$ to spotlight $f_1(x,y,t)$, the amount of light on the stage, $A(x,y,t)$, is given by equation 1 in figure 10.7. In the more general case, there is a very large number of successive episodes that could extend (for mathematical simplicity) from $-\infty$ to $+\infty$, as formalized by equation 2 in figure 10.7. Because different power transfers may have different transition functions, the temporal function $G_i$ in equation 2 is subscripted with episode $i$.

The extension of the stage illumination model to visual attention is quite straightforward. Illumination in the theater model is analogous to attention in an attention model. In the theater, information is available primarily from illuminated portions of the stage. In visual tasks, information is available primarily from areas of the visual field in which there are significantly nonzero values of attention $f_i(x,y,t)$. In the theater, the positions of the spotlights are fixed during rehearsals. Actors learn to move to where the lights will appear or the actors will find themselves in the dark. Similarly, in attention experiments, observers learn the typical sequence of events during a practice period that is often quite

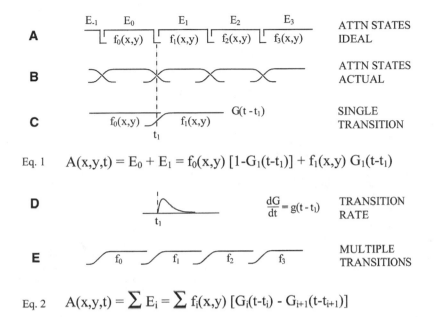

Eq. 1 $\quad A(x,y,t) = E_0 + E_1 = f_0(x,y) [1-G_1(t-t_1)] + f_1(x,y) G_1(t-t_1)$

Eq. 2 $\quad A(x,y,t) = \sum E_i = \sum f_i(x,y) [G_i(t-t_i) - G_{i+1}(t-t_{i+1})]$

**Figure 10.7**
Attention as a sequence of space–time separable episodes. (A) A sequence of ideal attention states (episodes), $E_0, E_1, E_2, E_3, \ldots$. Each episode $E_i$ is characterized by an onset time $t_i$, an offset time $t_{i+1}$, and a function $f(x,y)$ that describes the spatial distribution of attention (salience) during $E_i$. (B) Actual attention episodes start and turn off gradually (not instantaneously). (C) An isolated, single attention transition from $E_0$ to $E_1$ that occurs with temporal transition function $G(t - t_1)$. For the example in (C), attention $A(x,y,t)$ is the sum of $E_0$ and $E_1$ (equation 1). (D) The rate of an attention transition is a probability density function. (E) A sequence of attention episodes showing the spatial attention distribution functions that are in effect during each episode. Equation 2 is the general formulation of attention as the sum of a sequence of episodes.

extended, so that during the experiment proper, the observer's performance is highly reproducible and stereotypic.

One intrinsic property of the discrete spotlight stage model is that switching time does not depend on where spotlights happen to be pointing. More specifically, switching time is independent of distance. That attention switches should be independent of the distance of the attention shift is counterintuitive, but it has been verified in different laboratories (Cheal and Lyon, 1989; Sperling and Weichselgartner, 1995).

The shape of the attention window (as in figure 10.5) comes about from three successive episodes: (1) wait for and detect the cue to switch attention; (2) switch attention to the next-to-be-attended stream and admit items to memory; (3) close the attention window to avoid memory overflow. The net outcome of these processes is illustrated in figure 10.7.

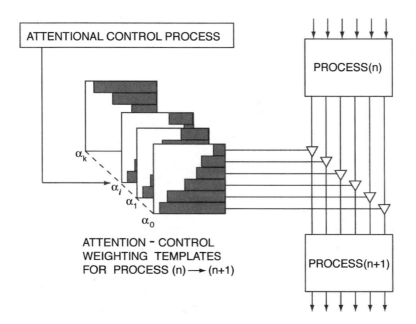

**Figure 10.8**
Attention in a neural network. Attention modifies the passage of signals from a neural process $n$ to $n + 1$. In well-practiced experimental subjects, a cue to shift attention causes a previously learned template of attentional weights $\alpha_0$ to be quickly put into place. This may occur simultaneously at several different levels $n$.

**Neural Implementation of Attention**   Neurally, attention is implemented as a control process that modulates the passage of information between neural processes ($n$) and ($n + 1$), as illustrated in figure 10.8. In the experimental situations in which attention is measured, there are typically thousands of trials, so performance becomes both optimal and, concurrently, quite stereotypic. The attention templates of weights (e.g., the $f_i(x, y, t)$) are well learned and quickly instantiated. Indeed, attention acts not only at the gateway to memory but also concurrently, at many levels. Attention determines, in perceptual stages, what information is passed on to pattern recognition processes or to memory; in decision stages it determines bias and sensitivity parameters; and in response selection and response execution stages, it determines the speed and accuracy with which particular responses are executed.

The model illustrated in figure 10.7 has been applied to four of the most widely used attention paradigms, and it quantitatively accounts for the results of quite diverse experiments. For more detail, the reader should consult Sperling and Weichselgartner (1995); the remainder of this chapter describes methods for examining the microstructure of attention processes.

## 10.3   The Salience Map: An Implementation of Attention

The logic behind this section is that apparent motion can be used as a delicate assay of attention. In particular, it is possible to construct third-order motion stimuli in which the direction of apparent motion is determined by attention. The fact that attention influences the direction of motion is itself diagnostic, and gives important insights into the mechanisms of attention. It is used here to develop a computational model of how attention to a feature, such as "red," is implemented via a salience map. To proceed, we need first to clarify what motion systems are, and in particular what a third-order motion system might be. This, in turn, requires the concepts of figure–ground segmentation and of a salience map.

### 10.3.1   Motion Systems, Flow Fields, Attention-Driven Apparent Motion

**First-Order Motion**   A motion system is a neurophysiological concept derived from psychophysical experiments; the essential ingredient is a flow field computation. To illustrate this, we consider the input to the first-order motion system, namely, the dynamic sequence of images that is formed on the retina and transformed by the early processing stages of the visual system. Processing by the retina removes the mean stimulus luminance from the signal (for nearly all neurons), so that only contrast signals (i.e., deviations from mean luminance) are transmitted to the lateral geniculate nucleus and cortex.

Let the stimulus luminance at a point with spatial coordinates $x,y$ at time $t$ be $l(x,y,t)$. Then the point contrast $c(x,y,t)$ is the normalized amount by which the luminance $l(x,y,t)$ differs from the mean luminance $l_0$:[5]

$$c(x,y,t) = (l(x,y,t) - l_0)/l_0 \qquad\qquad (3)$$

Positive values of $c(x,y,t)$ are carried by retinal ganglion cells and lateral geniculate cells with ON-center receptive fields, and negative values by OFF-center cells (Kuffler, 1953). The first-order motion system takes point contrast as its input and produces the first-order flow field as its output. The flow field $F_1(x,y,t)$ is a vector function that indicates the direction and velocity of motion in the neighborhood of location $x,y$, at time $t$.

A flow field does not directly indicate what may have caused the motion; it represents only the motion itself. And though we do not know exactly how the brain computes velocity, we do know that the first-order motion flow field is used to compute 3D structure from 2D motion (kinetic depth effect), and that it contributes to the control of locomotion, balance, orientation, and all the other functions usually attributed to motion perception (Dosher et al., 1989). Subsequent processing stages combine the information from a motion flow field with contour, color, texture, and other features to serve object and scene perception.[6]

**Second-Order Motion**   The second-order motion system computes a flow field analogously to the first-order system except that it discards the sign of $c(x,y,t)$ before the flow field computation, that is, it rectifies the point contrast and uses the absolute value (or squared value) instead of the point contrast directly. In neural terms, the outputs of ON-center and OFF-center cells are treated identically instead of oppositely.

As with first-order motion, there are complications. In second-order motion processing, rectification is preceded by spatiotemporal filtering, a combination that has been called texture grabbing (Chubb and Sperling, 1988). Spatial filtering followed by rectification means that the second-order system is sensitive to the amount of texture in each neighborhood of the stimulus, which is closely related to the luminance *variance* within the neighborhood. Whereas while the first-order motion system reports on the movement of areas that have fewer or more photons than their surround, the second-order system reports the movement of areas that have fewer or more texture features than their surround.

**Salience Map, Third-Order Motion**   The third-order system generates its flow field from figure–ground information. Most visual images can be segmented by the perceptual system into figure (the important parts that are designated for further processing) and ground (the remainder). According to Lu and Sperling (1995a, 1995b), Sperling and Lu (1998), and Blaser et al. (1999), the results of the figure–ground computation are stored in a salience map where figure is represented, for example, by 1 and ground by 0.

Not every point in every image can be unambiguously classified as figure or ground. Therefore, it is useful to define a real-valued variable, *salience,* to indicate the relative importance (or ''figureness'') of each image point in space and time. The instantaneous

**Figure 10.9**
How attention influences ambiguous motion displays via a salience map. (*A*) Five frames of an ambiguous motion display (1, 2, 3, 4, 5) with alternating features: odd frames modulate texture, even frames modulate binocular depth. Consecutive frames are shifted in phase by 90°, so that a motion signal arises only from the combination of odd and even frames (i.e., no motion within only the odd, or only the even, frames). (*B*) Three frames of the display (*a, b, c*) with their salience map representations, $M_a$, $M_b$, $M_c$, (*ellipses*) immediately to the right of each frame. When a subject attends the coarse texture patches, these patches acquire a higher salience value, as indicated by the X marks in the salience map ($M_a$, $M_c$). Areas with less binocular depth are automatically perceived as foreground, as indicated by the X marks ($M_b$). The dotted lines indicate the two possible directions of apparent motion (downward when attention selects the coarse texture, upward when it selects the fine texture). (*C*) Outputs of the salience map go to subsequent processes that compute motion, shape, and texture. (*D*) Left-eye and right-eye images (L, R) of one frame of the dynamic random-dot stereogram used to create a translating corrugated surface in depth (as shown schematically in *A* and *B*). (*E*) Five frames of an ambiguous third-order motion display. In the texture frames (2,3), salience is unambiguosly high in the high-contrast regions. In the other frames (1,3,5), the black-spot and white-spot regions have equal salience when there are no attentional instructions. Thus, no motion is seen without such instructions. Attention to white spots produces upward apparent motion; attention to black spots produces downward apparent motion.

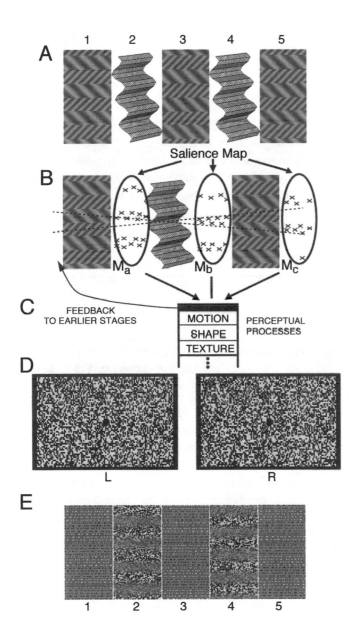

Salience Map

values of salience at each point of the visual field constitute a *salience map* of the visual field. The third-order motion system uses the time-varying salience map as its input, and computes a flow field that gives the direction and the magnitude of salience movement at each point as a function of time.

The third-order motion system computes the motion of those parts of the visual field which are designated as ''figure.'' This can be demonstrated by producing a succession of images in which the distinguishing features of the ''figure'' change from image to image. Figure may be defined by stereo depth in one image, by an area of greater texture contrast in the next image, and so on. If the areas defined as figure are displaced in a consistent direction from image to image, then observers perceive motion in that direction. It is worth noting that observers do not discriminate between motion that is produced by first-, second-, or third-order computations: they merely report ''apparent motion.''

The term ''salience map'' was first popularized by Koch and Ullman (1985), who used the concept to describe a winner-take-all network that determines a region in space from which information from various topographic feature maps is combined and directed to a central processor. Related concepts have emerged independently as an attention map (Mozer, 1991), a priority map (Ahmad and Omohundro, 1991), a selective tuning mechanism (Tsotsos et al., 1995; Tsotsos et al., chapter 14 in this volume), a hierarchical pruning mechanism (Burt, 1988), and under other names, with different authors giving somewhat different interpretations to these concepts.

**Attention to Feature**   A remarkable aspect of third-order motion is that attention can strongly influence the direction of motion perception (Lu and Sperling, 1995a), but this is not true for first- or second-order motion (Solomon and Sperling, 1994). Lu and Sperling arranged ambiguous motion displays (figure 10.9) so that when observers attended to one feature (e.g., coarse stripes [figure 10.9A] or white spots [figure 10.9E]), the display appeared to move in one direction; when they attended to the other feature (fine stripes or black spots), the display appeared to move in the opposite direction. Attention to a feature determined the direction of apparent motion even when the sequence of displays occurred so rapidly (five displays in 333 ms) that observers were unable to track any specific elements.[7] That attention can determine motion direction even when feature tracking is impossible implies that there must be another mechanism by which attention operates in these displays. Lu and Sperling (1995a) proposed that attention enhances the attended features at a level prior to conscious perception, and that these enhanced features are recorded as figure (versus ground) in the salience map. By influencing the input to the salience map, attention can determine third-order motion.

## 10.3.2 Selective Attention to Color

To investigate the proposed role of attention in increasing the salience of features, Blaser et al. (1999) used a third-order motion display involving attention to a color, red or green. Their experiment was designed to answer the following question: To what extent is selective attention to red (or green) equivalent to increasing the redness (or greenness) of a motion stimulus? Ultimately, this enabled them to measure the amount by which attention to a feature amplifies its salience.

**Stimulus Sequence**   The procedure used by Blaser and colleagues (1999) is shown in figure 10.10 (see also plate 6). A motion sequence consisted of five consecutive frames. In figure 10.10, the even frames (numbers 0, 2, 4 . . .) contain a contrast-modulated texture grating, and the odd frames (numbers 1, 3, 5 . . .) contain an isoluminant red–green grating. There is a 90° phase shift between consecutive frames. The phase shift between two color frames is 180°, so there is no directional motion signal within the color frames. Similarly, the phase shift between consecutive texture frames also is 180°, so there is no directional motion signal within the texture frames, either. To perceive a direction of motion, information from the color and texture frames must be combined.

The luminance is the same (average luminance in the case of texture areas) in all parts of all frames, both color and texture, so there is no usable first-order motion signal. This was verified by a sensitive calibration procedure (Anstis and Cavanagh, 1983; Lu and Sperling, 1999). Similarly, there is no significant texture in the isoluminant grating to stimulate the second-order motion system. Indeed, without attention instructions, observers usually do not report motion from this stimulus sequence.

To create the isoluminant color grating, the red gun of the display monitor was set to maximum intensity, and the green gun was adjusted to be of equal luminance. When the red and green stimulus colors were mixed 50/50, the result was a yellow that was equal in luminance to both the red and the green. The background was formed of this yellow. To create desaturated stripes of a color, say red, between 0 and 50% of the red was exchanged for green.

**Varying Salience: Red Advantage**   In the isoluminant color grating, the salience of a stripe (red or green) is assumed to be monotonically related to the amount by which it differs from the background (Lu et al., 1999). Blaser and colleagues (1999) called this the "chromaticity difference," which here is defined as follows: Let $r$ and $g$ represent the intensities of the red and green guns, respectively ($r, g \leq 1$). To maintain isoluminance, $r + g = 1$ at every location and point in time. The chromaticity difference $|R|$ of a red stripe from a yellow background is $|R| = r - g (r > g)$; the chromaticity difference of a green stripe is $|G| = g - r (g > r)$.

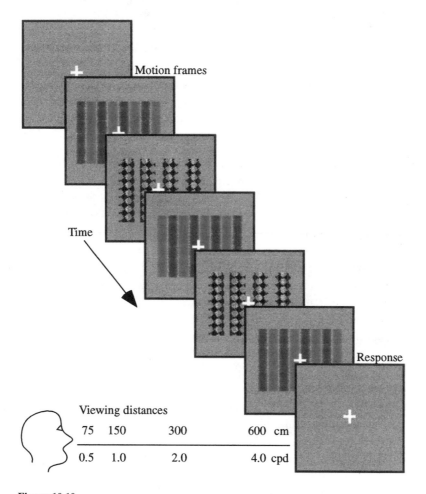

**Figure 10.10**
Procedure using amplification principle in third-order motion to measure the attentional amplification of salience. Even frames are texture-contrast gratings, with unambiguously high salience in the high-contrast texture bands. Odd frames are red–green color gratings, characterized by separate red-saturation and green-saturation values. Motion strength (e.g., as measured by Reichardt and motion energy detectors) is determined by the product of the modulation amplitudes in even and odd frames. When the texture modulation in the even frames is far above threshold, even weak salience modulations in the odd frames can produce apparent motion. Different viewing distances determine the spatial frequency (cycles per degree) of the gratings on the retina. (See plate 6 for color version.)

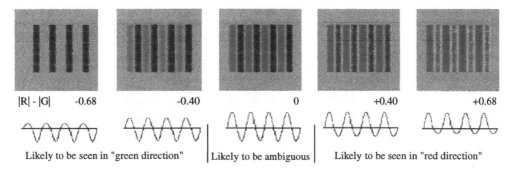

**Figure 10.11**
Five stimuli with different red advantages. From top to bottom: −0.68, −0.32, 0, +0.32, +0.68. For the displays of figure 10.11, attending to green (or red) produces apparent motion equivalent to a stimulus approximately one level higher (or lower). (See plate 7 for color version.)

It is critical whether red or green differs more from the background, because the stimulus will appear to move in one direction (the red direction) when red differs more, and in the other direction (the green direction) when green differs more. This aspect of the stimulus is characterized by a quantity called *red advantage,* which is simply $|R| - |G|$. For example, a stimulus that has only red stripes on a neutrally yellow background without green stripes (i.e., $|R| = 1$ and $|G| = 0$) would have a red advantage of 1. A stimulus that has only green stripes on a neutrally yellow background without red stripes (i.e., $|G| = 1$ and $|R| = 0$) would have a red advantage of $-1$. Finally, a stimulus with $|R| = |G|$ has a red advantage of 0. Stimuli actually used in the experiment had red advantages of −0.68, −0.4, 0, +0.4, and +0.68 (see figure 10.11, plate 7).

**Experimental Procedure**    In all sessions, a trial consisted of 0.5 s of a blank frame with a fixation point, followed by a five-frame stimulus at 100 ms/frame, and the observers simply judged the direction of movement. The stimulus grating was four cycles wide, and it was embedded in a much larger yellow background. There were many possible stimuli: five different chromatic gratings with various degrees of red advantage, randomized spatial phase, and randomly chosen direction of movement. The assignment of color gratings to odd frames and texture to even frames was reversed randomly from trial to trial. There were four different viewing distances, blocked by session, to produce four different stimulus spatial frequencies. Initially, observers were not given any attention instructions and ran through the whole sequence of trials. Subsequently, they were told to attend to the red (green) stimulus, and the entire procedure was repeated. Then the observers were told to attend to the previously unattended color and the entire procedure was repeated again.

**Results and Discussion**   Results are shown here for two observers, both practiced psychophysical observers. One was naive about the purpose of this experiment; the other was one of the experimenters. In the neutral condition (without attention instructions), when the red and green stripes both had maximum chromatic difference from the background ($|R| = |G|$), motion responses were random for one observer and showed a slight bias in favor of the red direction for the other. However, when there was a large red advantage ($|R| = 1.0$, $|G| = 0.32$, so $|R| - |G| = +0.68$), the direction of perceived motion was almost 100% in the red direction. For the same stimulus sequences, but with green advantage ($|R| = 0.32$, $|G| = 1.0$), the perceived motion direction was almost 100% in the opposite direction. For a spatial frequency of 4 cycles per degree (cpd), the resolution of the salience system for these stimuli is exceeded for one observer and his motion direction responses are almost random. The other observer's performance is impaired but remains far above chance.

The psychometric functions for the three resolvable gratings, in neutral attention conditions, go from 0 to 100% of apparent movement in the red direction as a function of red advantage (top three rows, figure 10.12, plate 8). This reflects the bottom-up control of salience. The greater the difference of a color stripe from the background, the greater its salience. In this kind of display sequence, when red is more salient, motion is in the red direction; when green is more salient, motion is in the green (opposite) direction; and when red and green are equally salient, there is no consistent apparent motion.

When observers pay selective attention to red, the psychometric functions appear to be shifted to the right; and when the observers attend to green, the opposite shift occurs. For example, under attention to red, direction judgments to the stimulus, $|R| = |G|$, are approximately the same as under neutral attention to a stimulus with a red advantage of $+0.3$, i.e., ($|R| - |G| = 0.3$).

**Attention Does Not Change Appearance**   An interesting, informal observation is that attending to red or to green does not make a stimulus sequence look different than in the neutral attention condition. Certainly, selective attention to color in a static display does not produce any noticeable change in the appearance of the static display. This is entirely consistent with previous observations that attention reduces the variance of various psychological judgments but does not alter the appearance of simple features (Prinzmetal et al., 1998). Indeed, one would expect selective attention to make judgments of a feature more accurate, not to bias the judgments in a particular direction. The difference in appearance between stimuli having red advantages of 0 and of 0.3 is very obvious, and if attention produced even 1/10 of this difference in appearance, it would be quite noticeable.

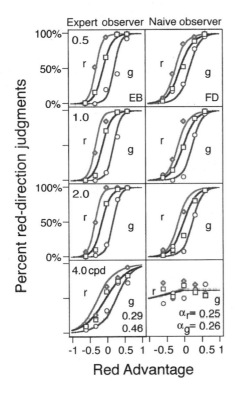

Expert observer  Naive observer

**Figure 10.12**
Results of the attention-amplification experiment. The percent of red-consistent motion judgments versus the red stimulus advantage, $|R| - |G|$ which is the difference $|R|$ of red from background yellow minus the difference $|G|$ of green from background yellow. As red advantage increases, the probability of perceiving motion in the red-consistent direction increases. Five data points are shown for each of four spatial frequencies (rows), three attentional conditions, and 2 observers (columns). Solid curves are model fits (see figure 10.13A). Middle curves indicate the baseline condition (no attention instructions); curves on right ($g$) and on left ($r$) are model fits for the attend-red and attend-green conditions, respectively. The estimated model parameters for the additional $|R|$ and $|G|$ amplification due to attention, $\alpha_r$ and $\alpha_g$, are indicated in the bottom panel for each observer. (See plate 8 for color version.)

### 10.3.3    A Dynamical Systems Model of Salience and Related Processes

The continuous curves drawn through the data in figure 10.12 account for 99% of the variance of the data for these observers. These curves are generated by the model of figure 10.13A. The "reduced" model of figure 10.13A includes just those components needed to generate the particular predictions in figure 10.12. Figure 10.13B shows these same components embedded in a larger system that illustrates how they relate more generally to attentional and perceptual processes.

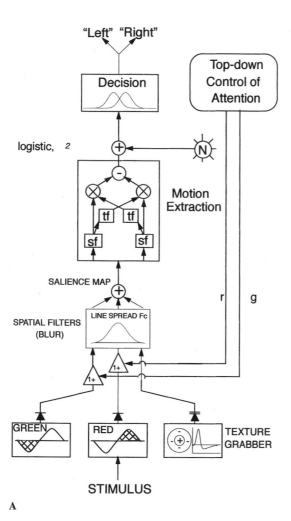

**Figure 10.13**

(*A*) A computational model of attention processes in third-order motion. The inputs are stimuli and attention instructions; the output is a direction-of-motion judgment. Stimuli are analyzed along the dimensions of texture and color. Instructions to attend to a color (red or green) are assumed to increase the gain of the attended color channel in the salience pathway by a factor of $\alpha$ to $1 + \alpha_r$ or $1 + \alpha_g$ depending on which color is attended. The texture channel produces output proportional to the amount of local texture. The salience map is the sum of all the stimulus inputs in the salience pathway; its output goes to the Motion III (third-order) computation. The third-order motion computation is represented as a Reichardt model (Reichardt, 1961; van Santen and Sperling, 1984); it produces a real-valued output that indicates a direction of motion and is perturbed by additive noise *N*. A decision processes outputs a response "right" if its input is greater than a criterion, and "left" otherwise. (*B*) A more comprehensive model of visual processing that shows sensory inputs bypassing the salience computation en route to subsequent processing. Although high salience does not seem to perturb the appearance of objects, it does eventually determine which signals are analyzed and remembered. The third-order motion signal is also available to subsequent perceptual processes, as indicated.

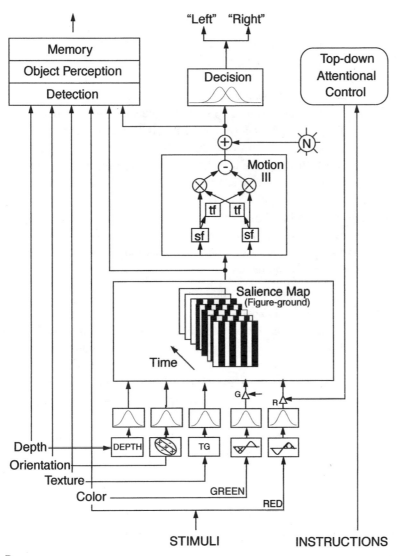

B

### 10.3.4   Components of the Computational Model

**Texture Grabber**   In the experiments, there are two kinds of inputs: visual stimuli and attention instructions. The stimuli are texture gratings and color gratings. To extract texture from the texture gratings requires a texture grabber (Chubb and Sperling, 1988, 1989a; Werkhoven et al., 1993). A texture grabber is composed of a linear bandpass filter (center-surround receptive field) that is most sensitive to spatial frequencies in a particular frequency range, a temporal filter, and a rectifier (figure 10.13). Because the output of a filter may be positive or negative, the filter output is rectified (absolute value or square) so that it represents the total quantity of texture. The texture grabbers of the second-order motion system are isotropic (circularly symmetric; see Werkhoven et al., 1993), but those of the third-order system are sensitive to orientation (Chubb and Sperling, 1991; Werkhoven et al., 1994). Although the filter could, in principle, process any texture, texture was not varied in this experiment. Therefore, for the present experiment, it is sufficient to assume that the output of the texture grabber is 1.0 in regions of maximum texture contrast and that it is 0 in regions where there is no texture.

**Color Grabber**   Extracting an arbitrary color that differs from an arbitrary background is a complex problem. For the present experiment, it is sufficient to extract red or green from a yellow background, and this is simple. In direct analogy to a texture grabber, a color grabber can be constructed from a wavelength-sensitive filter responding positively to red and negatively to green (or vice versa) followed by a rectifier. It is assumed that when red or green areas of the stimulus are at maximum intensity, the output of the color grabber is 1, whereas the output is 0 for a yellow stimulus, and is between 0 and 1 for intermediate stimuli.

In the visual system, positive and negative signals are carried by separate neurons (e.g., ON-center and OFF-center neurons). The red (positive) and green (negative) outputs are assumed to be carried by separate neurons. This is critical for the attention amplification, which acts separately on the red and green outputs.

**Attention Amplification**   Attention amplification is determined by instructions that have to be interpreted (a high-level cognitive process) and implemented (at a lower level). Under instructions to attend to red, the red amplifier is turned on and the output of the red channel is amplified, that is, multiplied by a factor of $1 + \alpha_r$, $\alpha_r > 0$, while $\alpha_g = 0$. Under instructions to attend to green, the green channel is amplified by $1 + \alpha_g$, $\alpha_g > 0$, while $\alpha_r = 0$. It is important to note that attentional amplification is independent of the stimuli being presented. An attention state is described by parameters $[\alpha_k]$ that represent the amplification of the various inputs. Once an attention state has been established, it determines the (altered) response to whatever stimuli may be presented.

**Spatial Filter**   The experiments do not distinguish the spatial resolution of the color and the texture systems, so limited spatial resolution arises from the same spatial filter for all inputs. Because the data are essentially the same for spatial frequencies of 0.5, 1.0, and 2.0 cpd, with a severe decline in performance only at 4 cpd, the spatial filter need have only a single parameter, $F_c$, the corner frequency at which resolution declines. For greater accuracy, spatial resolution could be modeled perfectly with three parameters. This would ensure that estimates of attention components are not contaminated by errors in estimating spatial resolution.

**Salience Map**   We assumed that in the brain, inputs from various sources sum at the salience map, and a complex figure–ground computation is performed. For the present experiment, it is sufficient to consider just the summing aspect of the computation, so in the block diagram (figure 10.13A) the salience map is represented by simple summation.

**Standard Motion Analysis**   For humans, the extraction of the direction of movement from dynamic (first-order and second-order) stimuli is very well modeled by a Reichardt detector (van Santen and Sperling, 1984). Other theories—based on Fourier motion energy (Adelson and Bergen, 1985), on Hilbert detectors (Watson and Ahumada, 1985), and on spatiotemporal gradients (Adelson and Bergen, 1986)—have been shown to be similar or indistinguishable (in terms of their overall computation) from an elaborated Reichardt detector (van Santen and Sperling, 1985). This overall computation has been called "standard motion analysis" by Chubb and Sperling (1989b), and it applies to both first- and second-order motion.

The third-order motion computation clearly is different from standard motion analysis because it fails the pedestal test (Lu and Sperling, 1995b) and because it seems to be more sensitive to displacement than to motion energy (Krauskopf et al., 1999). Whether this is due to an intrinsically different motion computation or to the preprocessing of the input (so that amplitude is only very coarsely quantized) has not been resolved. So, the motion component is represented simply as standard motion analysis. It produces a positive output for motion in one direction and a negative output for motion in the opposite direction.

**Noise and the Decision Process**   Psychophysical data are not deterministic; the same stimulus evokes different responses on repeated presentations. This is taken into account by adding Gaussian noise to the output of the motion detector. The variance of this noise determines the slope of the psychometric functions in figure 10.12. The decision process simply determines whether the net output is greater or less than zero, which represent the two permissible directions of motion in the experiment.

**Parameters and Efficiency of Prediction**    There are four data panels representing the four stimulus sizes (spatial frequencies), and each panel has five data points for each of three attention conditions: sixty data points per observer. The model has two attention parameters, $\alpha_r$ and $\alpha_g$, and one noise parameter, $\sigma$, that determines the slope of the psychometric function. Just one parameter is needed to describe the spatial filter for observer FD, but three are needed for the other observer. The four- and six-parameter predictions account for 99% of the variance of the data. This is efficient prediction.

The actual values of the attention amplification for the two observers in figure 10.12 are the following: observer EB: $\alpha_r = 0.29$, $\alpha_g = 0.46$; observer FD: $\alpha_r = 0.25$, $\alpha_g = 0.26$. The average value of 0.32 represents an attentional amplification of over 30%, which is quite significant.[8]

### 10.3.4    The "Full" Model

The computational model described above sufficed to fit the motion-direction data of the experiments. However, it deals neither with the observation that attention does not seem to change the appearance of stimuli, nor with the issue of how the processes described above relate to the more general functioning of a salience map. The full model links salience-related attentional processes to more general attentional processes.

**Three Pathways**    Modeling the attention-motion experiment requires three conceptual pathways. The first is a pathway for the instructions to attend to a color. These instructions are interpreted at a high cognitive level. In the model, these high level processes then send a control signal that modulates the inputs to the salience map, that is, it controls amplification prior to the salience computation. The second pathway conveys the stimulus to the salience map. The third pathway conveys the stimulus directly to other perceptual processes, such as motion perception, shape recognition, object perception, memory, and subsequent cognitive processes. The direct pathway is suggested by the informal observations that attention has no effect on appearance even though it produces a large effect on salience as determined by the direction of apparent motion of ambiguous stimuli.

In addition to color and texture, which were investigated in the experiment described here, previous studies of third-order motion showed sensitivity to depth and to texture orientation, so these inputs to the salience map are also represented in figure 10.13B. And surely there will be others as well.

The salience map has outputs that control detection, object perception, access to memory, and other perceptual and cognitive processes. For example, the salience map is assumed to generate the temporal attention window, described in the first part of this chapter, that controls access to short-term visual memory.

**Two Kinds of Amplification in Attention Processing**   One kind of amplification is the modulation of inputs to the salience map. The other kind is the actual implementation of salience. For example, in controlling memory access, the salience map may determine what input information is to be stored; the actual control of access is a different process, and it is useful to maintain the distinction.

**Salience Theories**   In the present model, the salience map has a privileged place in the processing hierarchy. A relatively small difference in the input to the salience map determines the figure–ground relations in the map, and these are assumed to ultimately determine the flow of information to other perceptual processes. In the neural network model of Koch and Ullman (1985), the salience map determined in which parts of the visual field features from other stimulus maps (e.g., color and shape maps) could be combined, and it embodied some of the computations envisioned here. At that time, it had not occurred to the authors that one might make direct measurements of salience.

In the neural network model of Tsotsos and colleagues (chapter 14 in this volume), control inputs modulate perceptual processing at various levels of a visual hierarchy. Once a particular area of the visual field is selected for further processing, the entire cone of information in the visual hierarchy that derives from the selected area is amplified relative to everything else. In this scheme, there is no privileged salience map per se; rather, salience is distributed throughout the visual hierarchy. Both of these models, as well as others that have been proposed, could be elaborated to take into account the experimental evidence and theoretical considerations reported here.

### 10.3.5   Salience Map: Applications to Other Paradigms

**Third-Order Motion**   The basis of the experiments at issue is that the output of the salience map can serve as an input to a third-order motion flow field. One of the useful features of the apparent motion paradigm is that it takes advantage of an amplification principle: the strength of apparent motion in a sequence of frames in which there is a spatial 90° phase shift from frame to frame is proportional to the *product* of the modulation amplitudes in each frame (van Santen and Sperling, 1984). Introducing high-contrast-texture stripes in a background of zero texture renders the textured regions highly salient. Introducing such high-amplitude salience modulation in the even frames of the Blaser et al. (1999) attention experiment enabled very sensitive measurement of attention-induced salience modulations that otherwise might have remained below threshold (Lu and Sperling, 1999). In the present case, the product amplification principle was applied to measuring attention-induced salience modulations in the red–green gratings of the odd frames. The same amplification principle in apparent motion offers the possibility of efficient and sensitive measurements of salience in other contexts, such as visual search and short-term memory.

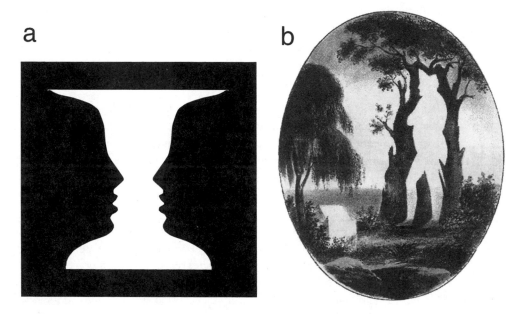

**Figure 10.14**
Figure–ground ambiguities. (*a*) Ambiguous profiles-vase, after Rubin (1915). (*b*) Forest scene with Napoleon. Normally, trees are seen as figure and the intervening space as ground. However, the intervening space can also be seen as figure when it is attended or has a meaningful shape. (Y&B Associates, after Currier and Ives, ca. 1835.) (See plate 9 for color version.)

**Figure–Ground and Pattern Recognition**    Much has been written about figure–ground segregation, much of it inspired by Rubin's (1915) famous illustration of a perceptually bistable vase—pair of face profiles (see figure 10.14, plate 9). Following his example, most of the literature has focused on the experiential nature of distinction between figure and ground. Figure is seen as more important than ground, it seems nearer in depth, boundaries seem to belong to the figure, and so on.

Lu and Sperling (1995a) suggested that the salience map is the mechanism that determines what parts of the visual field are sent to shape-recognition processes. For example, when mapmakers produce maps of the continents, they use little graphic devices that cause the continents to be seen as figure and the oceans as ground. The continents have lots of details; the oceans are plain. The continents have varieties of colors and features; oceans are homogeneous in color. Consequently, in the United States, most persons feel they know the shapes of North and South America, but very few know or would recognize the shapes of the oceans. Maps designed for sailing and oceanography practice just the opposite principle, keeping land areas very plain and putting the detail and livelier colors in the ocean.

Mapmakers take advantage of bottom-up salience processes. However, top-down processes also have a strong influence on salience. A good example is a forest scene. Normally, the trees are perceived as figure, and the space between the trees as ground. That is, the shape system computes the shape of the trees and not of the spaces between the trees. However, when running away from something, it becomes essential to compute the shape of the space between the trees: Will we fit? Will what is chasing us fit? The salience map interpretation of this process is that there is top-down enhancement in the middle of the space between the trees. This enhancement needs only to be sufficiently precise to cause the salience map to mark the space between the trees as figure and, consequently, for the shape system to compute its shape. A nice example of computing the shape between the trees is illustrated in figure 10.14B.

The example of "Napoleon in the trees" (figure 10.14B) embodies a well-documented principle of figure–ground segmentation: familiar shapes are more likely to be perceived as figure. This in turn suggests a top-down influence of figure–ground segmentation, which is more complex than anything considered in the present salience model but is the kind of vertical interaction in the processing hierarchy encompassed by the model of Tsotsos and colleagues (chapter 14 in this volume).

**Guided Search**    Perhaps most work on attention theory has been undertaken in the context of visual search tasks. In these tasks, an observer views an array of items comprising one or more targets and several distractors (nontargets). The search process is assumed to control the access of the to-be-searched items to pattern recognition processes either serially or in parallel, or in some more complex combination of both. Theories of search involve the strategic allocation of processing resources (Cave and Wolfe, 1990; Koopman, 1957; Sperling and Dosher, 1986). The sequence of items searched is determined by priorities that are assigned to spatial locations, to features, and to other stimulus properties that discriminate between stimuli and targets. Automatic, bottom-up factors are very important in locating targets that differ greatly from their surround (Cave and Wolfe, 1990); top-down factors may be equally important, such as the known probability of finding targets in particular locations. Because it combines both bottom-up and top-down influences, the salience map would provide an ideal mechanism to implement this kind of guided search.

**Access to Memory**    Of all the processes discussed, access to memory is the most restrictive. The partial report paradigm (Sperling, 1960) offers a simple example. Observers were briefly exposed to 3 × 3 or 3 × 4 arrays of letters and asked to report just one, (randomly) selected row. The cue to report a row was coded as a high-, medium-, or low-pitched tone, so that it could be interpreted very quickly. The cued row was reported quite accurately, even when the instruction occurred several hundred milliseconds after the exposure was terminated.

Performance is nicely accounted for by a model that assumes there is an initial, default state of attending to the middle row, and that there is a quick transition to the row indicated by the tone when it occurs (Gegenfurtner and Sperling, 1993). The salience map provides an obvious mechanism for this spatial shift of attention, which controls access of visual input to visual short-term memory. It is quite analogous to the temporal attention window that was the subject of the first part of this chapter, and to the attentional amplification of color that was the subject of the second part. Just like a cue to attend to a particular color, which must be interpreted at a higher, cognitive level but takes effect at a much lower, perceptual level, a tonal cue to attend to a particular region in space also ultimately takes effect at a lower level to control inputs to the salience map.

**Constraints on Top-Down Control of Salience**   With the eyes fixated, observers nevertheless can attend selectively to areas of visual space according to attention instructions. This is well known and has been amply confirmed. What are the constraints on the shape of the area to which observers can attend? The attention-modulation functions obtained from experiments on attention to motion provide one means of answering this question. Suppose that attention-modulation functions are determined primarily by limitations of the salience map, rather than by the specific stimuli used in our experiments. In this case, the spatial frequency filter functions of the model of Blaser and colleagues (1999) would describe the attentional constraints. That is, any request to distribute attention according to a particular spatial function, could be executed only to the level of accuracy permitted by the attentional filters. Whether the attention system could actually achieve this resolution limit is an empirical question.

A related question concerns the concurrent action of attention to color and attention to space. The attention system would be much simpler if there were two separate, independent attention processes—one allocating attention to a particular color in all of visual space, and the other allocating attention to a particular part of visual space. But this would imply that attention to location and to color are separable. One could attend to red in a certain location, but one could not attend to red in one location and to green in another. Results of preliminary experiments by Tse, Lu, and Sperling (2000) suggest that this is indeed true, implying that attention to color and to location are indeed separable. Obviously, such constraints and their dynamics need to be embodied in more detailed attention models than the ones proposed here.

## 10.4   Summary and Conclusions

Two models of attention have been proposed, each accounting for a significant set of experimental data and for important incidental observations. The first model shows how attention windows are constructed in successive attention episodes and how such attention windows control access to short-term memory. Once they are in memory, items acquired within a single attention episode lose their time stamp, and their order is coded simply in terms of their memory strength. It takes about 100 to 200 ms to self-generate an attention window in response to an attention cue, and the window width is several hundred milliseconds.

The second model describes the salience map, one of the most important mechanisms by which attention exerts its effects. This model is derived from experiments using a sensitive assay method involving third-order motion. Attention was found to amplify the salience of attended colors by, typically, about 30%. The model draws an important distinction between attentionally amplifying the salience of an attended color while leaving the appearance of the color itself unchanged. The salience map was proposed as the probable mechanism for a variety of tasks, including access to short-term memory, guided search, and pattern perception mechanisms. Both models made accurate and efficient predictions of significant data sets.

### Acknowledgment

This research was supported by AFOSR, Life Science Directorate, Visual Information Processing Program.

### Notes

1. In fact, pairs in which only one member of the pair is reported were included in the analysis because it was assumed that the other member would eventually have been reported if the response had not been artificially truncated after four reported numerals. Except for having more data to analyze by including partnerless items in an implicit pairing, there was no difference in any comparison or conclusion that depended on including or not including single-item pairs.

2. There also are measurement-theoretic inequalities involving $iBj$s that prove the data can be described by a strength model (see Reeves and Sperling, 1986: p. 189ff.).

3. In a later, more detailed model, the time to detect and interpret the attention-shift cue is represented not merely by the mean detection time but also by a distribution with a mean and variance. The same variance accounts for the variance of motor reaction times and for internal correlations in attention-shift data (Sperling and Shih, 1998).

4. This kind of attention hardware has some interesting difficulties in making accurate judgments of intermodal temporal order, like those baseball umpires attempt to make when judging the order of occurrence of a runner's foot touching a specific point and the sound of a baseball striking the fielder's glove.

5. How the mean luminance $l_0$ is computed and what constitutes the spatiotemporal neighborhood in which it is computed are complex questions that are of considerable interest in deriving an accurate theory of visual processing, but they are secondary to issues of attention. To simplify the estimation of mean luminance in the experiments described here, the stimuli were constructed so that the expected luminance was locally and globally the same everywhere in every frame.

6. Complications: (1) First-order vision is organized into channels, computations that are carried out within a particular spatial frequency band, typically one to two octaves wide. First-order motion is computed in all channels (spatial frequency bands), and each has a flow field. How these channel outputs are ultimately combined has not yet been resolved. (2) The Reichardt model—as well as all other equivalent or nearly equivalent models of first-order motion—computes only direction, not velocity directly. There are two proposed classes of velocity theories (temporal frequency counting and detector combination), but the brain's algorithm for computing velocity has not been determined.

7. Cavanagh (1992) presented observers with two superimposed gratings, a first-order (luminance) grating and an isoluminant color grating, moving in opposite directions. Observers perceived motion in the first-order direction. However, selective attention to an area of the colored grating could produce apparent motion consistent with the color-grating direction. The apparent motion of the color grating was assumed to be produced by the movement of attention in the process of tracking the moving area. The displays produced by Lu and Sperling (1995a) were much too quick to permit attentional tracking. Third-order motion is a more primitive process than attentional tracking, perhaps even a necessary precursor to the attentional tracking of moving objects.

8. A third observer, who was able to complete only half the experiment, had a red amplification factor $\alpha_r$ of 1.17, which indicates that selective attention to red more than doubled her red salience.

# References

Adelson, E. H., and Bergen, J. R. (1985). Spatiotemporal energy models for the perception of motion. *J. Optical Soc. America* A2: 284–299.

Adelson, E. H., and Bergen, J. R. (1986). The extraction of spatio-temporal energy in human and machine vision. In *Motion: Representation and analysis* (pp. 151–155). Washington, DC: IEEE Computer Society Press.

Ahmad, S., and Omohundro, S. (1991). *Efficient visual search: A connectionist solution.* International Computer Science Institute Technical Report tr-91-040. Berkeley: University of California.

Anstis, S., and Cavanagh, P. (1983). A minimum motion technique for judging equiluminance. In J. D. Mollon and E. T. Sharpe (eds.), *Colour vision* (pp. 155–166). New York: Academic Press.

Blaser, E., Sperling, G., and Lu, Z.-L. (1999). Measuring the amplification of attention. *Proc. Nat. Acad. Sci. USA* 96: 8289–8294.

Burt, P. (1988). Attention mechanisms for vision in a dynamic world. In *Proceedings ninth international conference on pattern recognition, Beijing, China* (pp. 977–987).

Cavanagh, P. (1992). Attention-based motion perception. *Science* 257: 1563–1565.

Cave, K. R., and Wolfe, J. M. (1990). Modeling the role of parallel processing in visual search. *Cog. Psychol.* 22: 225–271.

Cheal, M. L., and Lyon, D. (1989). Attention effects on form discrimination at different eccentricities. *Q. J. Exp. Psychol.* 41A: 719–746.

Chubb, C., and Sperling, G. (1988). Drift-balanced random stimuli: A general basis for studying non–Fourier motion perception. *J. Optical Soc. America* A5: 1986–2006.

Chubb, C., and Sperling, G. (1989a). Second-order motion perception: Space–time separable mechanisms. In *Proceedings: Workshop on visual motion. (March 20–22, 1989, Irvine, California.)* (pp. 126–138). Washington, DC: IEEE Computer Society Press.

Chubb, C., and Sperling, G. (1989b). Two motion perception mechanisms revealed by distance driven reversal of apparent motion. *Proc. Nat. Acad. Sci. USA* 86: 2985–2989.

Chubb, C., and Sperling, G. (1991). Texture quilts: Basic tools for studying motion-from-texture. *J. Math. Psychol.* 35: 411–442.

Dosher, B. A., Landy, M. S., and Sperling, G. (1989). Kinetic depth effect and optic flow: I. 3D shape from Fourier motion. *Vis. Res.* 29: 1789–1813.

Gegenfurtner, K., and Sperling, G. (1993). Information transfer in iconic memory experiments. *J. Exp. Psychol. Hum. Percep. Perf.* 19: 845–866.

Koch, C., and Ullman, S. (1985). Shifts in selective visual attention: Towards the underlying neural circuitry. *Hum. Neurobiol.* 4: 219–227.

Koopman, B. O. (1957). The theory of search. III. The optimum distribution of searching effort. *Oper. Res.* 5: 613–626.

Krauskopf, J., and Li, X. (1999). Effect of contrast on detection of motion of chromatic and luminance targets: Retina-relative and object-relative movement. *Vis. Res.* 39: 3346–3350.

Kuffler, S. W. (1953). Discharge pattern and functional organization of mammalian retina. *J. Neurophysiol.* 16: 37–68.

Lu, Z.-L., Lesmes, L. A., and Sperling, G. (1999). The mechanism of isoluminant chromatic motion perception. *Proc. Nat. Acad. Sci. USA* 96: 8289–8294.

Lu, Z.-L., and Sperling, G. (1995a). Attention-generated apparent motion. *Nature* 377: 237–239.

Lu, Z.-L., and Sperling, G. (1995b). The functional architecture of human visual motion perception. *Vis. Res.* 35: 2697–2722.

Lu, Z.-L., and Sperling, G. (1999). The amplification principle in motion perception. *Invest. Ophthalmol. Vis. Sci.* 40: S199.

Mozer, M. (1991). *The perception of multiple objects: A connectionist approach.* Cambridge, MA: MIT Press.

Prinzmetal, W., Amiri, H., Allen, K., and Edwards, T. (1998). Phenomenology of attention: I. Color, location, orientation, and spatial frequency. *J. Exp. Psychol. Hum. Percep. Perf.* 24: 261–282.

Reeves, A. (1977). The detection and recall of rapidly displayed letters and digits. Unpublished doctoral dissertation, City University of New York.

Reichardt, W. (1961). Autocorrelation, a principle for the evaluation of sensory information by the central nervous system. In W. A. Rosenblith (ed.), *Sensory communication.* New York: Wiley).

Rubin, E. (1915). *Edgar Rubin synsoplevede figurer: Studien i psykologisk analyse.* Copenhagen: Gyldendalske Boghandel. German trans.: *Visuell wahrgenommene Figuren: Studien in psychologischer Analyse.* Copenhagen: Gyldendalske Boghandel, 1921.

Shih, S., and Sperling, G. (2000). Measuring and modeling the trajectory of visual spatial attention. *Psychol. Rev.,* in press.

Solomon, J. A., and Sperling, G. (1994). Full-wave and half-wave rectification in 2nd-order motion perception. *Vis. Res.* 34: 2239–2257.

Sperling, G. (1960). The information available in brief visual presentations. *Psychol. Monog.* 74, no. 11 (whole no. 498). Pp. 1–29.

Sperling, G., and Dosher, B. (1986). Strategy and optimization in human information processing. In K. Boff, L. Kaufman, and J. Thomas (eds.), *Handbook of perception and performance,* vol. 1, Chapter 2 (pp. 1–65). New York: Wiley.

Sperling, G., and Lu, Z.-L. (1998). A systems analysis of visual motion perception. In T. Watanabe (ed.), *High-level motion processing* (pp. 153–183). Cambridge, MA: MIT Press.

Sperling, G., and Weichselgartner, E. (1995). Episodic theory of the dynamics of spatial attention. *Psychol. Rev.* 102: 503–532.

Sperling, G., and Reeves, A. (1980). Measuring the reaction time of a shift of visual attention. In R. Nickerson (ed.), *Attention and Performance VIII* (pp. 347–360). Hillsdale, NJ: Erlbaum.

Tse, C.-H., Lu, Z.-L., and Sperling, G. (2000). Attending to red and green concurrently in different areas reduces attentional capacity. *Invest. Ophthalmol. Vis. Sci.* 41: S42.

Tsotsos, J. K., Culhane, S. M., Wai, W. Y. K., Lai, Y., Davis, N., and Nuflo, F. (1995). Modeling visual attention via selective tuning. *Art. Intell.* 78: 507–545.

van Santen, J. P. H., and Sperling, G. (1984). Temporal covariance model of human motion perception. *J. Optical Soc. America* A1: 451–473.

van Santen, J. P. H., and Sperling, G. (1985). Elaborated Reichardt detectors. *J. Optical Soc. America* A2: 300–321.

Watson, A. B., and Ahumada, A. J. (1985). Model of human visual-motion sensing. *J. Optic. Soc. Am. A* 1: 322–342.

Werkhoven, P., Sperling, G., and Chubb, C. (1993). The dimensionality of texture-defined motion: A single channel theory. *Vis. Res.* 33: 463–485.

Werkhoven, P., Sperling, G., and Chubb, C. (1994). Perception of apparent motion between dissimilar gratings: Spatiotemporal properties. *Vis. Res.* 34: 2741–2759.

# 11 Perceptual Consequences of Multilevel Selection

**Jochen Braun, Christof Koch, D. Kathleen Lee, and Laurent Itti**

## 11.1 Introduction

Recent developments in neurobiology leave little doubt that visual attention can modulate neural activity throughout all levels of visual cortex, including primary visual cortex (area V1). In area V1 of human observers, functional imaging reveals a dramatic attentional modulation of hemodynamic activity that is comparable in size to the effect of visual stimulation (Brefczynski and DeYoe, 1999; Heeger et al., chapter 2 in this volume). Attentional modulations are evident also at the level of individual neurons, and have been observed in neuronal responses of areas V1, V2, V4, and MT/MST (Moran and Desimone, 1985; Motter, 1993; Treue and Maunsell, 1996; Luck et al., 1997; Roelfsema et al., 1998; Reynolds and Desimone, chapter 7 in this volume). Given an appropriate stimulus and task, the effect of attention can be quite large. For example, the response of in area V1 may double in size (Ito and Gilbert, 1999; Ito et al., chapter 5 in this volume).

How does the attentional modulation of all cortical levels mesh with psychological theories of attention? The two principal ways in which attention may operate, according to these theories (e.g., Pashler, 1998), are to select one or a few attended stimuli from the visual scene for perceptual processing (early selection) or, subsequent to perceptual processing of the entire visual scene, to mediate access of ''attended'' stimuli to a limited capacity for semantic processing (late selection). Although historically much effort has been devoted to demonstrating that attention is limited to one function or the other, it seems increasingly likely that attention performs a selective function at both early and late levels of processing (e.g., Pashler, 1997; Lavie, chapter 3 in this volume). If that is so, this would agree nicely with the neurobiological findings mentioned above. In fact, computational studies that take into account the architecture of visual cortex argue that attentional selection must necessarily involve all levels of the visual cortical hierarchy (Tsotsos, 1990; Olshausen et al., 1995; Tsotsos et al., chapter 14 in this volume). In short, there are now several good reasons to consider attention in terms of *multilevel selection,* that is, in terms of selective modulation of all visual cortical levels.

If selection takes place at multiple cortical levels, this should have some repercussions for the psychology of attention. First of all, because different cortical levels presumably make different contributions to perception, there should be multiple perceptual consequences of attention. In other words, there should be several different ways in which attention alters visual perception and, furthermore, each of these ways should correspond to a particular cortical level (or set of levels) modulated by attention.

Taking a ''natural history'' approach, we investigated the effect of attention on a wide range of visual discriminations, using a sensitive psychophysical paradigm involving *concurrent tasks* (Braun, 1994; Braun and Julesz, 1998; Lee, Koch, Braun, 1999; Lee et al., 1999). The results suggest that visual experience derives from both the focus of attention and an ambient awareness of poorly attended parts of the visual scene. The well-known ''pop-out'' phenomenon is an example of this ambient vision. The results show further that attention enhances or augments ambient vision in several qualititative and quantitative ways, as predicted by multilevel selection. First we will show how attentive and ambient vision can be distinguished with the help of concurrent-task experiments, and next we will examine their qualitative and quantitative differences more closely.

A *qualitative* contribution of visual attention appears to be the discrimination of spatial relationships of elementary stimulus attributes. This harks back to feature-integration theory and the notion that attention links each attribute to its proper location (Treisman, 1993). Tentative evidence suggests that this qualitative change in perception may reflect attentional modulation at intermediate cortical levels such as area V4 (Connor et al., 1996). A *quantitative* effect of attention is to lower thresholds for spatial vision, that is, for discriminating elementary stimulus attributes such as contrast, orientation, and spatial frequency. Here, detailed psychophysical measurements reveal some interesting limitations of attention, in that attention affects some thresholds (e.g., contrast) far less than others (e.g., orientation, spatial frequency). These results may reflect attentional modulation of the early cortical levels, at or near area V1, that are thought to determine spatial vision thresholds (e.g., Geisler and Albrecht, 1997; Carandini et al., 1997).

Another important implication of multilevel selection is that attention must be considered in the context of bottom-up processing. If attentional selection takes place within and through the visual hierarchy that mediates bottom-up processing, then the architecture of bottom-up processes should constrain the ways in which attention can act. Indeed, psychologists have long argued that what attention can and cannot select is to some extent governed by bottom-up factors such as visual segmentation and grouping (object-based attention; e.g., O'Craven et al., 1999; Roelfsema et al., 1998). This raises the possibility that attentive vision may be understood in largely the same terms as *bottom-up* processing, rather than requiring a qualitatively different, *top-down* approach.

Finally, we will investigate the extent to which attention can be understood in terms of bottom-up processing. To this end, we combine our measurements of how attention changes spatial vision thresholds with neural modeling of bottom-up processing. Like several other groups (e.g., Foley, 1994; Zenger and Sagi, 1996; Carandini et al., 1997), we model spatial vision in terms of a response normalization among neurons with overlapping receptive fields (Lee et al., 1999). The results suggest that attention modulates response normalization in a rather stereotypical fashion: the underlying interactions are intensified so as to accentuate response differences, without altering the qualitative response distribution. That is, strong responses are strengthened further, and weak responses are weakened further, than in the absence of attention. Note that this effect of attention is not specific to each psychophysical task, but seems to be the same for all five tasks studied. These results are consistent with the notion that attentional effects are constrained by the bottom-up architecture of visual cortex, as predicted by multilevel selection.

## 11.2 Attentive Vision

From the very beginnings of research on visual attention (e.g., Helmholtz, 1850/1962; James, 1890/1981; Neisser, 1967), it has been understood that attention is an essential component of many, if not most, aspects of visual performance. This premise is borne out by a large body of work that shows visual discrimination performance to be disrupted to varying degrees, up to complete abolition of performance, when attention is lacking or somehow compromised (e.g., Sperling and Melchner, 1978; Duncan, 1984; Nakayama and Mackeben, 1989; Duncan et al., 1994). Over the last several years, we have developed methods to quantify "attentional demand", that is, the extent to which a given discrimination depends on attention (Braun, 1994; Braun and Julesz, 1998; Lee et al., 1999). Here we present a summary of this work, beginning with discriminations that exhibit a high degree of dependence on attention.

All experiments reported here involve concurrent visual tasks and displays of almost identical layout (figures 11.1–11.5). In general, they combine a central task, which concerns five target elements near fixation, and a peripheral task, which concerns a single target appearing at varying locations but always at the same eccentricity (approximately 4.5°). An important aspect of the design is that the target of the peripheral task is visually salient, in other words, it is the most prominent stimulus in the periphery of the display. This minimizes positional uncertainty of the peripheral target and largely eliminates effects of lateral masking, crowding, or stimulus competition. By restricting ourselves to visually salient targets, we focus the investigation on the perception of single, well-localized objects, and on how their perception is altered by attention.

To prevent the observer from attending sequentially first to one part of the display and then to the other, the display is presented briefly and visual persistence is curtailed by masking (stimulus-onset-asynchrony, SOA, 100 to 250 ms). This means that each part of the display is visible just long enough to be discriminated on its own. The point of the experiment is to determine the extent to which one part of the display can still be discriminated when attention focuses on the other.

When a practiced observer is confronted by two visual tasks that each demand full attention, he or she is generally able to trade off performance of one task against performance of the other. For example, if asked to attend equally to both parts of the display, the observer performs both tasks comparably poorly. If asked to attend primarily to one part of the display, the observer performs better on this part and even worse on the other. By varying observer instructions in this way, one can extrapolate reliably to the situation in which attention is fully focused on the other task. Of course, this procedure is sensible only if observers divide attention during each trial, rather than attending in some trials to one part of the display and in other trials to the other. Fortunately, one can verify that observers maintain a reasonably stable division of attention during each block of trials by performing a contingency analysis and testing for a significant anticorrelation in the correctness of the two responses (Sperling and Dosher, 1986; Lee et al., 1999).

A typical experiment of this kind is illustrated in figure 11.1A. The experiment combines a central and a peripheral task, both of which involve discriminating between T- and

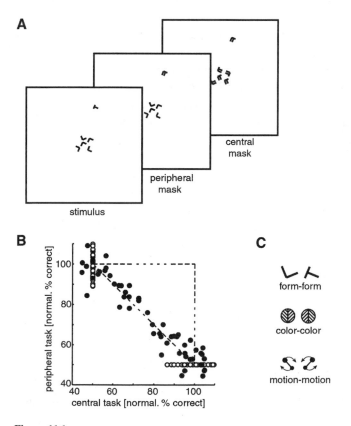

**Figure 11.1**
Concurrent tasks involving similar features. (*A*) Sequence of stimulus, peripheral mask, and central mask displays (schematic, not to scale). The stimulus contains five central targets and one peripheral target. (*B*) Performance of central and peripheral tasks alone (single-task, open circles) and together (double-task, filled circles). Results for two observers (10,200 trials total). Performance is normalized such that each task by itself is performed at 100% correct. Chance performance is 50% correct. (*C*) Alternative task types. Observers discriminate either form (T or L), color configuration (red–green or green–red), or sense of rotation (clockwise or counterclockwise).

L-shaped elements. In the central task, observers inspect the 5 central elements, which appear in various locations and rotations within 1° of fixation, and report whether they are the "same" (five Ts or five Ls) or "different" (four Ts and one L, or four Ls and one T). In the peripheral task, observers report whether the peripheral element, which appears at various locations of 4.3° eccentricity, is a T or an L. Analogous experiments can be conducted with other kinds of stimulus elements that require the discrimination of color or motion instead of form (figure 11.1B). For example, we have substituted bisected disks that are either red–green or green–red in order to study color discrimination, or "dumbbell" shapes rotating either clockwise or counterclockwise to study motion discrimination with and without attention (Lee et al., 1999).

The outcome is essentially the same in all three experiments (form, color, and motion discrimination). Figure 11.1B shows the results of individual blocks of fifty trials for various observer instructions. Open circles represent performance when observers perform only one task and produce only one response (single-task). Filled circles show performance when observers attempt to combine both tasks (double-task). In all cases, double-task performance is characterized by a linear trade-off between tasks: better performance of one task comes at the expense of worse performance of the other. The critical finding is that when either task is performed at its best, performance of the other is reduced to chance. In other words, each task is impossible when attention is fully focused on the other, implying that attention makes a qualitative difference in the perception of the attributes in question.

In view of this rather extreme outcome, the question arises of whether the results are specific to combinations of *similar* discriminations (i.e., form–form, color–color, or motion–motion), or whether they would be the same for combinations of *dissimilar* discriminations (i.e., color–form, color–motion, motion–form, or motion–color). To address this question, we repeated the experiment with four further task combinations. Because all three types of central discriminations produced comparable psychometric functions (i.e., similar performance at all presentation times or SOAs), they were readily interchangeable. The same was true for the three types of peripheral discriminations. The results for combined color–form, color–motion, motion–form, and motion–color discrimination are shown in figure 11.2. As before, double-task performance was characterized by a linear trade-off, and optimal performance of one task entailed chance performance on the other. The fact that the outcome of these experiments is the same no matter how attention is engaged (i.e., which concurrent discrimination is used) shows that different visual discriminations engage visual attention to the same extent. Thus, visual attention can be considered a unitary process. As an aside, we note that a concurrent *auditory* discrimination would *not* have engaged visual attention in this way (Lee et al., 1995; Duncan et al., 1997). Therefore, the fact that attention is a unitary

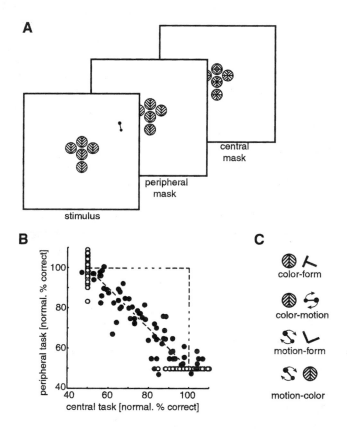

**Figure 11.2**
Concurrent tasks involving dissimilar features. (*A*) Sequence of stimulus, peripheral mask, and central mask displays (schematic, not to scale). The stimulus contains five central targets and one peripheral target. (*B*) Performance of central and peripheral tasks alone (single-task, open circles) and together (double-task, filled circles). Results for two observers (13,200 trials total). Performance is normalized such that each task by itself is performed at 100% correct. (*C*) Alternative task combinations. Observers discriminate either color and form, color and motion, motion and form, or motion and color.

process within the visual modality does not imply that the same is true across other sensory modalities.

## 11.3 Ambient Vision

Not every visual discrimination resembles those of the previous section and displays the same high degree of dependence on attention. Intuitively, it seems obvious that the richness of visual experience does not derive exclusively from a narrow focus of visual attention, but also includes a simultaneous awareness of poorly attended parts of visual space. The psychophysical results summarized below show that focusing attention narrowly on one location reduces, but does not eliminate, visual performance with respect to other locations in a visual scene. Thus it appears that observers enjoy a significant visual awareness of poorly attended stimuli, especially when these are salient and pop out from the scene. We propose the term "ambient vision" to describe this visual performance with respect to poorly attended but salient stimuli. As we shall see, ambient vision is robust and supports performance levels far above chance. In other words, there is nothing subliminal or implicit about ambient vision, at least in trained observers (see below).

In order to study ambient vision, one has to induce observers to focus attention on one part of the display, and thus at least partially withdraw attention from other parts of the display. In addition, one has to be able to verify that attention was indeed distributed in this unequal way, at least for a certain amount of time. Much ink has been spilled over the question of whether a stimulus can ever be *completely* unattended, especially when it involves a sudden visual onset, or is expected by the observer, or is the target of an observer response. Here we sidestep this issue and assume only quantitative (rather than qualitative) differences of attention. It should be understood, however, that this cautious position reflects the methodological limitations of psychophysics, not necessarily the underlying neural reality.

We manipulate the observer's distribution of attention with the same concurrent-task paradigm used in the previous section. Typically, observers view displays composed of two parts that pose two independent visual tasks, and perform either one task or the other, or both (depending on instructions). The objective is to determine the extent to which one part of the display can still be discriminated when attention focuses on the other. The results of the previous section show that such a highly unequal allocation of attention can be achieved reliably. Another crucial aspect of this paradigm is that the eyes remain fixated at the center of the display at all times. This ensures that the physical stimulus is the same, no matter which task or tasks are being performed.

A typical experiment is illustrated in figure 11.3A (Braun and Julesz, 1998). The *central task* requires discriminating whether five central elements are the same (five Ts or five Ls) or different (four Ts and one L, or four Ls and one T). The periphery of the display is covered by a dense texture of Gabor elements (background elements). A single peripheral target element appears briefly at varying locations of 4.3° eccentricity, either above or below the midline, and observers report whether the target had been in the upper or lower display half. The performance of this *peripheral task* depends on the orientation difference between target and background elements. When this difference is reduced from 45° to 15°, performance decreases substantially (d' falls by an order of

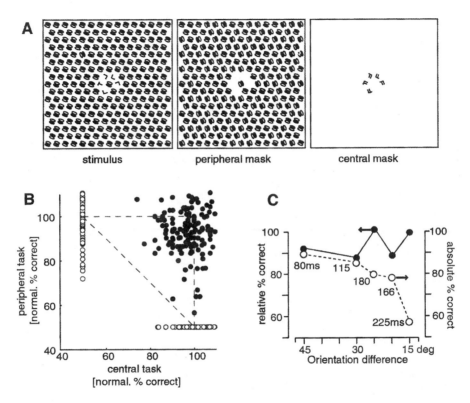

**Figure 11.3**
Evidence for ambient vision: pop-out localization. (*A*) Display sequence (schematic) including stimulus, peripheral mask, and central mask. The stimulus contains five central targets (Ts and Ls) and one peripheral target
(upper left quadrant), as well as numerous background elements. Observers report whether the central targets
are the "same" or "different" and, independently, whether the peripheral target appears in the upper or lower
half of the display. In the actual display, the peripheral target "pops out" from the background. (*B*) Central
and peripheral task performance of individual blocks of trials in which each task is performed by itself (single-
task, open circles) or both tasks are performed together (double-task, filled circles). Results for six observers
and various degrees of difficulty of the peripheral task (orientation difference 15°, 20°, 25°, 30°, and 45°; 27,000
trials total). Performance is normalized such that each task by itself is performed at 100% correct. Chance
performance is 50% correct. (*C*) Double-task performance of the peripheral task in absolute numbers (% correct,
filled circles) and relative to single-task performance (normalized % correct, open circles).

magnitude). In other words, far from being trivial, this peripheral task can be quite ''difficult,'' in fact, just as difficult as the attention-demanding peripheral tasks of the previous section.

Figure 11.3B shows the results of individual blocks of 100 trials for various observer instructions. Open dots represent performance when observers perform only one task and produce only one response (single-task). Closed dots represent performance when observers perform both tasks and give two independent responses (double-task). Performance is given as ''nominal % correct,'' which compensates for any differences in absolute performance, and reflects only the relative difference between single- and double-task performance (as explained in the caption of figure 11.3B). Although performance varies considerably between individual blocks of trials, the overall pattern is clear: both tasks are performed about comparably well together and alone. As far as the central task is concerned, this simply reflects the fact that observers treated it as the primary task, and focused attention on the central targets under both single- and double-task conditions. In the case of the peripheral task, however, this outcome is far from trivial, for it implies that peripheral targets were readily perceived even when attention was focused on the central targets. Note that the outcome does not depend on the absolute performance of the peripheral task, so that even barely detectable peripheral targets continue to be (barely) detected when attention is focused elsewhere (figure 11.3C).

To further investigate ambient vision, we combined the same central task with a variety of other peripheral tasks (Braun and Julesz, 1998). One goal was to ascertain whether observers are able to discriminate elementary stimulus attributes such as contrast, color, orientation, and spatial frequency in poorly attended parts of the display. Another goal was to determine whether ambient vision lives up to its name and extends to multiple stimuli at different locations. An experiment that is relevant to both issues is illustrated in figure 11.4A. Here the peripheral task involves two chromatic target elements embedded in a texture consisting of isoluminant but achromatic background elements. The targets again appear at 4.3° eccentricity, one in the upper half and the other in the lower half of the display. Observers must independently report the hue of both the upper (pink/orange) and lower (green/turqoise) target element. The difference between hues is subtle, and all chromatic targets are equally detectable in this background, so that hues cannot be distinguished on the basis of differential salience. The results are shown in figure 11.4B. Both peripheral hue discriminations are carried out well above chance, even in the triple-task situation in which attention focuses fully on the central task. This shows that observers are able to discriminate the hues of poorly attended targets at two separate locations of the display. Analogous experiments support similar conclusions with respect to the discrimination of other elementary stimulus attributes, such as contrast, orientation, and spatial frequency (Braun and Julesz, 1998; Lee et al., 1999).

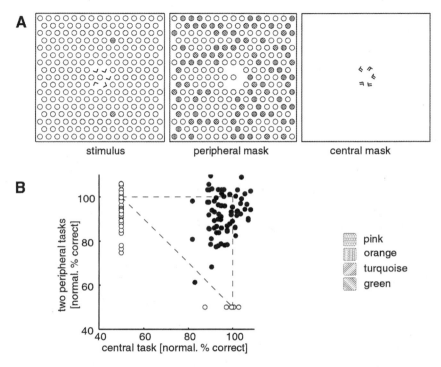

**Figure 11.4**
Hue discrimination with ambient vision. (*A*) Display sequence (schematic): stimulus, peripheral mask, and central mask. The stimulus contains five central targets (Ts or Ls) and two peripheral targets (upper half and lower half), as well as background elements. Observers independently discriminate the hue of each peripheral target (pink/orange and green/turqoise). (*B*) Performance of central and peripheral tasks alone (single-task, open circles), and central and peripheral tasks together (double-task, filled circles). Results for two observers and two degrees of difficulty of the peripheral task (7,100 trials total). Performance is normalized such that each task by itself is performed at 100% correct.

To illustrate the general validity of this conclusion, we mention one further experiment of this kind (figure 11.5). This experiment once again combines the central task with two peripheral targets, but this time the peripheral targets have two different orientations and four different colors. To simplify responses, observers report a particular combination of orientation and color by means of a memorized nickname (figure 11.5A). Observers readily report both attributes of both peripheral targets, even when these are poorly attended (because attention is engaged by the central task) (figure 11.5B). The point to emphasize is not that performance with poor attention is *identical* to that with full attention (which, as we shall see, it is not), but that performance with poor attention is far *above chance*. The results of this experiment show a significant effect of response order, in that performance

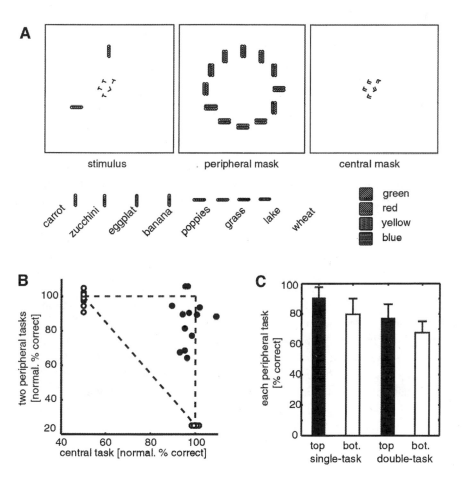

**Figure 11.5**

Object identification with ambient vision. (*A*) Display sequence (schematic): stimulus, peripheral mask, and central mask. The stimulus contains five central targets (Ts or Ls) and two peripheral targets, each of which is oriented horizontally or vertically, and colored red, green, blue, or yellow. Observers report the orientation and color of peripheral targets with the help of memorized nicknames. (*B*) Performance of central and peripheral tasks alone (single-task, open circles), together (double-task, filled circles). Results for three observers (3,700 trials total). Performance is normalized such that each task by itself is performed at 100% correct. Peripheral chance performance is 12.5% correct. (*C*) Effect of response order. Performance is consistently higher on the first-reported (top) than on the second-reported (bottom) peripheral target.

on the first-reported peripheral target is significantly superior to that on the second-reported target (figure 11.5C). Presumably, this difference reflects the difficulty of holding information about multiple targets in short-term memory, from the time at which the display is masked to the time at which a manual response can be made.

The experiments described above represent a small cross section of the cumulative evidence for ambient vision (Braun and Sagi, 1990, 1991; Ben-Av et al., 1992; Braun, 1993, 1994, 1998; Braun and Koch, 1995; Braun and Julesz, 1998). Collectively, these findings establish that visual perception derives from both fully attended and poorly attended parts of a visual scene. It goes without saying that the perception of fully attended stimuli is very different from, and far richer than, that of poorly attended ones. Indeed, the perceptual difference between poor and full attention is precisely what interests us (see next two sections). In the present context, the importance of ambient vision lies less in whatever role it may play in everyday vision (although this may well be substantial) than in its giving us psychophysical access to visual processing in the absence (or near absence) of attention. If it were not for ambient vision, all psychophysical experiments with voluntary reports would necessarily concern attentive vision. In short, ambient vision provides a psychophysical equivalent to recording from a single unit while the animal directs attention away from the receptive field.

A final point may be in order on whether our conclusions depend on the method by which attention is engaged. It has been suggested that ambient vision disappears when attention is engaged with the help of an attentional blink paradigm (Joseph et al., 1997). The idea was that an attentional blink may engage attention more completely than the concurrent tasks used in the present experiments. However, a direct comparison of the attentional-blink and concurrent-task situations shows that the two paradigms produce identical results, as long as one distinguishes between novice (<500 trials), trained (>2000 trials), and expert (<500 trials but prior experience from unrelated experiments) observer populations (Braun, 1998). Thus, the ambient vision of trained and expert observers proves robust, no matter how attention is engaged and no matter how high the concurrent attentional demands are raised.

## 11.4 Qualitative Difference Between Attentive and Ambient Vision

The two preceding sections described visual discriminations that cannot be performed at all (section 11.2) or are performed rather well (section 11.3) with poor attention. Although intermediate outcomes are of course possible, it is instructive to focus on the extremes of the range. Figure 11.6 juxtaposes discriminations requiring full attention (T- or L-shape, color order of two-colored disks, clockwise or counterclockwise rotation) with those re-

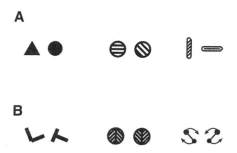

**Figure 11.6**
Attentional requirements of various discrimination tasks. (*A*) Discrimination of simple shapes (e.g., triangle/ circle), target hue (e.g., pink/orange), and object identity (e.g., orientation and color) is readily possible with ambient vision. (*B*) Discrimination of letter shape, color configuration, and sense of rotation requires attentive vision. These results suggest that a task requires attention when it involves discriminating the precise spatial relationship of more elementary features.

quiring little or no attention (triangular and circular form, orientation, color). What might distinguish the two types of discrimination? As mentioned before, the difference certainly does not lie in the psychometric function (i.e., how easy or difficult a particular discrimination is at any given presentation time). An obvious alternative possibility is that attention-demanding discriminations, though not necessarily more difficult, are somehow more complex in nature. However, as we saw in section 11.3, even discriminations that do not demand attention can be complex enough to involve several independent decisions (figure 11.5). Thus, a rather specific kind of complexity seems to be required to generate high attentional demand.

From the evidence gathered so far, it would seem that attentional demands arise whenever a task involves discriminating the *relative position* of more elementary attributes. For example, the T/L task requires discriminating the relative position of two line elements, the two-color-disk task hinges on the relative position of the two colors, and the sense-of-rotation task involves discriminating the relative positions of two dots moving in opposite directions. For the reasons mentioned, the demand for attention does not seem to arise from the fact that each of these tasks involves two components (line elements, colored half-disks, dots in opponent motion). Rather, attention seems required to know the relative position of the two components.

This interpretation is consistent with the recent finding that neural responses in visual cortical area V4 are modulated by attention in such a way that they "carry information about the spatial relationship between visual stimuli and [the focus of] attention" (Connor et al., 1996; Salinas and Abbott, 1997). These single-unit results further strengthen the hypothesis that the relative spatial position of stimulus attributes remains ill-defined unless and until visual attention focuses in the vicinity. The intimate connection between attention and relative spatial position proposed here is also consistent with the large body of work by Treisman and others on visual search (e.g., Treisman, 1993). One of the central tenets of Treisman's influential feature-integration theory is that attention is required to link attributes (color, orientation, etc.) to a particular spatial location. We reach similar conclusions based on rather different experimental methods.

## 11.5 Quantitative Differences Between Attentive and Ambient Vision

In section 11.3, we saw that shifting attention away from a visual stimulus does not completely eliminate visual performance, and interpreted this observation in terms of ambient vision. We now take a closer look at the discrimination of elementary stimulus attributes such as contrast, orientation, and spatial frequency under these conditions (Lee et al., 1999). The behavioral thresholds for these stimulus attributes collectively characterize spatial vision. Our goal is to compare and contrast behavioral thresholds with ambient vision and poor attention, on the one hand, and with normal vision and full attention, on the other. This comparison should reveal in detail how attention alters the early levels of processing that underlie spatial vision.

To establish thresholds when stimuli are poorly attended, we once again used a concurrent-task paradigm (figure 11.7). In the double-task situation, observers focus attention near fixation in order to perform a central task (i.e., report whether the five central targets are the "same" or "different"), which they are instructed to treat as their primary task. Thus, little or no attention remains for peripheral stimuli (see section 11.2). Nevertheless, practiced observers reliably perform a secondary task with respect to a peripheral target, especially when the display is uncluttered and the target in question is visually salient (double-task thresholds). In the single-task situation, observers view the same display (with identical eye fixation) but ignore the central task. In this situation, attention is free to focus on the peripheral task (single-task thresholds). The comparison of single- and double-task thresholds reveals if and how attention alters spatial vision.

We conducted five separate experiments to compare thresholds under single- and double-task conditions (figure 11.8A–E). When peripheral targets are fully attended, contrast detection thresholds (zero mask contrast) are about 20% lower and contrast discrimination thresholds (mask contrast greater than zero) are about 40–50% lower than when peripheral targets are poorly attended (figure 11.8A). In addition, the *decrease* of the discrimination threshold as mask contrast increases from zero (the well-known "dipper") is evident only when targets are fully attended. Note that the target position varies from

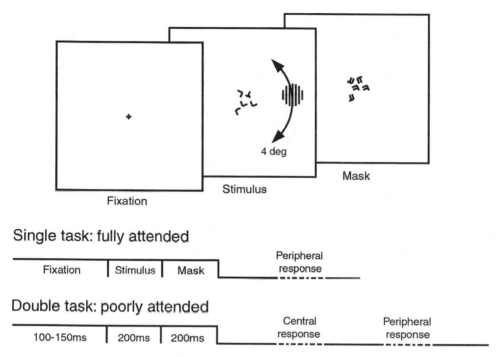

Single task: fully attended

Double task: poorly attended

**Figure 11.7**
Spatial vision thresholds measured with either full or poor attention. (*Top*) Sequence of fixation, stimulus, and mask displays (schematic). The stimulus contains five central targets (Ts or Ls) and one peripheral target. With respect to the peripheral target, observers perform a threshold judgment (see figure 11.8), and thresholds are determined with an adaptive staircase procedure. (*Middle*) Single-task (peripheral target fully attended): observers fixate the center but respond only to the peripheral target. (*Bottom*) Double-task (peripheral target poorly attended): observers fixate the center and respond to both tasks, treating the central task as their primary task.

trial to trial (in order to forestall eye movements) and that positional uncertainty of this kind is known to reduce the dipper. Therefore, our data may well underestimate the true depth of the dipper.

The effects of attention on spatial frequency and orientation discrimination are even more pronounced (figure 11.8B, C). Spatial frequency thresholds are about 60% lower and orientation thresholds are about 70% lower when peripheral targets are fully attended, compared to when they are poorly attended. Both types of thresholds remain essentially constant for contrast values above 20%. Although this is typical for orientation and spatial frequency thresholds, it is quite unlike the behavior of contrast discrimination thresholds, which continue to improve markedly with increasing stimulus contrast.

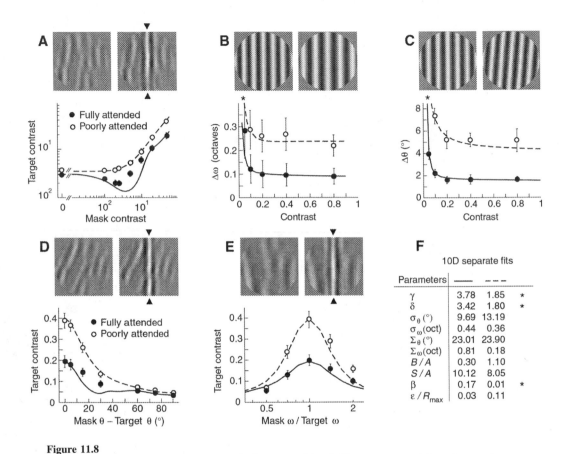

**Figure 11.8**
Single- and double-task thresholds compared. Five types of thresholds were measured. In each case, observers discriminated between two forms of the peripheral (4° eccentricity) target. Filled and open symbols represent fully attended (single-task) and poorly attended (double-task) thresholds, respectively (mean and standard error of two observers). Solid and dashed curves represent the corresponding model predictions. (A) Contrast detection and discrimination: Observers report the presence (arrows) or absence of a vertical target stripe on a circular masking pattern (contrast range 0.0–0.5). (B, C) Spatial frequency and orientation discrimination: Observers report whether a circular target grating (contrast 0.2–0.8) exhibits higher or lower spatial frequency (B), or whether its orientation is vertical or tilted clockwise (C). (D, E) Orientation and spatial frequency masking: Observers report the presence (arrows) or absence of a vertical target stripe on circular masking patterns (contrast 0.5) of different orientation (difference range 0° to 90°, in D) or different spatial frequency (difference range −1 to +1 oct, (E). (F) Model parameters: Solid and dashed curves represent plausible fits computed separately for single- and double-task data, respectively (all ten parameters are permitted to differ). (*) indicates further data points off scale.

Interactions between superimposed stimuli of different orientation or spatial frequency (target and mask; figure 11.8D, E) also are altered by attention. When target and mask have similar orientation or spatial frequency, attention lowers the maximal threshold by about 50% (consistent with figure 11.8A, mask contrast 0.5). As target and mask become progressively more different, fully and poorly attended thresholds decrease toward the same baseline level. The baseline is comparable to thresholds without mask (figure 11.8A, mask contrast 0.0), indicating minimal interactions between targets and masks of very different orientation or spatial frequency.

Collectively, these observations reveal how attention affects the mechanisms underlying spatial vision. In the next section, we will present a computational model of bottom-up processing at or near the level of area V1 to fully interpret these findings. Even without such a model, however, we can draw some qualitative conclusions about the way in which attention appears to alter the neural representation of contrast, orientation, and spatial frequency. For example, attention evidently does not act primarily by reducing background noise. This follows from the data in figure 11.8A, which show that the smallest effects of attention are obtained for stimuli with the lowest contrast. A reduction of background noise would produce the opposite result, in that stimuli with the lowest contrast would exhibit the largest effects of attention.

Another qualitative conclusion concerns the contrast gain of the neural response. The data in figure 11.8A, D, and E show that attention reduces the threshold elevation caused by a superimposed mask by about 50%. The easiest way to account for the reduced threshold elevation is to postulate higher contrast gain, because this would increase the incremental response obtained when the target is added to the mask. A strong qualitative conclusion can also be drawn about the orientation- and spatial-frequency tuning of neural responses. The data in figure 11.8B and C show a substantial *vertical* shift in thresholds with attention. Since increased contrast gain can produce only a *horizontal* shift, it follows that attention *also* sharpens the tuning for orientation and spatial frequency. Finally, the data in figure 11.8D and E suggest that the range of orientation and spatial frequency over which differently tuned mechanisms interact is fairly constant with attention. This is implied by the fact that threshold elevation retains the same *relative* size with both full and poor attention, no matter how similar or different the orientation and spatial frequency of target and mask may be. If attention would produce a substantial change in the range of interactions, we would not expect this simple proportionality of the results.

## 11.6   Bottom-Up Model of Quantitative Attention Effects

Perceptual thresholds for stimulus contrast, orientation, and spatial frequency have been studied for several decades (Nachmias and Sansbury, 1974; Wilson, 1980; Legge and

Foley, 1980). Quantitative accounts of these spatial vision thresholds have become increasingly refined and usually involve a population of noisy filters tuned to different orientations and spatial frequencies. Typically, psychophysical models assume that individual filter responses are normalized relative to the total response of the local filter population, and for this purpose postulate divisive inhibition (Wilson and Humanski, 1993; Foley, 1994; Zenger and Sagi, 1996).

The presumed neural basis of spatial vision thresholds is neural responses at or near the level of area V1 (e.g., De Valois and De Valois, 1990; Geisler and Albrecht, 1997). These responses are thought to be shaped by recurrent iterations (Somers et al., 1995; Shapley and Sompolinsky, 1998) that seem to accomplish a response normalization consistent with divisive inhibition (Carandini and Heeger, 1994; Carandini et al., 1997). Thus, perceptual studies and single-unit recordings lead to essentially the same model of bottom-up processing at this level: divisive inhibition among a local population of filters (neurons) tuned to different orientations and spatial frequencies. In fact, the similarities between perceptual and neural models of bottom-up processing at this level go beyond overall architecture and extend to functionality. Thus, divisive inhibition reproduces the qualitative and quantitative effects of response normalization at both the perceptual and the neural level. This includes the initial decrease and later increase of contrast discrimination thresholds with increasing stimulus contrast (dipper function), the sharper tuning of responses to orientation and spatial frequency, and the relative constancy of orientation and spatial frequency tuning over a wide range of stimulus contrasts (Bowne, 1990; Somers et al., 1995).

Our model of bottom-up processing at or near the level of area V1 is similar to several others (Wilson and Humanski, 1993; Foley, 1994; Zenger and Sagi, 1996; Carandini et al., 1997) and comprises three stages: (1) a local population of filters responsive to different orientations and spatial frequencies at one visual location, (2) divisive inhibition within this population to carry out response normalization, and (3) an ideal observer decision that discriminates between stimulus alternatives on the basis of the maximum likelihood and is limited only by noise (figure 11.9).

The first stage of the model consists of a population of visual filters that are selective for stimuli of different orientations and spatial frequencies. The linear response $E_{\theta\omega}$ of such filters to a sinusoidal grating stimuli of contrast $c_s$, orientation $\theta_s$, and spatial frequency $\omega_s$ is given by

$$E_{\theta\omega} = A \, c_s \exp\left(\frac{(\theta - \theta_s)^2}{2\sigma_\theta^2}\right) \exp\left(\frac{(\omega - \omega_s)^2}{2\sigma_\omega^2}\right) + B. \tag{1}$$

Here, $A$ is the contrast gain, $B$ is the background activity, $\theta$ and $\omega$ are the preferred orientation and spatial frequency, and $\sigma_\theta$ and $\sigma_\omega$ are the sharpness of tuning. The response to

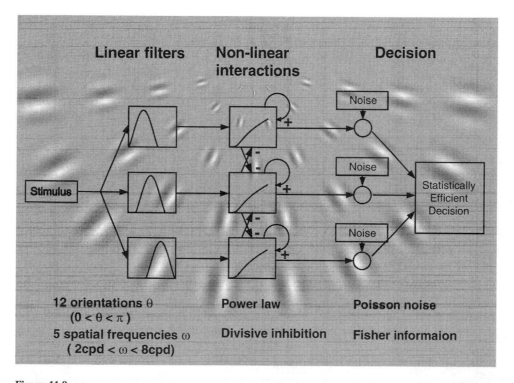

**Figure 11.9**
Computational model of spatial vision thresholds (schematic). At the first level, the stimulus is analyzed by a local population of independent and linear filters, tuned to different orientations $\theta_i$ and spatial frequencies $\omega_i$ (linear responses $E_{\theta\omega}$). Some of these linear filters are shown in the background. At the second level, filters interact via a power law and divisive inhibition (nonlinear responses $R_{\theta\omega}$). At the third level, noise is added to the nonlinear responses and thresholds are computed, assuming a statistically efficient decision (ideal observer).

stimuli other than sinusoidal gratings is obtained by applying appropriate corrective factors to $A$, $\sigma_\theta$ and $\sigma_\omega$.

The second stage of the model assumes that the linear filter responses interact so as to normalize individual responses relative to the filter population. Specifically, the nonlinear response $R_{\theta\omega}$ is obtained by subjecting the linear response $E_{\theta\omega}$ to a power law followed by divisive inhibition:

$$R_{\theta\omega} = \frac{(E_{\theta\omega})^\gamma}{S^\delta + \sum_{\theta'\omega'} W_{\theta\theta'\omega\omega'} (E_{\theta'\omega'})^\delta}. \tag{2}$$

The exponents $\gamma$ and $\delta$ are of particular consequence, inasmuch as they govern the strength of the interaction between filters, and their difference determines the saturation of responses at high contrast. The semisaturation constant, $S$, determines the response at low stimulus contrast. The distribution of weight factors, $W_{\theta\theta'\omega\omega'}$,

$$W_{\theta\theta'\omega\omega'} = \exp\left(-\frac{(\theta - \theta')^2}{2\Sigma_\theta^2}\right) \exp\left(-\frac{(\omega - \omega')^2}{2\Sigma_\omega^2}\right), \tag{3}$$

whose Gaussian widths are given by $\Sigma_\theta$ and $\Sigma_\omega$, determines whether the inhibitory pool includes the entire filter population or only filters tuned to similar orientations and spatial frequencies.

The third stage of the model discriminates between stimulus alternatives on the basis of the maximum likelihood of the nonlinear responses. The nonlinear responses $R_{\theta\omega}$ are assumed to be corrupted by Gaussian noise, the variance $V_{\theta\omega}^2$ of which increases with the mean response according to

$$V_{\theta\omega}^2 = \beta(R_{\theta\omega} + E), \tag{4}$$

where $\beta$ is the "light noise" and $\varepsilon$ is the "dark noise." This approximates the response variance of visual cortical neurons (e.g., Geisler and Albrecht, 1997). This corresponds to an ideal observer whose performance is limited only by the variance of the nonlinear responses. Further details about the decision stage can be found elsewhere (Itti et al., 1997).

When we fit this model (10 free parameters: $\gamma$, $\delta$, $\sigma_\theta$, $\sigma_\delta$, $\Sigma_\theta$, $\Sigma_\omega$, $\beta$, $\varepsilon$) separately to single- and double-task data, we obtain excellent agreement between predicted and observed threshold values (solid curves in figure 11.8A–D). Moreover, this agreement is obtained with physiologically plausible parameter values (figure 11.8F). Note in particular the realistic widths of filter tuning, with half-widths at half-maximum between 12° and 15° for orientation and 0.42$oct$ and 0.52$oct$ for spatial frequency—which compares to 20±9° and 0.76±0.30$oct$ for neurons in monkey visual cortex (Geisler and Albrecht, 1997)—and the distribution of the weights with which different filters contribute to divisive inhibition, with a half-width at half-maximum of approximately 28° for orientation and approximately 0.5$oct$ for spatial frequency.

To assess the significance of a change in a parameter value, we determined whether or not this change would degrade the overall quality of the fit by more than 10% (allowing the other nine parameters to assume their optimal values in each case). By this criterion, we found that only three parameters—the exponents $\gamma$ and $\delta$, and the light noise $\beta$— are significantly affected by attention. Further analysis showed that changes in only two parameters—the exponents $\gamma$ and $\delta$—account fully for the observed effects of attention. Specifically, good fits are obtained when attention is permitted to alter *only* the exponents $\gamma$ and $\delta$, and all other parameters remain unchanged (12-dimensional fit). As for the light noise $\beta$, our results are inclusive and neither rule out nor require that this parameter be changed by attention. Returning to the exponents $\gamma$ and $\delta$, we can say that an increase in value from approximately 1.8 to approximately 3.5 alters the effect of filter interactions from a very "soft" max-operation to an almost "hard" max-operation. In effect, larger exponents imply *intensified competition among visual filters.*

To summarize, a model of bottom-up processing allows us to interpret attentional changes in spatial vision thresholds. To a very good approximation, attention seems to alter exactly one aspect of bottom-up processing, the intensity of competition among visual filters.

This is illustrated in figure 11.10 (also plate 10), which shows how attention alters the response distribution across a population of filters tuned to different orientations. By intensifying competition, attention enhances relatively large responses and suppresses

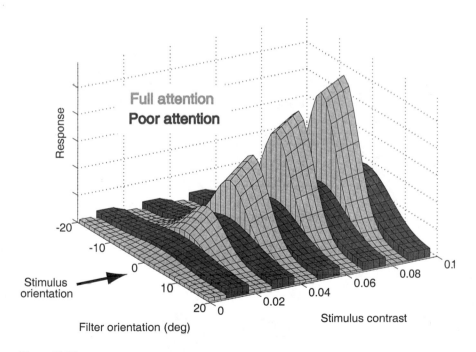

**Figure 11.10**
Attentional change in the response distribution. Nonlinear responses $R_{\theta\omega}$ of filters tuned to orientations between $-20°$ to $+20°$, with a grating stimulus of orientation $0°$ and contrasts between 0 and 5% (threshold regime). Responses to fully and poorly attended stimuli are represented by the red and blue surfaces, respectively (shown interleaved for clarity). By strengthening a winner-take-all competition among visual filters, attention emphasizes the filters that respond best to the stimulus at hand. This both increases the gain and sharpens the tuning of the filters in question. (See plate 10 for color version.)

relatively small ones, so that existing response differences are accentuated without changing qualitative aspects of the response distribution. As by-products of intensified competition, the contrast gain of the most responsive filters (neurons) increases approximately
threefold, and the orientation tuning sharpens by approximately 30%.

Perhaps the most surprising implication of these findings is that attention seems to be
*task-independent* and to alter bottom-up processing in the same manner during all five
investigated tasks. This is surprising because it appears to be far from optimal. Different
subsets of the filter population carry information about the contrast, orientation, or spatial
frequency of a given stimulus (figure 11.11), and consequently one might have expected
attention to emphasize the most informative subset of filters for each particular task. Instead, our results are consistent with the possibility that attention is unable to select an
appropriate subset of filters, and is restricted to selecting the entire filter population at the
attended location (i.e., an entire hypercolumn in neuronal terms).

If these inferences about the limitations of attention are correct, there should be a substantial downside to attention. In particular, the ability of attention to enhance perception
of more intense stimulus components should come at the expense of degrading the perception of less intense components. This is illustrated in figure 11.12 (also plate 11), which
shows responses to a composite stimulus with a low-contrast and a high-contrast component. Although the effect depends on the relative contrast and orientation of the two components, attention generally *suppresses* the response to the low-contrast component. Thus,

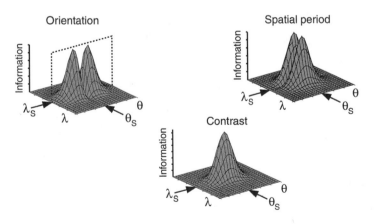

**Figure 11.11**
Fisher information with respect to each attribute is shown as a function of filter orientation $\theta$ and spatial period
$\omega$ (see also Pouget et al., chapter 13 in this volume). The stimulus pattern has orientation $\theta_s$ and spatial period
$\omega_s$. Information about stimulus orientation, spatial period, and contrast is carried by different subpopulations of
filters. This implies that the effect of attention would have to be task-dependent in order to be optimal.

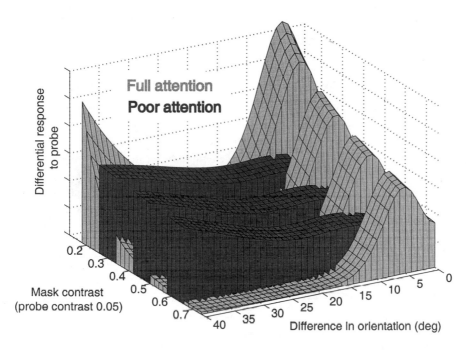

**Figure 11.12**
Attentional change in the response to a weak stimulus component. Incremental response $\Delta R_{\theta\omega}$ of the filter tuned optimally to a weaker stimulus component ("probe," orientation 0°, contrast 0.05), in the presence of a superimposed stronger stimulus component ("mask," orientation 0° between 40°, contrast between 0.1 and 0.75). Response values are given in multiples of the response without mask. For many mask parameters, attention *reduces* the incremental response. This predicts that attention can be counterproductive (i.e., lowers performance of tasks concerning the weaker stimulus component). (See plate 11 for color version.)

our model predicts a wide range of situations in which attention should adversely affect perception (see also Yeshurun and Carrasco, 1998).

## 11.7   Discussion

Although attention undoubtedly exercises a profound influence over visual perception, it is not equally important to all aspects of visual performance. This is demonstrated by concurrent-task experiments, in which observers focus attention on one part of the display and leave other parts of the display unattended or poorly attended. For example, visual discriminations of elementary stimulus attributes such as contrast, orientation, spatial frequency, and color are readily performed even in unattended or poorly attended parts of the display. On the other hand, more complex discriminations, especially those involving spatial relationships, are performed well only with full attention. Contrary to a widely held belief, the extent to which a visual discrimination depends on attention is unrelated to task difficulty. In other words, discriminations with comparable psychometric functions (e.g., performance as a function of stimulus presentation time) may exhibit wildly different requirements for attention.

These results suggest that phenomenal visual experience derives from two sources, one that depends critically on attention (attentive vision) and another that does not (ambient vision). Ambient vision is limited in scope, and provides information only about the salient stimuli of a display and, furthermore, only about elementary attributes of such stimuli. Nevertheless, a wide range of demanding visual discriminations are readily possible on the basis of ambient vision. Thus, there is nothing subliminal or implicit about ambient vision.

Attention enhances and augments ambient vision in both qualitative and quantitative ways. The multiplicity of the perceptual consequences of attention may reflect multilevel selection, that is, the observation that potentially attention can modulate all levels of visual cortex. An important *qualitative* contribution of attention is the discrimination of spatial relationships. Discriminations involving relative position (e.g., green–red vs. red–green, T vs. L) require full attention and are performed at chance when attention is focused elsewhere in the display. These results are consistent with ''feature-integration theory,'' according to which attention associates stimulus attributes and stimulus location (Treisman, 1993). The neural basis of this aspect of attention remains unclear, although some single-unit results suggest that neurons in area V4 encode the spatial relationship between a visual stimulus and the focus of attention (Connor et al., 1996). How attention might enable visual cortex to represent spatial relationships is illustrated by a computational model of attentional gain fields (Salinas and Abbott, 1997).

The *quantitative* effects of attention are evident in visual thresholds for elementary stimulus attributes (i.e., attributes that are discriminable with both attentive and ambient vision). In detailed psychophysical measurements, we characterized how attention alters visual thresholds for contrast, orientation, and spatial frequency. These spatial vision thresholds are thought to reflect processing at or near the level of area V1 and can be modeled in terms of bottom-up interactions among filters (neurons) with overlapping receptive fields. The effect of these interactions is to normalize the response of each filter (neuron) relative to the total response of the population. The threshold changes we observe are consistent with the possibility that attention alters one particular aspect of bottom-up processing, namely, that it accentuates response differences by intensifying competition among a local population of filters. Surprisingly, the effect of attention appears to be the same in all five tasks investigated, which implies that attention does not optimize processing according to the requirements of each particular task. Although the general effect of attention—accentuation of response differences—is beneficial for most tasks (i.e., lowers thresholds), it is expected to be harmful for many others (i.e., to raise thresholds). In particular, tasks involving the discrimination of the weaker components in multicomponent displays should be harmed by attention. The overriding conclusion, however, is that the effect of attention at or near the level of area V1 is best described as a modulation of bottom-up processing.

In summary, we have characterized the perceptual consequences of attention by using concurrent-task psychophysics. We find that attention alters perception in several qualitative and quantitative ways. This is consistent with a hierarchical theory of attention in which selection takes place at multiple processing levels, each of which accounts for some of the perceptual consequences of attention. We further find that attention is unable to fully optimize processing for different visual tasks, and appears to be constrained by the architecture of bottom-up processing. This is also consistent with the notion that attention modulates multiple levels of bottom-up processing. We further believe that the combination of psychophysics and computational modeling can contribute significantly to our understanding of visual attention and its neural substrate.

## Acknowledgment

This research was supported by NIMH, NSF, NSF-ERC for Neuromorphic Engineering, the Office of Naval Research, and the Institute of Neuroinformatics at the ETH Zürich.

## References

Ben-Av, M. B., Sagi, D., and Braun, J. (1992). Visual attention and perceptual grouping. *Percep. Psychophys.*, 52: 277–294.

Bowne, S. F. (1990). Contrast discrimination cannot explain spatial frequency, orientation or temporal frequency discrimination. *Vis. Res.* 30: 449–461.

Braun, J. (1993). Shape-from-shading is independent of visual attention and may be a "texton". *Spatial Vis.* 7: 311–322.

Braun, J. (1994). Visual search among items of different salience: Removal of visual attention mimics a lesion in extrastriate area V4. *J. Neurosci.* 14: 554–567.

Braun, J. (1998). Vision and attention: The role of training. *Nature* 393: 424–425.

Braun, J., and Julesz, B. (1998). Withdrawing attention at little or no cost: Detection and discrimination tasks. *Percep. Psychophys.* 60: 1–23.

Braun, J., and Koch, C. (1995). Stimulus competition and nonattentive selection: Interactions between motion and orientation contrasts. *Invest. Ophthalmol. Vis. Sci.* (supp.) 36: 3926.

Braun, J., and Sagi, D. (1990). Vision outside the focus of attention. *Percep. Psychophys.* 48: 45–58.

Braun, J., and Sagi, D. (1991). Texture-based tasks are little affected by second tasks requiring peripheral or central attentive fixation. *Perception* 20: 483–500.

Brefczynski, J. A., and DeYoe, E. A. (1999). A physiological correlate of the "spotlight" of visual attention. *Nature Neurosci.* 2: 370–374.

Carandini, M., and Heeger, D. J. (1994). Summation and division by neurons in primate visual cortex. *Science* 264: 1333–1336.

Carandini, M., Heeger, D. J., and Movshon, J. A. (1997). Linearity and normalization in simple cells of the macaque primary visual cortex. *J. Neurosci.* 17: 8621–8644.

Connor, C. E., Gallant, J. L., Preddie, D. C., and Van Essen, D. C. (1996). Responses in area V4 depend on the spatial relationship between stimulus and attention. *J. Neurophysiol.* 75: 1306–1308.

De Valois, R. L., and De Valois, K. K. (1990). *Spatial vision.* New York: Oxford University Press.

Duncan, J. (1984). Selective attention and the organization of visual information. *J. Exp. Psychol. Gen.* 113: 501–517.

Duncan, J., Martens, S., and Ward, R. (1997). Restricted attentional capacity within but not between sensory modalities. *Nature* 387: 808–810.

Duncan, J., Ward, R., and Shapiro, K. (1994). Direct measurement of attentional dwell time in human vision. *Nature* 369: 313–315.

Foley, J. M. (1994). Human luminance pattern-vision mechanisms: Masking experiments require a new model. *J. Optical Soc. America* A11: 1710–1719.

Geisler, W. S., and Albrecht, D. G. (1997). Visual cortex neurons in monkeys and cats: Detection, discrimination, and identification. *Vis. Neurosci.* 14: 897–919.

Helmholtz, H. (1850/1962). In J. P. C. Southall (ed.), *Handbuch der physiologischen Optik.* New York: Dover. (First published 1850.)

Ito, M., and Gilbert, C. D. (1999). Attention modulates contextual influences in the primary visual cortex of alert monkeys. *Neuron* 22: 593–604.

Itti, L., Braun, J., Lee, D. K., and Koch, C. (1997). A model of early visual processing. In M. C. Mozer, M. I. Jordan, and T. Petsche (eds.), *Advances in neural information processing systems,* vol 9 (pp. 173–179). Cambridge, MA: MIT Press.

James, W. (1890/1981). *The principles of psychology.* Cambridge, MA: Harvard University Press. (First published 1890.)

Joseph, J. S., Chun, M. M., and Nakayama, K. (1997). Attentional requirements in a "preattentive" feature search task. *Nature* 387: 805–807.

Lee, D. K., Itti, L., Koch, C., and Braun, J. (1999). Attention activates winner-take-all competition among visual filters. *Nature Neurosci.* 2: 375–381.

Lee, D. K., Koch, C., and Braun, J. (1995). Visual tracking of multiple moving objects requires modality-specific attention. *Invest. Ophthalmol. Vis. Sci.* (supp.) 36: 4133.

Lee, D. K., Koch, C., and Braun, J. (1999). Visual attention is undifferentiated: Concurrent discrimination of form, color, and motion. *Percep. Psychophys.* 61: 1241–1255.

Legge, G. E., and Foley, J. M. (1980). Contrast masking in human vision. *J. Optical Soc. America* 70: 1458–1471.

Luck, S. J., Chelazzi, L., Hillyard, S. A., and Desimone, R. (1997). Neuronal mechanisms of spatial selective attention in areas V1, V2, and V4 of macaque visual cortex. *J. Neurophysiol.* 77: 24–42.

Moran, A. J., and Desimone, R. (1985). Selective attention gates visual processing in the extrastriate cortex. *Science* 229: 782–784.

Motter, B. C. (1993). Focal attention produces spatially selective processing in visual cortical areas V1, V2, and V4 in the presence of competing stimuli. *J. Neurophysiol. 70: 909–919.*

Nachmias, J., and Sansbury, R. V. (1974). Letter. Grating contrast: Discrimination may be better than detection. *Vis. Res.* 14: 1039–1042.

Nakayama, K., and Mackeben, M. (1989). Sustained and transient components of focal visual attention. *Vis. Res.* 29: 1631–1647.

Neisser, U. (1967). *Cognitive psychology.* New York: Appleton-Century-Crofts.

O'Craven, K. M., Downing, E., and Kanwisher, N. G. (1999). fMRI evidence for objects as the units of attentional selection. *Nature* 401: 584–587.

Olshausen, B. A., Anderson, C. H., and Van Essen, D. C. (1995). A multiscale dynamic routing circuit for forming size- and position-invariant object representations. *J. Comput. Neurosci.* 2: 45–62.

Roelfsema, P. R., Lamme, V. A., and Spekreijse, H. (1998). Object-based attention in the primary visual cortex of the macaque monkey. *Nature* 395: 376–381.

Salinas, E., and Abbott, L. F. (1997). Invariant visual responses from attentional gain fields. *J. Neurophysiol.* 77: 3267–3272.

Shapley, R., and Sompolinsky, H. (1998). Orientation tuning in striate cortex. *Curr. Opin. Neurobiol.* 38: 743–761.

Somers, D. C., Nelson, S. B., and Sur, M. (1995). An emergent model of orientation selectivity in cat visual cortical simple cells. *J. Neurosci.* 15: 5448–5465.

Sperling, G., and Dosher, B. (1986). Strategy and optimization in human information processing. In K. Boff, L. Kaufman, and J. Thomas (eds.), *Handbook of perception and performance,* vol. 1 (pp. 1–65). New York: Wiley.

Sperling, G., and Melchner, M. J. (1978). The attention operating characteristic: Some examples from visual search. *Science* 202: 315–318.

Treisman, A. (1993). The perception of features and objects. In A. Baddeley and L. Weiskrantz (eds.), *Attention: Selection, awareness, and control* (pp. 1–35). Oxford: Clarendon Press.

Treue, S., and Maunsell, J. H. R. (1996). Attentional modulation of visual motion processing in cortical areas MT and MST. *Nature* 382: 539–541.

Tsotsos, J. K. (1990). A complexity level analysis of vision. *Behav. Brain Sci.,* 13: 423–455.

Wilson, H. R. (1980). A transducer function for threshold and suprathreshold human vision. *Biol. Cybern.* 38: 171–178.

Wilson, H. R., and Humanski, R. (1993). Spatial frequency adaptation and contrast gain control. *Vis. Res.* 33: 1133–1149.

Yeshurun, Y., and Carrasco, M. (1998). Attention improves or impairs visual performance by enhancing visual resolution. *Nature* 396: 72–75.

Zenger, B., and Sagi, D. (1996). Isolating excitatory and inhibitory nonlinear spatial interactions involved in contrast detection. *Vis. Res.* 36: 2497–2513.

# 12 The Resolution of Ambiguous Motion: Attentional Modulation and Development

Shinsuke Shimojo, Katsumi Watanabe, and Christian Scheier

## 12.1 Introduction

Two identical visual targets moving across each other can be perceived in two ways: they either bounce off or stream through each other (figure 12.1; Metzger, 1934). In spite of this theoretical ambiguity, the perception is typically not ambiguous: observers usually have a strong bias to see the streaming percept (Goldberg and Pomerantz, 1982; Bertenthal and Kramer, 1988; Bertenthal et al., 1993). This is equally true whether the two targets move on a plane (i.e., on paths that cross each other like an X) or on a line (i.e., directly toward each other).

The streaming/bouncing ambiguous motion phenomenon is often considered to be the result of local motion integration (Bertenthal and Kramer, 1988; Bertenthal et al., 1993; Sekuler et al., 1995; Gorea and Labarre, 1997a, 1997b). The basic account along this line is that cooperative interactions among local motion detectors favor continued motion and bias perception toward streaming (temporal integration or temporal recruitment; Lappin and Bell, 1976; Nakayama and Silverman, 1984; McKee and Welch, 1985; Anstis and Ramachandran, 1986; Casco and Morgan, 1987; Bowne et al., 1989; Snowden and Braddick, 1989a, 1989b; 1991; Zanker, 1992; Watamaniuk et al., 1995). The temporal recruitment hypothesis is consistent with the observation that a brief pause (15–45 ms) at the moment of coincidence tends to reverse the perceptual dominance (Berthental et al., 1993), so that the bounce percept becomes dominant. Presumably, the pause stops the recruitment process and the streaming perception is no longer facilitated.

Whereas the temporal recruitment hypothesis postulates integration of motion signals along a continuous trajectory, a set of independent studies demonstrates how attention can modulate motion perception. In fact, most ambiguous motion perceptions are known to be modulated (Ramachandran and Anstis, 1983; Gogel and Tietz, 1976; Gogel and MacCracken, 1979; Gogel and Sharkey, 1989; Chaudhuri, 1990; Hock and Balz, 1997), or even caused, by attention (Cavanagh, 1992; Hikosaka et al., 1993a, 1993b, 1996; Lu and Sperling, 1995a, 1995b). Thus, one may suspect that attention will also affect the bouncing/streaming perception.

Yet another intriguing aspect of the bouncing/streaming display is that it is also susceptible to nonvisual sensory inputs. For example, when a brief sound occurs at the moment of visual coincidence, the streaming percept no longer dominates, and the vast majority of observers report the bouncing event (Sekuler et al., 1997). However, when the sound is not synchronized with the visual coincidence by a margin larger than 150 or 250 ms, the bounce-inducing effect disappears.

In summary, it appears that temporal recruitment favors the streaming percept as long as recruitment is not disrupted by salient stimulus such as a pause or a synchronous sound. Thus we can use the streaming/bouncing display to explore visual–visual and visual–auditory interactions. Our working hypothesis is that the salient nature of a pause or a sound disrupts attentional processes that promote the streaming perception. This chapter summarizes our latest results along these lines.

In addition to generic perceptual processes such as recruitment, saliency, and attention, the stream/bounce percept may also reflect acquired knowledge about collision events in the real world. Real collisions tend to cause simultaneous visual and auditory events, and this might be used by cross-modal perceptual systems to disambiguate the bounce/stream percept. Under this associative learning hypothesis, the bounce percept would dominate whenever the situation resembles a real-world collision, rather than being governed by generic factors such as saliency or attention. Another implication of this hypothesis is that the bounce/stream percept of newborns or infants should differ from that of adults, because of their limited exposure to real-world collisions.

The first set of experiments reported below demonstrates that auditory context and saliency are crucial in determining the effect of a synchronous sound. The second set of experiments uses either exogenous or endogenous cues to draw attention away from the visual coincidence. The results show that reduced attention favors the bouncing percept, suggesting that the normal bias in favor of the streaming percept may reflect some forms of attentional processes. In the last part of this chapter, we report that there is a major difference between four-month-olds and six-month-olds in terms of perceiving the bounce/stream display in categorically different ways, depending on the relative timing of sound and collision. From at least the age of eight months, infants appear to have qualitatively the same bounce/stream percept as adults.

## 12.2   Effect of Auditory Context and Saliency

### 12.2.1   Background and Purpose

A single sound synchronized with the moving targets' coincidence leads to a bias toward bouncing perception, as already described (Sekuler et al., 1997). However, the underlying mechanism remains an open question.

In the reaction time literature on cross-modal interaction, cross-modal facilitation from the nontarget modality has been explained by either (a) energy (Reynolds, 1964) or probability summation (Raab, 1962), or (b) "preparation enhancement" (Nickerson, 1973). "Energy" refers to the strength of some neural signal; "probability summation," to the probability of making a particular response; and "preparation summation," to the fact that stimuli in various modalities can serve as a warning signal. Unfortunately, these accounts are specifically tailored to explain the shortening of reaction times, and do not explain the change from a streaming to a bouncing percept. Although it may be true that a sound increases arousal, alertness, or readiness, none of the hypotheses predict which percept—streaming or bouncing—will be facilitated.

So, what is so special about the sound synchronized with the visual coincidence? How could it bias the perception toward bouncing? As the initial step toward fully answering these questions, we raised an experimentally more feasible question, as follows: (a) What is the temporal range of audiovisual interaction? (b) Does the saliency of sound matter? Especially, does the saliency in temporal context of sound(s) matter?

### 12.2.2  General Methods

The visual stimulus was generated with a computer and presented on a CRT display, and was identical in experiments 1.1 and 1.2. Two disks appeared above a fixation cross, and moved laterally toward the center of the display, where they coincided, then reached the other end. In experiment 1.1 (*single/double sound*), either a single sound was presented at various onset times with regard to the visual coincidence (*single sound*), or an additional sound was presented either before or after the synchronized sound (*double sound*). The observers viewed the display and reported their percept by pressing appropriate keys in a two-alternative, forced-choice procedure: whether the targets appeared to stream through or to bounce against each other. (See figures 12.1 and 12.2.)

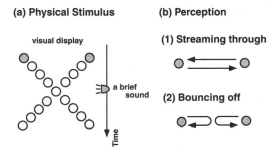

**Figure 12.1**
Ambiguous motion display for the "stream/bounce" percept. (*A*) Visual stimulus (schematic). Two objects appear at one side of the display and move with constant velocity toward the other side, crossing at the midline (visual coincidence). (*B*) Two possible percepts (schematic). Subjects perceive the two targets either as moving continuously and without interacting at the point of coincidence (streaming through), or as colliding and reversing their motion at the point of coincidence (bouncing off). Surprisingly, this visual percept is strongly influenced by sound: although normally the streaming percept is dominant, the bouncing percept dominates when a sound is synchronized with the visual coincidence.

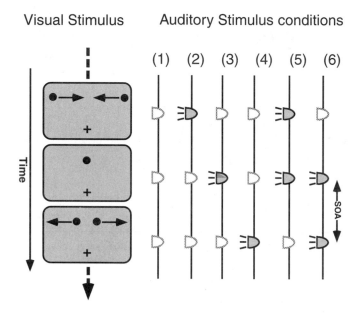

**Figure 12.2**
Single and double sound experiment (experiment 1.1). (*Left*) Time course of visual stimulation. In addition to a fixation cross, one target appeared on each side of the upper field, each moving smoothly toward the other side; they crossed at the midline (visual coincidence). Subjects reported whether targets appeared to "stream" through or "bounce" off each other. (*Right*) Time course of auditory stimulation. Six sound conditions were investigated, varying randomly from trial to trial: (1) no sound; one sound before (2), at (3), or after (4) the visual coincidence; two sounds before and at (5), or at and after (6) the visual coincidence. The display was presented on a computer screen in a dimmed room. The moving targets (diameter 0.13°) appeared 1.5° above fixation, with an initial separation of 3.3° and a velocity of 1.6°/s. Sound bursts were characterized by 1.8 kHz frequency, 3 ms duration, and 58 dB pressure.

In experiment 1.2 (*multiple sound*), the same tone burst was presented seven times, with the fourth one (i.e., the middle sound) synchronized to the visual coincidence. This middle sound was either the same as, or differed from, the other sounds in pitch or intensity. In addition, there were two further conditions: *no sound* and middle sound omitted (*sound omission*). Otherwise, the procedure was identical to that in experiment 1.1. (See figure 12.3.)

The same nine adult subjects participated in both experiments.

### 12.2.3  Results and Discussion

Figure 12.4A shows the results in the *no sound* and *single sound* conditions of experiment 1.1. The mean percentage of "bouncing" judgments is plotted against the timing of the sound with regard to the visual coincidence. As is obvious from the figure,

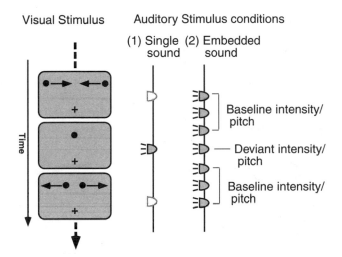

**Figure 12.3**
Multiple sound experiment (experiment 1.2). (*Left*) Time course of visual stimulation; note visual coincidence of moving targets (middle). Stimulus configuration and parameters were identical to experiment 1.1 (figure 12.2). (*Right*) Time course of auditory stimulation. In the single sound condition, a tone burst was precisely synchronized to the visual coincidence. In the embedded sound condition, six additional sound bursts were presented before and after the coincidence. These additional sounds could differ in pitch (higher, lower, or same) or intensity (higher, lower, or same) from the synchronized sound. Not shown are two further conditions: no sound and sound omitted (i.e., no synchronized sound). The parameters for each sound were identical to those in experiment 1.1, though the sequence of sounds was different. The tone burst was presented either once (single) or seven times (embedded), with the middle (i.e., the fourth) one always synchronized with the visual coincidence. This middle sound was either the same as, or differed from, all the other sounds in one of two features: (*A*) pitch (high, same, or low) or (*B*) intensity (high, same, or low). There were two additional conditions: no sound and sound omission (the fourth sound, at the synchronous position, was omitted).

the single sound has a strong effect of inducing the bounce percept, but only within a certain window around the time of visual coincidence. The size of this time window was from −250 ms to +150 ms, a range roughly consistent with previous findings (Sekuler et al., 1997). That this time window is rather narrow and includes times *after* the visual coincidence clearly argues against the idea of preparation enhancement. Figure 12.4B shows the results in the *double sound* conditions of experiment 1.1. Here, the mean percentage of "bouncing" judgments is plotted against the timing of the *asynchronous* sound with regard to the visual coincidence (and the onset of synchronous sound). There was only one dip in the curve (i.e., there was only one time period of significant attenuation of the bounce perception, which was from −450 to −250 ms. Thus, an additional sound presented about 300 ms before the synchronous sound significantly attenuated the bounce-inducing effect of the synchronous sound, but an additional sound afterward did not.

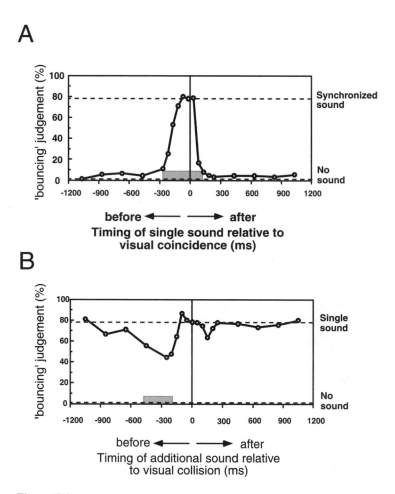

**Figure 12.4**
Results of single and double sound experiment (experiment 1.1; see also figure 12.2). Mean percentage of "bouncing" judgment as a function of sound timing, relative to the visual coincidence of the moving targets. (*A*) Single sound, presented at various times before and after the visual coincidence. A bounce percept is induced only during a relatively narrow time window around the visual coincidence (gray zone). Dashed lines indicate results for a precisely synchronized sound and no sound, respectively. (*B*) Double sound, one precisely synchronized to the visual coincidence and another presented at various times before and after the visual coincidence. The additional sound disrupts the bounce percept if presented shortly before the coincidence (gray zone). Dashed lines indicate results for a single sound and no sound.

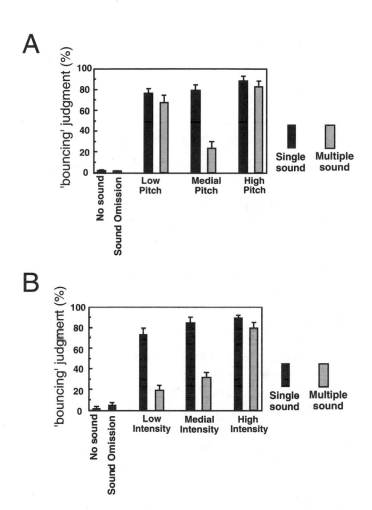

**Figure 12.5**
Results of multiple sound experiment (experiment 1.2; see also figure 12.3). Mean percentage of "bouncing" judgment and standard errors are plotted as a function of various conditions: no sound, sound omission, single sound, and multiple sound. (*A*) Effect of sound frequency (pitch). (*B*) Effect of sound intensity.

Figure 12.5A shows the effects of pitch change in experiment 1.2 (*multiple sound* experiment). They can be summarized as follows:

• *Single sound* always showed a strong bounce-inducing effect, regardless of its pitch.

• The sound that was synchronized with the visual coincidence, but embedded in the other sounds, showed an almost comparable bounce-inducing effect as long as it was salient in terms of pitch. When it was at the baseline pitch, so that it was not discernible from the other sounds, the bounce-inducing effect was significantly attenuated, though still significantly above the results in the *no sound* and the *sound omission* conditions.

• *Sound omission* produced the same effects as *no sound,* and showed no bounce-inducing effect.

Figure 12.5B shows the effects of intensity change. They can be summarized as follows:

• *Single sound* showed a strong bounce-inducing effect, though there was a tendency to increase with higher intensity.

• The embedded sound showed an almost comparable bounce-inducing effect only with the higher intensity. At lower and the same (baseline) intensities, the bounce-inducing effect was significantly attenuated, though still significantly above the results in the *no sound* and *sound omission* conditions.

• *Sound omission* produced almost the same results as *no sound,* and showed little bounce-inducing effect.

To summarize, an additional sound of equal quality (intensity and pitch) presented immediately before the synchronized sound (with 150–450 ms range of sound onset interval) significantly attenuated the bounce-inducing effect of the synchronized sound (experiment 1.1). Further, when the synchronized sound was embedded in a series of sounds, the effect was very attenuated, yet recovered to some extent if the synchronized sound was an "oddball" in its pitch or intensity, and thus salient among the others in the sequence (experiment 1.2). The overall patterns of results were similar for the pitch and the intensity manipulation, except for the lower intensity of the synchronized sound (see figure 12.5A), where the recovery of the bounce-inducing effect was not as clear as at the higher intensity (figure 12.5B) or the lower pitch (figure 12.5A).

The results of *sound omission* are somewhat at odds with the literature on mismatch negativity in EEG, where one finds a "surprise" component in response to the omission of a sound from a sequence (e.g., Naeaetaenen et al., 1978). Likewise, the dependence on sound intensity seems to require some factor other than perceptual grouping. Yet, the overall pattern of results can be understood in terms of saliency, which depends on the context as well as on the presence and saliency of the synchronous sound. In other words, a synchronous sound must be prominently salient in order to induce the bouncing percept. Prominently salient are (1) single sounds, (2) the first of two sounds, (3) sounds with a distinctive pitch, and (4) sounds with higher intensity relative to the others in the repeated sounds. Not prominent or salient are (1) no sound, (2) the second of two sounds, (3) sounds whose pitch and intensity are identical to the others,

(4) sounds with a lower intensity, and (5) omission of the sound at the time of visual coincidence.

## 12.3  Effect of Visual Distractors

### 12.3.1  Background and Purpose

Experiments 1.1 and 1.2 suggested that a synchronous sound must be prominently salient in order to induce the bouncing percept. This leads to the question of whether the same effect could be achieved by presenting something, other than a sound, that is also prominently salient as well as synchronous with the visual coincidence of the streaming/bouncing display. A related question is whether the simultaneous occurrence of a salient event, per se, is what matters or the fact that such an event draws attention away from the visual coincidence. In other words, one would like to know whether the streaming/bouncing percept is determined purely by passive motion integration or is modulated by other factors, such as attention. A sudden visual event automatically attracts visual focal attention (attention capture; Jonides and Yantis, 1988; Hillstrom and Yantis, 1994; Yantis and Egeth, 1994; Yantis and Jonides, 1996). The transient sensory event that draws attention (away from the motion display, in this case) can be termed an *exogenous* cue of attention, according to the classical literature of attention (e.g., Posner, 1980; Muller and Findlay, 1988). The specific prediction would be that any other sensory events, as far as they draw attention away from the motion display, would have the same effect of inducing the bounce perception. We first test this hypothesis by replacing the sound with a visual distracter (experiment 2). If it also leads to bounce perception, then the second main question would be whether we can obtain the same bounce-inducing effect by *endogenous* distraction of attention from the visual coincidence (experiment 3). (Endogenous, as opposed to exogenous, attention stands for task-driven, voluntary attention.)

In experiment 2, a visual distracter was presented at various times and locations while subjects observed the ambiguous motion display in the peripheral visual field, and judged whether it appeared as bouncing or streaming. The timing and location were manipulated partly to examine the effectiveness of the distracter as an exogenous attention cue, but also to see if the results would be consistent with predictions from the associative learning hypothesis, mentioned earlier. It would explain the sound effect on the ambiguity-solving process by claiming that synchrony between visual and auditory events would be highly unlikely or accidental in the real world, unless they are caused by the same physical event, such as a collision. The observed effect of synchronized sound biasing perception toward bouncing may reflect a generic interpretation principle adopted by the cross-modal perceptual system: interpret synchronous events as caused by a single physical event (a generic interpretation) and avoid interpreting them as caused by two independent physical events (an accidental interpretation).

The associative learning hypothesis, at least the stringent version in the literal sense, predicts that the transient sensory event should not only occur synchronously but also at the same location as the visual coincidence in order to induce the bouncing percept.

### 12.3.2   General Methods

We used a stream/bounce display similar to that in experiment 1. However, a visual distracter (a ring) was briefly presented instead of a sound. It appeared either at various timings but always at the location of the visual coincidence (experiment 2.1; *same location*), or always at the moment of the visual coincidence but at various vertical locations (experiment 2.2; *same timing*).

The configuration and time course of the stimulus are illustrated in figure 12.6. The subject observed the stimulus display, and judged whether the two squares appeared to stream through or bounce off each another by pressing the mouse buttons accordingly (a two-alternative, forced-choice task). (For more details of stimuli and procedures in this and in experiments 2 and 3, see the caption of figure 12.6 and Watanabe and Shimojo, 1998).

### 12.3.3   Results and Discussion

The average percentage of ''bouncing'' judgments across all subjects is shown in figure 12.7A (*same location*) and 12.7B (*same timing*). When the distracter appeared at the same time as the coincidence, the frequency of the bouncing percept significantly increased (figure 12.7A). This increase in the bouncing percept with the simultaneous presentation of the distracter was observed uniformly, irrespective of the location of the distracter relative to the motion event (figure 12.7B).

Thus, the abrupt presentation of a visual distracter increased the frequency of the bouncing percept. Given the phenomenon of attentional capture (exogenous distraction of attention), this suggests that an attentional process may be involved in the streaming/bouncing percept, and that the effect of attention is to promote the streaming percept. On the other hand, we cannot exclude the possibility that the distractor effect in experiment 2.1 is mediated by a passive, stimulus-driven mechanism, or perhaps by associative learning (based on synchrony), rather than by attention.

The results of experiment 2 do not support a strong version of the associative learning hypothesis. Specifically, they do not support a version that associates events which coincide in both time *and* space. However, the results are consistent with a weaker version, which associates events coinciding in time but not in space. It would be interesting to see if this

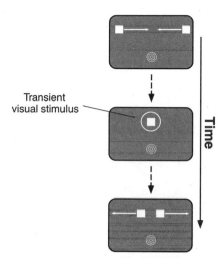

**Figure 12.6**
Distracting attention with a salient event (experiment 2). In addition to the fixation mark (bull's-eye pattern) and the moving targets of the bounce/stream display, a salient distractor (white circle, 0.8° diameter, 14 ms duration) appeared at varying times and locations (relative to the time and location of the visual coincidence of the moving targets). In experiment 2.1, the distractor appeared at varying times (−139, −69, 0, 69, or 139 ms temporal offset), but always at the same location (0.0° spatial offset). In experiment 2.2, the distractor appeared at varying locations (−3.2°, −1.6°, 0.0°, 1.6°, 3.2° above or below), but always at the same time (0 ms temporal offset). Both experiments included control trials without distractors. Stimuli were displayed on a computer monitor in a dimmed room (size 20° × 20°, viewed binocularly from 70 cm). The diameter of the bull's-eye was 0.58°, the size of moving targets 0.2°, and their trajectory 4.9° above fixation. Targets started 3.6° to the left and right of fixation, then moved laterally and smoothly toward the other side, meeting briefly at the center (speed 3.2°/s, duration 1.1 s). For further details, see Watanabe and Shimojo (1998).

pattern of results generalizes to auditory distracting events. Note also that this insensitivity to distracter location argues strongly against cognitive penetration or demand characteristics, that is, the possibility that the subject implicitly infers what the experimenter expects, and responds accordingly. This is because a transient sensory event (a sound or a flash) is caused by a collision only if it coincides in both space and time with the collision event. In other words, the generic principle should apply to both space and time.

## 12.4 Distracting Attention with a Concurrent Task

### 12.4.1 Purpose

The importance of visual distractors in experiment 2 shows that the streaming/bouncing percept is not simply the result of motion integration. Instead, the streaming/bouncing percept of moving targets seems to be modulated either by attention (drawn away

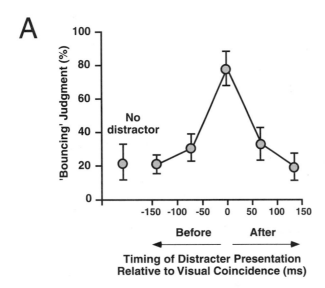

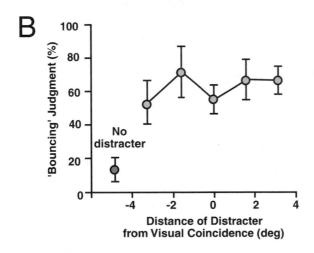

**Figure 12.7**
Results of distracting attention with a salient event (experiment 2). Mean percentage of ''bouncing'' judgment and standard errors as a function of distractor location and timing. (A) Distractors with variable timing and constant location (experiment 2.1). (B) Distractor with variable location and constant timing (experiment 2.2).

*exogenously* by the distractors) or directly by the presence of distracters. To establish attentional modulation, we must show that the bouncing percept is also favored when attention is drawn away *endogenously* by a concurrent visual task (i.e., in the absence of salient distracters).

To manipulate attention without introducing salient visual events, we combined the bouncing/streaming judgment with a visual discrimination task at the center of the display. (See Lavie, chapter 3 in this volume, and Braun et al., chapter 11 in this volume, for the method of concurrent tasks and related theoretical issues.) For this purpose, the stimulus of the concurrent discrimination task was designed not to be visually salient. We expected the streaming/bouncing percept to be altered as long as the concurrent task engages attention until the visual coincidence or thereafter, but not if the concurrent task is completed prior to the visual coincidence (this would free attention to focus on the moving targets). To test this prediction, we manipulated the timing of the concurrent task (experiment 3.1).

We also manipulated the spatial location (eccentricity) of the moving targets relative to the concurrent task (experiment 3.2). In this case, we predicted that the streaming/ bouncing judgment would remain unchanged, because the attentional distraction would be equally effective. This prediction is consistent with the results of experiment 2, which indicated that the effect of the exogenous distracter is sensitive to temporal timing, but insensitive to its location. More details about experiments 3.1 and 3.2 can be found in Watanabe and Shimojo (1998).

### 12.4.2  General Methods

The stimuli were similar to those used in experiment 1, with one critical exception: instead of presenting the visual distracter, a small spatial gap appeared for 13.9 ms on either the left or right side of the bull's-eye pattern at the center of the display (figure 12.6), around the time when the two visual targets (squares) coincided (figure 12.8). The width of the gap was determined for each subject such that he or she was not able to discriminate the position of the gap without a firm fixation and focal attention on the bull's-eye pattern. In experiment 3.1 (*same eccentricity*), the timing of the gap presentation was randomized around the moment of the visual coincidence, whereas the eccentricity of the motion event was fixed. In experiment 3.2 (*same timing*), the eccentricity of the motion event was varied, whereas the gap was always presented at the same time as the targets' coincidence. Each of the two subexperiments consisted of four sessions. Two sessions were run with the concurrent (gap) task (*with task*), in which the subject was asked to report which side of the bull's-eye pattern had a gap and also to judge whether the two squares appeared to stream through or bounce off one another. In the other two sessions, the central task stimulus was still presented, but the subject was instructed to ignore it and to report only the streaming/bouncing percept (*without task*).

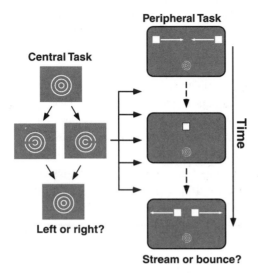

**Figure 12.8**
Distracting attention with a concurrent task (experiment 3). (*Left*) The concurrent task concerns a bull's-eye pattern at fixation, which has to be monitored until a small gap appears briefly (14 ms) in either the left or the right side of the pattern. Gap width is chosen for each subject (mean 1.8′) such that the task requires direct fixation and focused attention. This task involves *no* visually salient event. (*Right*) Spatial configuration and time course of the display (schematic). In experiment 3.1, the timing of the appearance of the gap was varied relative to the visual coincidence of the moving targets (−139, −69, 0, 69, 139 ms), but the moving targets were always at the same eccentricity (4.9° above or below fixation). In experiment 3.2, the gap always appeared at the same time (0 ms), but the moving targets were placed at varying eccentricities (0.8°, 2.9°, 4.9°, 6.9°, 8.9° above or below fixation). In the "with task" condition, subjects reported on both the gap (left or right side?) and the moving percept (stream or bounce?). Subjects concentrated on the gap task and maintained at least 90% correct performance. In the "without task" condition, subjects ignored the gap task and reported only on the moving percept. However, subjects still fixated the bull's-eye pattern, so that physical stimulus conditions remained the same.

## 12.4.3   Results and Discussion

The mean performance on the central task was at or above 95%, and there was no statistical difference in the central task performance among the different timing conditions in experiment 3.1 and different eccentricities in experiment 3.2.

The results of the perceptual judgment in experiment 3.1 are presented in figure 12.9A. When the concurrent, central task was not required, the percentages of bouncing judgment were at relatively low levels, and there was no difference among the different central task timing conditions (dashed curves). If the central task was required *before* the time of the targets' coincidence (solid curves), no significant difference was found between *with task* and *without task* conditions (left side of figure 12.9A). In contrast, when the central task took place *at* or *after* the time of the targets' coincidence, the frequency of the bouncing

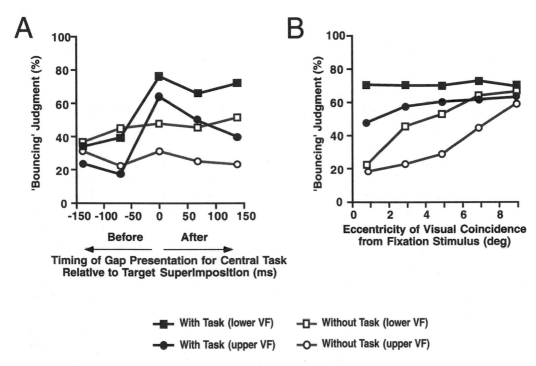

**Figure 12.9**
Results of distracting attention with a concurrent task (experiment 3). Results with and without the concurrent task and for upper and lower visual fields are plotted separately. (*A*) Mean percentage of "bouncing" judgment as a function of the timing of the gap in the bull's-eye pattern (i.e., the stimulus relevant to the concurrent task). The bouncing judgment is enhanced if the gap appears at or after the visual coincidence. (*B*) Mean percentage of "bouncing" judgment as a function of the visual eccentricity of the moving targets. A dependence on eccentricity is evident only when attention is *not* engaged by a concurrent task.

percept increased significantly (right side of figure 12.9A). Additionally, the subjects reported the bouncing percept significantly more often when the event was presented in the lower visual field than in the upper visual field (see Watanabe and Shimojo, 1998).

The results show that attentional resources for processing the moving targets and facilitating the streaming perception are reduced significantly when subjects perform the concurrent central task. As expected from the results of experiment 2 and from the attentional modulation hypothesis, the bouncing percept then became dominant.

The results of experiment 3.2 are shown in figure 12.9B, which plots the mean percentage of bouncing judgments against the eccentricity of the moving target's coincidence. When the central task was not required, the percentage of bouncing judgments increased with eccentricity (dashed curves). When the central task was required, however, the overall bouncing percentage became significantly higher, but the dependency on eccentricity diminished (solid curves).

In short, the presence of the attentional demand for the central task at the time of the targets' coincidence facilitated the perception of bouncing and suppressed that of streaming, as we had expected. Without the central task, the effect of the gap appearance was minimal (presumably because it was not salient). This strongly indicates direct involvement of attention, as opposed to stimulus-driven factors.

The frequency of the bouncing percept increased with eccentricity, but only when attention was free to focus on the moving targets (*without task* condition). This sheds new light on an anecdotal finding by Bertenthal and colleagues (1993), who reported that the dominance of streaming diminished with increasing target eccentricity. Whereas Bertenthal and colleagues reasoned that the density of local motion operators is responsible (which decreases with eccentricity; Fredericksen et al., 1993; van de Grind et al., 1983), our results suggest that the eccentricity dependence reflects the spatial distribution of visual attention. If detector density mattered, we would have observed an eccentricity dependence in both *with task* and *without task* conditions.

The overall pattern of results in experiment 3.2, as well as those in experiment 3.1, are consistent with the following assumptions:

• The normal distribution of attentional resources across the visual field peaks at the fovea (Sagi and Julesz, 1986; Balz and Hock, 1997).

• An attention-demanding task concentrates attentional resources at the relevant location, leaving uniformly sparse resources at other locations.

• Attention facilitates the streaming (and suppresses the bouncing) percept by enhancing the temporal recruitment of local motion signals.

• This does not exclude the possibility that salient events may contribute to the bouncing percept independently of attention (see next section).

## 12.5    Developmental Aspects

### 12.5.1    Background and Purpose

Because the stream/bounce perception integrates transient and sustained sensory events both across and within modalities, and also is modulated by spatial attention, it provides us with a powerful tool to investigate early development of these functions. In particular, it permits us to ask when and how the infant becomes able to utilize sensory synchronization and/or spatial attention for bounce perception.

Although the insensitivity of the bounce-inducing effect to location/eccentricity in both exogenous and endogenous distractions of attention (experiments 2 and 3) made the strict version of the associative learning hypothesis unlikely, it may be still consistent with the weaker version of it (temporal coupling only; see section 12.3.3). Early development can also contribute indirectly to this ambiguity-solving capability via its contribution to maturation of attentional control mechanisms. Thus, a developmental progression could be due either to associative learning or to the maturation of attentional control. We examined responses of human infants to the cross-modal stream/bounce display, and found evidence that infants' perception changes during the first year of life.

### 12.5.2  Experiments

We have been employing two different methods while applying the stream/bounce display: the habituation/dishabituation paradigm to assess the infant's perceptual categorization, and eye movement recording to assess the nature of perception and behavioral responses.

The stimulus was almost the same in both experiments (see figure 12.10). After a looming circle was presented to draw the infant's attention and to facilitate gaze fixation, one disk was presented on the left side and one on the right side, which then started moving toward one another, superimposed, and further moved to the other side. A sound was presented at various onset times (see the caption of figure 12.10 for more details of the stimuli).

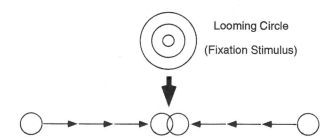

**Figure 12.10**
The stream/bounce display employed in the developmental studies. The overall display extended about 6° of visual angle while the infant subject was sitting on a baby chair 30 cm from the display. The objects moved toward one another at a speed of 34°/s. (repeating at 0.42 Hz). The sound intensity was 68 dB (SPL) as measured at the infant's head, and it was randomized across three frequencies: 500, 1500, and 3000 Hz. The infant was first presented with a fixation figure. As soon as the infant fixated, the experimenter started the *habituation* stimulus (sound at the visual coincidence). Whenever the infant looked away for more than 1 s, the trial was terminated, and the fixation point was shown again. This was repeated until the gaze time decreased to a predetermined habituation threshold, at which time the three dishabituation stimuli were presented: (1) sound 2 s before the visual coincidence, (2) sound at the visual coincidence (same as habituation stimulus), and (3) sound 2 s after visual coincidence. More than ten infants were tested in each age group.

**Habituation/dishabituation**   This is a common technique in developmental studies of perception and memory to assess the infant's ability to discriminate, categorize, and memorize percepts. It is based on the robust observation that repeated or prolonged exposure to perceptually identical stimuli leads to habituation, and thus a decrease of gazing time, whereas presentation of novel stimuli leads to an immediate recovery (dishabituation), and thus a sudden increase of gazing time. However, this is true only if the infant can discriminate the difference between the old and the new stimuli. Thus, the dishabituation can be taken as evidence that infants perceive a categorical difference between old and new stimuli.

An infant-controlled habituation procedure was used in the present study. In the habituation phase, the stream/bounce display *and* the sound synchronized with the visual coincidence, which lead to the bouncing percept in adults, were repeatedly presented until the infant's gazing time was reduced (i.e., until the infant got bored) to a predetermined habituation threshold. In the testing phase, three dishabituating displays were presented in this order: the sound was presented (1) at the beginning of the moving targets' trajectory (2 s before the visual coincidence), (2) at the time of the visual coincidence (as in the habituation stimulus), and (3) at the end of the trajectory (2 s after the visual coincidence). Because condition (2) was identical to the habituation stimulus, the prediction was longer looking times to (1) and (3) and shorter looking times to (2). Of course, this prediction assumes that the infant experiences the bouncing perception only when the sound is synchronized, as adults do.

Figure 12.11 shows the total looking time in seconds during each of the three test trials in each age group. The expected pattern of test results is apparent only in the six-months-olds and the eight-month-olds.

**Eye Movement Recording**   Identical stimuli were employed for the eye-tracking experiment. We used an infrared eye-tracking system that was specifically designed in our laboratory to monitor infants' eye movements. This video-based system is noninvasive and relatively accurate in tracking the eyes, the head, and any other body parts without yoking the infant's body and head. Figure 12.12 shows sample recordings from an eight-month-old male infant (*sound* in the left, and *no sound* in the right). In his case, there were fifteen runs in total where we could obtain a complete trajectory, seven with sound and eight without sound. Four of the seven runs with sound and six of the eight runs with no sound showed eye-movement patterns similar to those in figure 12.12. The remaining runs (three with sound and two without sound) were unclear, and intermingled tracking and saccadic eye movements.

The results from the habituation/dishabituation experiment suggests that by five or six months of age, infants perceive the streaming/bouncing display differently, depending upon the timing of the sound. Furthermore, some infants can track moving targets according to

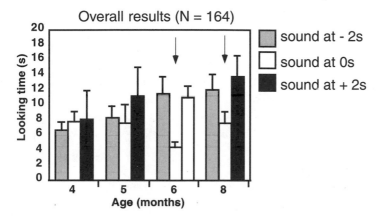

**Figure 12.11**
Results of the habituation/dishabituation experiment (see figure 12.10). Mean gaze times and standard errors are plotted for each of the three dishabituation stimuli and each age group. The arrows indicate low gaze times for the second dishabituating stimulus, indicating that this stimulus now appears familiar to the infant, presumably because at this age the synchronous sound induces a bounce percept.

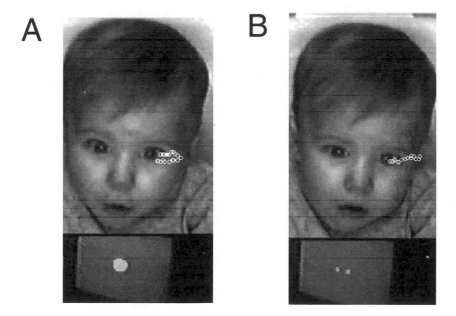

**Figure 12.12**
Examples of spatial tracking records obtained from the same infant (8 month-old male) are shown. (*Left*) Evidence for bouncing percept. This pattern was observed only with a sound at the visual coincidence. (*Right*) Evidence for streaming percept. This pattern of tracking was typically observed in the absence of a sound.

stream/bounce distinction as much as an adult would by the age of eight months, at the latest. The onset age estimated here for cross-modal integration is somewhat later than those presented in the literature on this topic. Prior studies have shown that younger infants can discriminate auditory-visual synchrony as long as the visual information is unambiguous (Lewkowicz, 1996). However, the mechanisms that allow a six-month infant to utilize sounds to disambiguate a visual display remain an open question, considering the main findings (attentional modulation) in experiments 2.1 and 2.2. One likely candidate for such a mechanism is a higher-level form of attention that is mediated by the posterior attention pathway.

## 12.6  Summary and Conclusions

There is perceptual ambiguity in the Metzger's (1934) original display of visual crossing. The observers typically and commonly report ''stream'' perception, although ''bounce'' perception becomes dominant in the peripheral visual field (Bertenthal et al., 1993). A sound synchronized with the visual coincidence (Sekuler et al., 1997), a visual flash (Watanabe and Shimojo, 1998), or a pause of movement at the time of coincidence (Bertenthal et al., 1993) commonly favors bounce perception. In addition, exogenous and endogenous distraction of attention from the visual coincidence also induces bounce perception (Watanabe and Shimojo, 1998). To induce bounce perception, exogenous distracters of attention have to occur near the time, but not near the location, of the visual coincidence (temporal but not spatial sensitivity). Endogenous distracters of attention need to pose a demanding concurrent task. Finally, perceptual categorization based on a synchronous sound seems to have its developmental onset at the age of five or six months. By the age of eight months, the infant becomes capable of tracking the perceived motion with his or her eyes.

All the results above can be understood in terms of the following general principles. First, temporal recruitment of motion signals leads to stream perception. Second, attention increases, and distraction decreases, the recruitment process. Third, these mechanisms mature somewhere between four and eight months of age. Considering the relatively limited variety of techniques available in the literature to study cross-modal interaction, and also that this is one of the very rare cases of auditory influence over vision, the streaming/bouncing display seems to have potential as a psychophysical tool to investigate cross-modal integration as well as mechanisms of spatial attention.

## References

Anstis, S. M., and Ramachandran, V. S. (1986). Entrained path deflection in apparent motion. *Vis. Res.* 26: 1731–1739.

Balz, G. W., and Hock, H. S. (1997). The effect of attentional spread on spatial-resolution. *Vis. Res.* 37: 1499–1510.

Bertenthal, B. I., Banton, T., and Bradbury, A. (1993). Directional bias in the perception of translating patterns. *Perception* 22: 193–207.

Bertenthal, B. I., and Kramer, S. J. (1988). Perceptual constraints on the direction of moving surfaces. *Invest. Ophthalmol. Vis. Sci. (Suppl.)*, 29: 250.

Bowne, S. F., McKee, S. P., and Glaser, D. A. (1989). Motion interference in speed discrimination. *J. Optical Soc. America* 6: 1112–1121.

Braun, J., and Sagi, D. (1990). Vision outside the focus of attention. *Percep. Psychophys.* 48: 45–58.

Casco, C., and Morgan, M. J. (1987). Detection of moving local density differences in dynamic random patterns by human observers. *Perception* 16: 711–712.

Cavanagh, P. (1992). Attention-based motion perception. *Science* 257: 1563–1565.

Chaudhuri, A. (1990). Modulation of the motion aftereffect by selective attention. *Nature* 344: 60–62.

Fredericksen, R. E., Verstraten, F. A. J., and van de Grind, W. A. (1993). Spatiotemporal characteristics of human motion perception. *Vis. Res.* 33: 1193–1205.

Gibson, B. S., and Egeth, H. (1994). Inhibition of return to object-based and environment-based locations. *Percep. Psychophys.* 55: 323–339.

Gogel, W. C., and MacCracken, P. J. (1979). Depth adjacency and induced motion. *Percep. Motor Skills* 48: 343–350.

Gogel, W. C., and Sharkey, T. J. (1989). Measuring attention using induced motion. *Perception* 18: 300–320.

Gogel, W. C., and Tietz, J. D. (1976). Adjacency and attention as determiners of perceived motion. *Vis. Res.* 16: 839–845.

Goldberg, D. M., and Pomerantz, J. R. (1982). Models of illusory pausing and sticking. *J. Exp. Psychol. Hum. Percep. Perf.* 8: 547–561.

Gorea, A., and Labarre, J. (1997a). A simplified, low level account of the bistable perception yielded by objects drifting toward and past one another. *Perception (suppl.)* 26: 90.

Gorea, A., and Labarre, J. (1997b). Streaming and bouncing: A low level account. *Invest. Ophthalmol. Vis. Sci.* 38: S693.

Hikosaka, O., Miyauchi, S., and Shimojo, S. (1993a). Focal visual attention produces illusory temporal order and motion sensation. *Vis. Res.* 33: 1219–1240.

Hikosaka, O., Miyauchi, S., and Shimojo, S. (1993b). Visual attention revealed by an illusion of motion. *Neurosci. Res.* 18: 11–18.

Hikosaka, O., Miyauchi, S., and Shimojo, S. (1996). Orienting spatial attention—its reflective, compensatory, and voluntary mechanisms. *Cog. Brain Res.* 5: 1–9.

Hillstrom, A. P., and Yantis, S. (1994). Visual motion and attentional capture. *Percep. Psychophys.* 55: 399–411.

Hock, H. S., and Balz, G. W. (1997). The effect of attention on the formation of self-organized motion patterns. *Invest. Ophthalmol. Vis. Sci.* 38: S372.

Jonides, J., and Yantis, S. (1988). Uniqueness of abrupt visual onset in capturing attention. *Percep. Psychophys.* 43: 346–354.

Lappin, J. S., and Bell, H. H. (1976). The detection of coherence in moving random-dot patterns. *Vis. Res.* 16: 161–168.

Lewkowicz, D. J. (1996). Perception of auditory-visual temporal synchrony in human infants. *J. Exp. Psychol. Hum. Percep. Perf.* 22: 1094–1106.

Logan, G. D. (1978). Attention in character-classification tasks: Evidence for automaticity of component stage. *J. Exp. Psychol. Gen.* 107: 32–63.

Lu, Z.-L., and Sperling, G. (1995a). Attention-generated apparent motion. *Nature* 377: 237–239.

Lu, Z.-L., and Sperling, G. (1995b). The functional architecture of human visual motion perception. *Vis. Res.* 35: 2697–2722.

McKee, S. P., and Welch, L. (1985). Sequential recruitment in the discrimination of velocity. *J. Optic. Soc. America* 2: 243–251.

Metzger, W. (1934). Beobachtungen über phänomenale Identität. *Psychologische Forschung* 19: 1–49.

Muller, H. J., and Findlay, J. M. (1988). The effect of visual attention on peripheral discrimination thresholds in single and multiple element displays. *Acta Psychol.* 69: 129–155.

Naeaetaenen, R., Gaillard, A. W. K., and Maentysalo, S. (1978). Early selective attention effect on evoked potential reinterpreted. *Acta Psychol.* 42: 313–329.

Nakayama, K., and Silverman, G. H. (1984). Temporal and spatial characteristics of the upper displacement limit for motion in random dots. *Vis. Res.* 24: 293–299.

Nickerson, R. S. (1973). Intersensory facilitation of reaction time: energy summation or preparation enhancement? *Psychol. Rev.* 80: 489–509.

Posner, M. I. (1980). Orienting of attention. *Q. J. Exp. Psychol.* 32: 3–25.

Raab, D. H. (1962). Statistical facilitation of simple reaction times. *Trans. N.Y. Acad. Sci.* 24: 574–590.

Ramachandran, V. S., and Anstis, S. M. (1983). Perceptual organization in moving patterns. *Nature* 304: 529–531.

Reynolds, D. (1964). Effects of double stimulation: Temporary inhibition of response. *Psychol. Bull.* 62: 333–347.

Sagi, D., and Julesz, B. (1986). Enhanced detection in the aperture of focal attention during simple discrimination tasks. *Nature* 321: 693–695.

Sekuler, R., Sekuler, A. B., and Brackett, T. (1995). When visual objects collide: Repulsion and streaming. *Invest. Ophthalmol. Vis. Sci.* 36: S50.

Sekuler, R., Sekuler, A. B., and Lau, R. (1997). Sound alters visual motion perception. *Nature* 385: 308.

Snowden, R. J., and Braddick, O. J. (1989a). The combination of motion signals over time. *Vis. Res.* 29: 1621–1630.

Snowden, R. J., and Braddick, O. J. (1989b). Extension of displacement limits in multiple-exposure sequences of apparent motion. *Vis. Res.* 29: 1777–1787.

Snowden, R. J., and Braddick, O. J. (1991). The temporal integration and resolution of velocity signals. *Vis. Res.* 31: 907–914.

Treue, S., and Maunsell, J. H. R. (1996). Attentional modulation of visual motion processing in cortical areas MT and MST. *Nature* 382: 539–541.

van de Grind, W. A., van Doorn, A. J., and Koenderink, J. J. (1983). Detection of coherent movement in peripherally viewed random-dot patterns. *J. Optical Soc. America* 73: 1674–1683.

Watamaniuk, S. N. J., McKee, S. P., and Grzywacz, N. M. (1995). Detecting a trajectory embedded in random direction motion noise. *Vis. Res.* 35: 65–77.

Watanabe, K., and Shimojo, S. (1998). Attentional modulation of perception of visual motion events. *Perception* 27: 1041–1054.

Yantis, S., and Egeth, H. E. (1994). Visual salience and stimulus-driven attentional capture. *Invest. Ophthalmol. Vis. Sci.* 35: S1619.

Yantis, S., and Jonides, J. (1996). Attentional capture by abrupt onsets—new perceptual objects or visual masking. *J. Exp. Psychol. Hum. Percep. Perf.* 22: 1505–1513.

Zanker, J. M. (1992). Noise thresholds of Fourier, drift-balanced and paradox theta motion. *Invest. Ophthalmol. Vis. Sci.* 33: S974.

# 13   The Relevance of Fisher Information for Theories of Cortical Computation and Attention

Alexandre Pouget, Sophie Deneve, and Peter E. Latham

## 13.1   Introduction

Many sensory and motor variables in the brain are represented by a population code, that is, by the joint activity of a large number of neurons. In these population codes, each neuron is only marginally informative about the values of the encoded variables; collectively, however, the values are represented with high precision. For example, in the medial temporal visual area (MT), neurons respond to the direction of motion according to bell-shaped tuning curves (Maunsell and Van Essen, 1983). Although neurons in MT respond to a relatively wide range of directions, the actual direction of motion is accurately represented by the population. Other examples of variables represented by a population code include stimulus contrast, the orientation of a line, and the direction of an intended movement in motor cortex. Often, a neuronal population represents several stimulus dimensions at the same time. A population of neurons in primary visual cortex (area V1), for instance, simultaneously represents the contrast, orientation, and spatial frequency of a particular stimulus.

Given their prevalence, it is important to study population codes and to understand how the brain can read them and piece together the distributed information they contain. What makes the problem particularly difficult is the noisy nature of neuronal activity. For example, a neuron responding on one occasion with twenty spikes to the presentation of a particular stimulus might respond on other occasions with fifteen or with twenty-four spikes. The problem faced by the brain, and by the theoretician trying to understand the brain, is how to estimate stimulus quantities such as contrast, orientation, and color, from the noisy responses of a large population of neurons during a single stimulus presentation.

Various estimation procedures, or "estimators," as they are called in statistics, have been proposed. One that has been used extensively in neuroscience is the "population vector" estimator (Georgopoulos et al., 1982). However, this estimator is not necessarily the best; others may be significantly more accurate. To assess the quality of a particular estimator, one can present the same stimulus many times, estimate the values of the encoded variables on each presentation, and then compute the mean and variance of the result. The best estimators are those which are accurate on average (i.e., the mean estimate equals the true value) and consistent from trial to trial (i.e., the variance of the estimate is as small as possible) (Papoulis, 1991). In this chapter, we consider only estimators for which the mean is equal to the true value, so the quality of an estimator will be measured solely by its variance. If the statistics of the neuronal responses are known—that is, the mean response and distribution of the noise—then the smallest possible variance that can be achieved by any estimator may be computed analytically (Papoulis, 1991). An estimator whose variance is equal to this analytically computed lower bound is optimal, and is said to be *efficient*.

The smallest possible variance of an estimator is the inverse of a quantity known as the *Fisher information*. In the context of a neural population code, where individual neurons are broadly tuned, the optimal algorithms are often equivalent to maximum-likelihood estimators (Paradiso, 1988; Seung and Sompolinsky, 1993). Maximum-likelihood estimators are also optimal for discriminating various stimulus alternatives on the basis of a noisy population response and, accordingly, are sometimes called ''ideal observer'' models (Hawken and Parker, 1990; Britten et al. 1992; Shadlen et al., 1996; Geisler and Albrecht, 1997; Lee et al., 1999).

A natural question to ask is whether a biologically plausible network can extract all the Fisher information contained in the noisy responses of a neuronal population. In other words, can it behave like an ideal observer? This question is addressed in the first part of our chapter. The answer turns out to depend on the neuronal noise, but for the types of noise considered here—Gaussian noise with either constant or stimulus-dependent variance—all or almost all of the Fisher information can be extracted. This result is based both on analytical arguments and on numerical simulations of networks of model neurons. In essence, we demonstrate that the kind of network found throughout cortex—nonlinear units with broad tuning and recurrent connectivity—can in many cases come close to behaving like a maximum-likelihood estimator.

The second part of the chapter uses these basic results about neuronal population codes to outline a conceptual framework for attention. Since attention improves behavioral performance, it is often argued that attention somehow enhances the neural representation of sensory information. In the context of a population code, this would mean that attention increases the Fisher information. Several studies of *individual* neurons and their responses suggest that attention improves the neural representation, either by sharpening neuronal tuning (Spitzer et al., 1988) or by improving the signal-to-noise ratio of their responses (McAdams and Maunsell, 1999; Martinez and Treue, 1988). Unfortunately, an improvement at the level of an individual neuron does not necessarily translate into an improvement at the level of the neuronal population. Our analysis will show that the Fisher information depends on the covariance matrix of the population response, and that it may remain constant even though individual neurons may exhibit sharper tuning or improved signal-to-noise ratios. Thus, in the absence of experimental measurements of the covariance matrix, we cannot know how attention affects Fisher information or, indeed, whether it affects Fisher information at all.

## 13.2   Neural Implementation of an Ideal Observer

An ideal observer of a neuronal population extracts all of the information encoded in that population. In this section we ask whether the brain can act as an ideal observer. In other words, is there a plausible network that can extract *all* the Fisher information from a population of neurons? To examine this question, we numerically simulated neural networks that take as their input a noisy pattern of activity and produce as their output a noise-free pattern of activity. From the noise-free activity, we estimate the values of the variables encoded by this population. By repeating the simulations many times (each time with different noise in the input), one can determine the variance of the output estimate and compare it to the variance of the ideal observer estimate computed from the Fisher information.

### 13.2.1   Network Architecture

We carry out this program using a highly simplified model of a cortical hypercolumn in area V1. In this model, a network encodes two dimensions of the visual stimulus—orientation, $\theta$, and spatial frequency, $\lambda$—at one spatial location. The network, which is described in detail in the Appendix, consists of one layer containing a two-dimensional array of units linked by lateral connections. The units are nonlinear, and their activation involves divisive normalization with respect to other units in the population (see Appendix). The latter choice is motivated by the fact that divisive normalization provides a good model for the nonlinearity found in neurons of area V1 (Heeger, 1992; Nelson, 1994; Carandini and Ringach, 1997).

The network receives input, denoted $a_{ij}(\theta,\lambda)$, which depends both on the stimulus (orientation, $\theta$, and spatial frequency, $\lambda$) and on the noise. The mean input, $f_{ij}(\theta,\lambda) \equiv \langle a_{ij}(\theta,\lambda) \rangle$, reflects the input tuning curves, which were chosen to be bell-shaped functions of orientation and spatial frequency (the angle brackets, $\langle \ldots \rangle$, indicate an average over many stimulus presentations). On any given trial, $a_{ij}(\theta,\lambda)$ is obtained by adding random noise to $f_{ij}(\theta,\lambda)$: $a_{ij}(\theta,\lambda) = f_{ij}(\theta,\lambda) + n_{ij}$, where $n_{ij}$ has a zero mean Gaussian distribution. Thus, the input consists of a two-dimensional distribution that is roughly bell-shaped but very noisy, as illustrated in the lower part of figure 13.1.

After the network is initialized to $a_{ij}(\theta,\lambda)$, activity propagates through the lateral connections. This causes the activity to evolve over time, eventually reaching the smoothly peaked distribution illustrated in the upper part of figure 13.1. The shape of the steady-state distribution reflects the lateral connection weights: the peaked distribution forms because the lateral connections are weighted in favor of nearby units. The position of the peak of the hill depends on the input pattern, and thus conveys information about the encoded variables, $\theta$ and $\lambda$. It is this property that allows us to use the network to estimate the encoded orientation and spatial frequency. Indeed, one can simply use the position of the peak of the smooth hill as en estimate of orientation and spatial frequency, which we denote $\hat{\theta}$ and $\hat{\lambda}$, respectively. One can assess the quality of this estimate by repeatedly exposing the network to the same stimulus (each time with different noise $n_{ij}$), and computing the variance of the resulting series of peak positions.

## OUTPUT

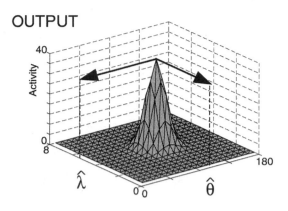

## INPUT

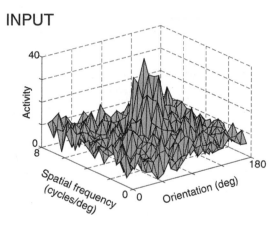

**Figure 13.1**
Activity distribution before (*lower panel*) and after (*upper panel*) network relaxation. Before relaxation, the distribution reflects the stimulus plus noise (input). After relaxation, it reflects the network attractor (output). The output distribution has a fixed shape, described by the output tuning curves, but variable position along the orientation and spatial frequency axes. The peak position, $\hat{\lambda}$ and $\hat{\theta}$, represents the network's estimate of stimulus orientation and spatial frequency.

Not all recurrent networks relax to a smoothly peaked activity distribution. In the present context, however, we are concerned only with networks that do possess this property. Details about how the activation function and the connection weights have to be chosen so that the steady-state distribution is smoothly peaked can be found elsewhere (Pouget et al., 1998; Deneve, Latham et al., 1999). Here we note only that the profile of the peak (i.e., the width of the output tuning curves) can be manipulated by adjusting the relative strengths of the lateral connections. As we will see, the quality (i.e., the variance) of the network estimate depends on this width.

### 13.2.2  Simulation Results

How well does the network perform? The answer depends on network parameters and on the structure of the input noise. To optimize the network for a given visual stimulus, we varied the widths of output tuning curves (this was done by adjusting lateral connection weights). The input noise of each unit was independent and sampled from a zero mean Gaussian distribution with variance either fixed or set to the mean activity of each unit, $f_{ij}(\theta,\lambda)$. The latter choice is more consistent with the noise that is observed experimentally in visual cortex (Tolhurst et al., 1983; Shadlen and Newsome, 1998; Gershon et al., 1998). We will refer to fixed variance as "flat noise" and to variance proportional to the mean as "proportional noise".

The networks we consider produce estimates that are accurate on average, that is, the means of the estimated values, $\langle \hat{\theta} \rangle$ and $\langle \hat{\lambda} \rangle$, are equal to the true values, $\theta$ and $\lambda$. The variance of the estimated values, which determines the quality of the estimate, depends on both network parameters and input noise. We denote the variance of $\hat{\theta}$ and $\hat{\lambda}$ as $\langle (\hat{\theta} - \theta)^2 \rangle$ and $\langle (\hat{\lambda} - \lambda)^2 \rangle$, respectively, and the covariance between these quantities as $\langle (\hat{\theta} - \theta)(\hat{\lambda} - \lambda) \rangle$. Because our network is invariant under interchange of $\theta$ and $\lambda$ (see Appendix), the variances of $\hat{\theta}$ and $\hat{\lambda}$ are identical and the covariance, $\langle (\hat{\theta} - \theta)(\hat{\lambda} - \lambda) \rangle$, vanishes. Thus, in the remainder of this chapter, we need to consider only the variance of $\hat{\theta}$, $\langle (\hat{\theta} - \theta)^2 \rangle$. To compare the network to an ideal observer, we must compare the variance of $\hat{\theta}$ with the minimum possible variance that is achieved by a maximum likelihood estimator. This minimum variance is the inverse of the Fisher information, also known as the Cramér-Rao bound.

Our simulations show that network comes very close to the Cramér-Rao bound. In its best configuration, the variance of the network estimator is within 1.6% of the Cramér-Rao bound for flat noise and within 5.1% for proportional noise. In each case, the smallest variance is obtained for a particular width of the output tuning curves. This is illustrated in figure 13.2, which shows the variance of the orientation estimates as a function of the width of the output tuning curves. For flat noise, the network performs best when the output tuning curve is about 30% narrower than the input tuning curve (figure 13.2A). For proportional noise, the situation is somewhat different. In this case, the network performs best when the output and input tuning curves are nearly identical (figure 13.2B). In both cases, network performance degrades smoothly as the width of the output tuning curve moves away from its optimal value. As long as the width remains within $\pm 10°$ of its optimal value, network performance remains within 10% of the Cramér-Rao bound.

These results indicate that there is an optimal ratio between the widths of the input and output tuning curves. This highlights a potential drawback of this kind of network: if

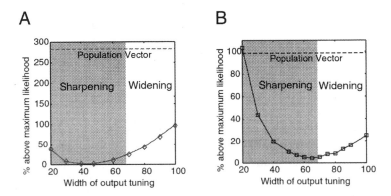

**Figure 13.2**
Performance of the network compared to an ideal observer. The variance of orientation estimates is plotted relative to the variance of an ideal observer (Cramér-Rao bound), for flat noise (*A*) and for proportional noise (*B*). In both cases, the lowest variance is reached for an output tuning curve of particular width. With flat noise, the optimal output tuning is only about 2/3 as wide as the input tuning. With proportional noise, the optimal output tuning is just about as wide as the input tuning. The width of the input tuning was kept constant at 69° (vertical line). The upper curve represents performance if the stimulus orientation is estimated directly from the (noisy) input pattern. In this case the variance remains constant, because it depends only on the width of the input tuning curve, which does not change.

different types of stimuli (e.g., gratings, bars, Gabor patches, natural scenes) produce different input tuning curves, the network will not always perform optimally. However, as long as the input tuning does not change much, performance should be only weakly affected (figure 13.2). Interestingly, cortical neurons often preserve the width of their tuning curves over a wide variety of stimulus types. For example, cells in area MT show similar tuning to a wide range of moving stimuli (Albright, 1992), and cells in area V1 exhibit the same tuning width over a large range of stimulus contrast (Skottun et al., 1987). It is therefore possible for a given network to be optimal for many different stimuli.

### 13.2.3  Analytical Results

Intuitively, these results can be understood as follows: both our network and maximum likelihood essentially fit a "template" to the noisy input, and use the position of the template to estimate the orientation and spatial frequency of a stimulus. Maximum likelihood uses an optimal template determined by the input tuning and by the structure of the noise (Pouget et al., 1998; Deneve, Latham, et al., 1999). In the case of our network, the template is determined by network parameters such as the input tuning and the relative weights of lateral connections. By adjusting these parameters, we alter the template until it is close to optimal.

To make these ideas more rigorous, we studied recurrent networks using a perturbation approach (Deneve, Latham, et al., 1999). Specifically, we studied networks that admit an $M$-dimensional attractor, every point of which is neutrally stable. By a neutrally stable $M$-dimensional attractor, we mean simply that the network asymptotes to a state that can be described by $M$ parameters. The network considered above falls into this category, because it relaxes to a state described by two parameters, $\hat{\theta}$ and $\hat{\lambda}$ (figure 13.1). We found that networks of this kind are guaranteed to reach the Cram'er-Rao bound, provided the input noise satisfies certain conditions. Although these conditions are somewhat technical, there are two common types of noise that allow the network to reach ideal observer performance. One is Gaussian noise with a constant covariance matrix, such as the flat noise considered here, and the other is Poisson noise.

In the case of flat noise, it is therefore always possible to specify a network that acts like an ideal observer. For the network described above, one can show numerically that performance is ideal when the width of the output tuning curve is 48°. This is indeed the value for which performance is closest to the Cramér-Rao bound (1.6% above). The reason the network does not exactly reach the bound is that we adjusted only the width of the output tuning curve. For fully optimal performance, we would have had to adjust the shape of the output tuning curve as well.

The situation is different with proportional noise. In this case, the covariance matrix is not constant but depends on orientation and spatial frequency. Thus no member of the class of networks we considered (i.e., networks that admit an M-dimensional attractor and are amenable to perturbation analysis) can reach the Cramér-Rao bound. Nevertheless, our analytical approach still permits us to predict which set of parameters yields the network that comes closest to the bound, and how close this will be. The result of this computation is that the optimal width of the output tuning curve should be 67° and should reach a variance 4.6% above the Cramér-Rao bound. Again, this is consistent with our simulation results, which were optimal when the width of the output tuning curve was 67°, at which point the variance was 5.1% above the bound. As before, the simulation remains slightly below the theoretical performance because we adjusted only the width (and not the shape) of the output tuning curves.

The kinds of networks we investigated—networks of nonlinear neurons with broad tuning curves and recurrent connections—are found throughout cortex. Our results show that for a broad class of noise distributions, cortical areas can compute a maximum-likelihood estimate of a variable, based on the noisy population activity in a preceding area. In short, cortical areas can behave like ideal observers. It is unlikely, however, that every input is always processed optimally by the visual cortex. For instance, human performance on simple discrimination tasks improves when the subject pays more attention to the relevant stimuli. It is therefore clear that the subjects are not ideal observers when they do not pay attention, but it is possible that attention brings the cortical circuitry closer to an optimal regime. This is the perspective that we explore in the next section.

## 13.3 Implications for Attention

Attention is often considered to be a process that selects those stimuli which are most relevant to the behavioral task at hand (Desimone and Duncan, 1995). Such a selection could be accomplished by boosting the representation of attended stimuli, suppressing the representation of unattended stimuli, or both. Here we focus on the first possibility, namely, on how the representation of attended stimuli can be enhanced by attention. Two neurophysiological mechanisms have been suggested: (1) sharpening of neuronal tuning curves and (2) increasing the gain of the neuronal response. The former possibility is consistent with evidence from Spitzer and colleagues, according to which attention sharpens orientation tuning in area V4 (Spitzer et al., 1988), but could not be confirmed by more recent work (McAdams and Maunsell, 1999). The latter possibility has the support of several recent studies, which find that the gain of neuronal responses in area V4 and MT increases as a result of attention (Spitzer et al., 1988; McAdams and Maunsell, 1999; Martinez and Treue, 1998; Maunsell and McAdams, chapter 6 in this volume; Reynolds and Desimone, chapter 7 in this volume).

The question is whether either of these mechanisms can enhance the representation of the attended stimulus. The answer depends, of course, on what is meant by "enhance." One possibility is to ask whether attention can increase the Fisher information with respect to the attended stimulus. Fisher information is an objective measure of the quality of a representation and, as we have shown in the previous section, it is a relevant bound for biological systems because it can be extracted by recurrent cortical networks (Pouget et al., 1998; Deneve, Latham, et al., 1999).

To address this question, we consider a simplified network consisting of $N$ neurons tuned to orientation. The mean response of each neuron is given by an orientation tuning curve, $f_i(\theta)$, but on any individual trial the response also reflects noise, which we will assume to be Poisson-distributed around the mean. Naturally, our conclusions are not specific to visual orientation but can be generalized to other sensory or motor variables.

### 13.3.1 Sharper Tuning

For a population of neurons with independent Poisson noise, the Fisher information with respect to stimulus orientation is given by

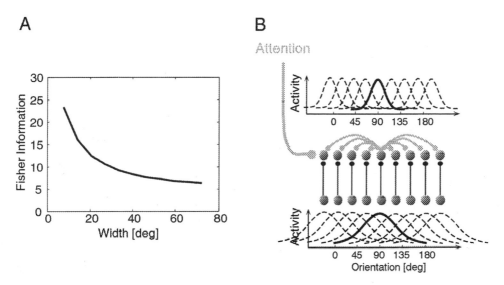

**Figure 13.3**

(A) Fisher information versus the width of the orientation tuning curves in a population of neurons with independent Poisson noise. Fisher information with respect to stimulus orientation increases as the orientation tuning of the neurons becomes sharper. This is true only if the noise remains independent for all tuning widths. (B) Two-layer network of neurons with variable output tuning. The projection from input to output neurons is one-to-one, but output neurons also receive recurrent projections from other output neurons. Due to the recurrent projections, output neurons are tuned more sharply than input neurons, which tends to increase Fisher information. However, recurrent projections also introduce noise correlations among output neurons, which tends to decrease Fisher information. Overall, Fisher information decreases or remains the same.

$$I = \sum_{i=1}^{N} \frac{f_i'(\theta)^2}{f_i(\theta)}, \tag{1}$$

where $f_i'(\theta)$ is the derivative of the tuning curve with respect to $\theta$. Consistent with the notion that attention can increase information by narrowing tuning curves (figure 13.3A), the Fisher information given by equation 1 increases with the derivative of the tuning curve, $f_i'(\theta)$ (which is larger with narrower tuning). There are, however, two problems with this observation. First, if the population encodes several stimulus variables, such as orientation and spatial frequency, sharpening the tuning in all dimensions no longer increases Fisher information. Sharper tuning in two dimensions leaves Fisher information unchanged, and sharper tuning in three or more dimensions *decreases* Fisher information (Zhang and Sejnowski, 1999). The reason is that sharper tuning reduces the number of neurons that respond to a given stimulus, and thus reduces the Fisher information of the population as a whole even though it increases the Fisher information of some individual neurons. In one dimension, the increase of information in the most responsive neurons dominates; in two dimensions, the two effects cancel each other; and in three or more dimensions, the decrease in the number of responsive neurons dominates.

Even if the tuning sharpens only in one dimension, there is a second problem. Equation 1 is valid only as long as the noise in each neuron is *independent*. If the mechanisms that sharpen tuning also introduce correlations into the noise, we can no longer rely on equation 1 to compute the Fisher information. For example, consider the network depicted in figure 13.3B. The input layer consists of neurons with broad tuning curves and independent Poisson noise. Each input neuron projects to one output neuron, and the output layer contains neurons linked by lateral connections. The effect of the lateral connections is to sharpen the output tuning curves, as has been proposed by several models (Somers et al. 1995; Carandini and Ringach, 1997; Lee et al., 1999; Braun et al., chapter 11 in this volume). We assume that lateral connections are deactivated in the unattended state (so that there is no sharpening) and activated in the attended state (so that sharpening occurs).

We can use equation 1 to compute Fisher information in the unattended state because the noise is independent in the output layer; this independence follows because, without the recurrent connections, the output layer is just a copy of the input layer, and the noise in the input layer is assumed to be independent. However, we cannot use equation 1 in the attended condition because the lateral connections, which sharpen the tuning curves, also introduce correlations among output units. Although we can no longer use equation 1, we can still use Fisher information to answer our original question: Does sharpening increase Fisher information at the population level? One could use a general equation for Fisher information valid for correlated noise (Abbott and Dayan, 1999). For this particular example, though, simple considerations about information transmission are sufficient to answer our question. Specifically, in the unattended condition, the output layer of this network conveys all the Fisher information present in the input layer because of the one-to-one connectivity (assuming also that the activation function of the output unit is monotonic). This is, of course, the best the network can possibly do with respect to information transmission. It is therefore impossible for attention to improve the representation in the output layer. In fact, if anything, sharpening is likely to *decrease* the amount of information available in the output layer.

This example shows that sharper tuning curves do not necessarily increase information at the population level. Even worse, it is possible for information to increase at the single-unit level but to decrease at the population level. This would be the case if the network in figure 13.3B involves spiking neurons whose firing rate follows Poisson statistics in both the attended and the unattended state (e.g., Shadlen and Newsome, 1998). In this case, the Fisher information of a *single* unit is given by

$$I = \int_{-\pi/2}^{\pi/2} \frac{f_i'(\theta)^2}{f_i(\theta)} \frac{d\theta}{\pi}.$$

This expression is proportional to the derivative of the tuning curve, $f_i'(\theta)$, which implies that Fisher information increases as the tuning becomes sharper. Yet, as we have just argued, the Fisher information has to decrease, or at best stay the same, at the population level.

Are there situations in which sharper tuning increases information at the population level? Yes, as long as the tuning width is suboptimal in the unattended state. For instance, this may occur in the network described above in section 13.2. Consider figure 13.2B, which shows network performance as a function of the width of the output tuning while input tuning is kept constant. Optimal performance is reached when input and output tuning curves have approximately the same width. For other output tuning widths, performance is no longer optimal, and this is particularly true when the output tuning is significantly wider than the input tuning. In this case, attention could improve information transfer by sharpening the output tuning, bringing its width closer to that of the input tuning. Note, however, that it is not the sharper tuning per se that is beneficial. If the initial output tuning is sharper than the input tuning, then attention would have to *widen* output tuning to improve information transfer. In short, attention may improve the performance of such networks by bringing the output tuning closer to the optimal value, but this may require *either* sharpening or widening.

The important conclusion of this section is that sharper tuning does not necessarily increase the Fisher information encoded in a population of broadly tuned neurons. Furthermore, it is possible that the information of some units increases but that of the entire population decreases. To assess the effect of attention at the population level, it is necessary to record from multiple units so that correlations among neurons can be studied.

### 13.3.2   Gain Increase

An increase of mean response levels is often called a ''gain increase''. In a population of neurons with uncorrelated Poisson noise, a gain increase increases the Fisher information. This is evident from the following, slightly modified expression for the Fisher information,

$$I = \sum_{i=1}^{N} G \frac{f_i'(\theta)^2}{f_i(\theta)}, \tag{2}$$

where $G$ is the gain of the tuning curve and $f_i(\theta)$ is a normalized tuning curve with gain 1. This expression implies that Fisher information is proportional to gain. In contrast to the situation with sharper tuning (see above), this is truly independent of the number of variables encoded. Noise correlations, however, are once again a concern. If the mechanisms responsible for higher gain also increase noise correlations, the information in the population will not necessarily increase. Such a situation could arise, for example, if the gain increase is due to an amplification mechanism involving lateral connections.

To estimate the effect of noise correlations on population information, we consider a simplified model in which neurons tuned to the same orientation are correlated but neurons tuned to different orientations are not. Specifically, we assume that $n$ neurons are tuned to each of $K$ orientations, so that the total number of neurons is $nK$, and denote the correlation coefficient among each group of $n$ neurons as $c$. We further assume proportional noise (i.e., a Gaussian distribution with a variance proportional to the mean). For this network it is straightforward to show that the $nK$ correlated neurons have the Fisher information

$$I = \frac{G}{c + (1 - c)/n} \sum_{i=1}^{K} \frac{f_i'(\theta)^2}{f_i(\theta)} + I_0, \tag{3}$$

where $I_0$ is a term that does not depend on gain. This expression implies that, for large $n$, the gain-dependent component of the Fisher information is proportional to $G/c$. Thus, if Fisher information is to increase, the gain has to grow faster than the correlation coefficient.

Biologically plausible networks that increase gain more than correlations are relatively easy to construct. Consider a two-layer network of integrate-and-fire neurons in which the input layer contains both excitatory and inhibitory neurons, all firing at a mean rate $\lambda_{in}$ (figure 13.4). In the output layer, each neuron receives projections from numerous input neurons. The projection pattern is sufficiently broad to ensure that any two output neurons share 25% of the projections they receive (on average) and that each output neuron receives an equal number of excitatory and inhibitory projections. Several groups have shown that, when excitation and inhibition are balanced in this way, the spike count of the output neurons is well approximated by a Gaussian distribution with variance proportional to the mean (Troyer and Miller, 1997; Shadlen and Newsome, 1998; van Vreeswijk and Sompolinsky, 1996).

What we need now is a mechanism that can increase the firing rate of the output units (i.e., the network gain) while the input rate is kept constant, and while (1) the output noise still follows a Gaussian distribution with variance proportional to the mean, and (2) the correlations increase more slowly than the gain. One way to do this is to increase the size of the postsynaptic potentials (PSPs). Our simulations show that increasing the PSP size

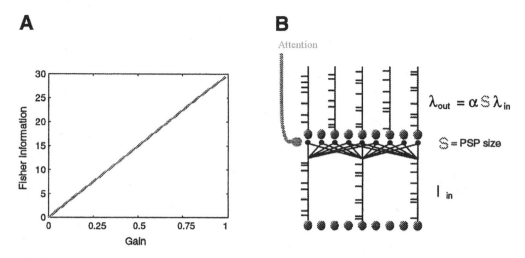

**Fig. 13.4**

(*A*) Fisher information versus gain in a population of neurons with independent Poisson noise. Fisher information increases linearly with the gain of the tuning curve, but only if the noise remains independent for all gain levels. (*B*) Network of integrate-and-fire neurons with balanced excitation and inhibition. With a suitable choice of parameters, one can obtain a regime in which the output neurons fire with Poisson statistics (mean rate $\lambda_{out} = \alpha S \lambda_{in}$), and the correlation between any two output neurons remains constant, for any value of $\alpha S$ between 0 and 1. Here, $S$ is the size of postsynaptic potentials (PSPs) and $\alpha$ is a scale factor. In this regime, gain is determined by PSP size, and Fisher information in the output layer increases monotonically with PSP size (see figure 13.5A). When PSP size grows beyond this regime, correlations between output neurons increase and Fisher information saturates.

produces an approximately linear increase in output firing rate without affecting input firing rate (see also Shadlen and Newsome, 1998). Moreover, the correlation coefficient turns out to be virtually independent of PSP size (figure 13.5B) and, accordingly, of gain as well. This makes intuitive sense: the PSP size increases for both common (i.e., shared by several output units) and noncommon inputs, so that the correlation coefficient remains approximately constant (note that the correlation coefficient reflects the balance between the two kinds of input).

Given that the gain increases with PSP size while the correlation coefficient remains nearly constant, we expect a commensurate increase in Fisher information. This expectation is confirmed by simulations, as shown in figure 13.5A. Of course, the Fisher information cannot increase indefinitely with PSP size, because this would lead to a situation where the output contains more information than the input. Indeed, Fisher information saturates when a single PSP becomes large enough to trigger a spike in the output layer. When this occurs, correlations become so strong that they neutralize any benefits of larger gain.

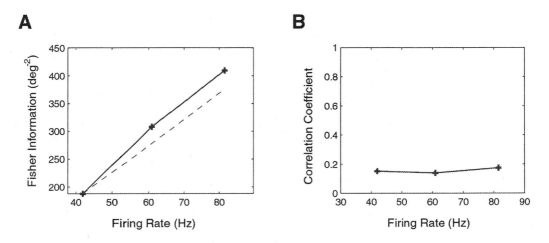

**Figure 13.5**
(*A*) Fisher information increases with gain when gain is modulated by changing PSP size (see Fig. 13.4B). Thus, attention could increase information transfer by modulating PSP size. (*B*) In the investigated regime, the correlation coefficient between pairs of output neurons remains almost constant. However, when PSP size grows even larger, correlation coefficients rise as well (not shown).

These considerations indicate that an increase in PSP size leads to an increase in the amount of Fisher information transmitted in a two-layer network of integrate-and-fire neurons. Whether attention uses this mechanism to increase gain remains to be established. However, such a mechanism is quite easy to implement in cortex. For instance, noradrenaline might be released in the attended state and potentiate postsynaptic receptors through a second messenger metabolic chain. This would lead to an increase in the output firing rate and, thus, in the network gain. Interestingly, it has been suggested that this is how noradrenaline could mediate the effects of attention (Servan-Schreiber et al., 1990).

Whether correlations in cortex are independent of gain or, at least, increase more slowly than gain, remains to be seen. Simultaneous recordings from multiple units would be particularly informative in this respect, but even a comparison of single-unit firing and local field potentials might yield valuable information on this issue.

## 13.4   Conclusions

We have argued that Fisher information is an important concept for the theory of attention. It provides a quantitative measure for the quality of the neural representation of a visual stimulus, and allows us to determine objectively whether or not attention improves this representation. One outcome of this analysis is that the structure of the noise, especially its correlational structure, is of crucial importance for the amount of information carried by a population of neurons. Thus, to determine whether or not attention enhances the quality of neural representation, we need to obtain information about noise correlations among two or more neurons.

### 13.4.1  Does Attention Mimic an Increase in Contrast?

Recently, several groups have pointed out that the effect of attention on neural responses appears to mimic an increase in the contrast of the attended stimulus or a decrease in the contrast of the unattended stimulus (Reynolds and Desimone, 1997; Martinez and Treue, 1998; McAdams and Maunsell, 1999; Maunsell and McAdams, chapter 6 in this volume). In particular, attention and higher contrast have been shown to produce comparable increments in the signal-to-noise ratio of single cells, raising the possibility that attention may be the equivalent of higher contrast, at least from a computational point of view. However, our analysis argues against equating attention with higher contrast. Contrast is a stimulus property, and higher contrast means that more information is available to the visual system. Higher contrast is expected to boost Fisher information at all levels of representation, beginning with the retina. Attention, on the other hand, does not increase Fisher information but merely controls what fraction is being transmitted. Attention can ensure that the available information is better utilized, but it cannot increase the total amount of available information, as higher contrast does.

At the circuit level, the difference between contrast and attention is also apparent. Consider the network in figure 13.4B, for example. Here, higher contrast raises firing rates in both input and output layers, and increases the total amount of Fisher information available to the network. Attention, on the other hand, merely increases firing rates in the output layer, by increasing the size of postsynaptic potentials. Although this may increase the Fisher information in the output layer, the total amount of information available to the network remains the same.

### 13.4.2  Implications for Ideal Observer Models

Ideal observer models are becoming the preferred method for relating neuronal responses to behavioral performance. Typically, these models are constructed as follows. First, the model neurons are characterized with deterministic equations, and predictions about mean response levels are obtained. Second, independent noise is added to the mean response of each model neuron. Finally, an ideal observer model is used to infer behavioral performance from the noisy responses of the model (Hawken and Parker, 1990; Britten et al., 1992; Shadlen et al., 1996; Geisler and Albrecht, 1997; Lee et al., 1999). In chapter 11 of this volume, Braun and colleagues use such a model to infer how cortical circuits would have to change to account for the effect of attention on visual thresholds (see also Lee et al., 1999). A key assumption of this approach is that attention modifies only the deterministic aspects of the model; independence of the noise and ideal observer decision are left intact. In this approach, sharper tuning and higher gain increase Fisher information, because the correlational structure of the noise remains unchanged.

As we have seen, more realistic models behave differently. In such models, there is no distinction between cortical circuits, on the one hand, and ideal observers, on the other. The cortical circuitry is the observer, and as information is transmitted from layer to layer, so is the associated noise. When noise propagation is taken into account, the consequences of sharper tuning and increased gain become less clear, because any increase in noise correlations can counteract, and even invert, their effect. Another difference is that, in a more realistic model, attention cannot increase the total amount of available information; it can only increase the fraction of information transmitted between input and output layers. An increase in the transmitted fraction can be accomplished in several ways, and does not necessarily require sharper tuning and/or higher gain.

In conclusion, relating neuronal responses to behavioral performance, and understanding the information flow through cortical circuits and how this flow is modulated through attention, will require a better understanding of the propagation of noise.

## 13.5  Appendix

The following gives the details of the network discussed in section 13.2.1. The dynamics of the network is governed by coupled, nonlinear evolution equations:

$$u_{ij}(t + 1) = \sum_{kl} w_{ij,kl} o_{kl}(t) \tag{4}$$

$$o_{ij}(t + 1) = \frac{u_{ij}^2(t + 1)}{S + \mu \sum_{kl} u_{kl}^2(t + 1)} \tag{5}$$

where $o_{ij}(t)$ is the "firing rate" and $u_{ij}(t)$ is the "membrane potential" of unit $ij$, and $S$ and $M$ are constants that determine the threshold and the relative importance of excitatory (numerator) and inhibitory (denominator) terms. The weights, $w_{ij,kl}$, determine the connectivity of the network, which in turn controls the extent to which activity from units tuned to similar orientations and spatial frequencies are pooled. The weights are given by

$$w_{ij,kl} = w_{i-k,j-l} = K_\omega \exp\left(\frac{\cos[2\pi(i - k)/P_\theta] - 1}{\delta_{\omega\theta}^2}\right) \exp\left(\frac{\cos[2\pi(j - l)/P_\lambda] - 1}{\delta_{\omega\lambda}^2}\right) \tag{6}$$

where $K_\omega$ is a constant and $\delta_{\omega\theta}$ and $\delta_{\omega\lambda}$ control the extent of pooling. These weights can easily be implemented with lateral connections, and it is quite likely that such pooling takes place in cortex (Shadlen et al., 1996).

The initial conditions, $o_{ij}(t = 0)$, of equations 4 and 5 are determined by the activity of the input layer, specifically, $o_{ij}(t = 0) = a_{ij}(\theta,\lambda)$. The input activity, $a_{ij}(\theta,\lambda)$, varies from trial to trial and is sampled from a Gaussian distribution with mean $f_{ij}(\theta,\lambda)$ and variance $\sigma^2_{ij}(\theta,\lambda)$,

$$P(a_{ij} - f_{ij} \mid \theta,\lambda) = \frac{1}{\sqrt{2\pi\sigma^2_{ij}}} \exp\left( - \frac{(a_{ij} - f_{ij})^2}{2\sigma^2_{ij}} \right).$$

The tuning curve of unit $ij$, which represents the deterministic part of the response to a stimulus with orientation $\theta$ and spatial frequency $\lambda$, is modeled as the sum of a circular normal function and a small amount of spontaneous activity,

$$f_{ij}(\theta,\lambda) = K \exp\left( \frac{\cos(\theta - \theta_i) - 1}{\sigma^2_\theta} \right) \exp\left( \frac{\cos(\lambda - \lambda_i) - 1}{\sigma^2_\lambda} \right) + v \tag{7}$$

where $K$, $\sigma_\theta$, $\sigma_\lambda$, and $v$ are constant and the units are arranged on a $P_\theta \times P_\lambda$ grid: $\theta_i = 2\pi i/P_\theta$, $i = 1, \ldots, P_\theta$ and $\lambda_j = 2\pi j/P_\lambda$, $j = 1, \ldots, P_\lambda$. To avoid edge effects, spatial frequency is treated as a cyclic variable (like orientation); this should not affect the results as long as $\lambda$ is far from $2\pi m$ where $m$ is an integer.

In all simulations, we use a $20 \times 20$ array of units ($P_\theta = P_\lambda = 20$), and the parameters are set to the following values: $K = 74$, $v = 3.7$, $\sigma_\theta = \sigma_\lambda = 0.38$, $M = 0.002$, $S = 10$, $K_\omega = 1$. For flat noise, we use $\sigma^2_{ij} = 25$, independent of $i$ and $j$. For proportional noise, we use $\sigma^2_{ij} = f^2_{ij}(\theta)$. The remaining parameters, $\delta_{\omega\theta}$ and $\delta_{\omega\lambda}$, which affect the extent of spatial pooling of the connection weights, and thus the width of the output tuning curves, are kept equal and are systematically varied within the interval of [0.14, 0.718].

Because we chose our noise distribution and connection weights to be symmetric with respect to the interchange of $\theta$ and $\lambda$ (equation 6 with $\delta_{\omega\theta} = \delta_{\omega\lambda}$ and equation 7 with $\sigma_\theta = \sigma_\lambda$), by symmetry the variance of $\hat{\theta}$ is equal to the variance of $\hat{\lambda}$; the covariance $\langle(\hat{\theta} - \theta)(\hat{\lambda} - \lambda)\rangle$ vanishes; and the network is unbiased, $\langle\hat{\theta}\rangle = \theta$ and $\langle\hat{\lambda}\rangle = \lambda$. Thus, the quality of the estimates produced by the network is measured solely by the variance, $\langle(\hat{\theta} - \theta)^2\rangle$. The variance can be computed from the standard formula, which is valid for unbiased estimators,

$$\langle(\hat{\theta} - \theta)^2\rangle = \frac{1}{N_T - 1} \sum_{i=0}^{N_T} (\theta - \hat{\theta}_i)^2$$

where $N_T$ is the number of trials.

The stimulus orientation, $\theta$, and spatial frequency, $\lambda$, affect the network solely through the input tuning curves, $f_{ij}(\theta,\lambda)$, which determine the initial conditions (together with the noise). For a given initial condition, equations 4 and 5 are iterated until a Gaussian distribution of activity emerges, as shown in figure 13.1. The peak of this distribution constitutes our estimate of $\theta$ and $\lambda$. We recover the peak position $\hat{\theta}$ and $\hat{\lambda}$ with the help of a complex estimator (Seung and Sompolinsky, 1993; Pouget et al., 1998), which is equivalent to a population vector estimate (Georgopoulos et al., 1982):

$$\hat{\theta} = phase\left( \sum_{kl} a_{kl} e^{i\theta_l} \right)$$

where $i$ stands as $\sqrt{-1}$.

## References

Abbott, L. F., and Dayan, P. (1999). The effect of correlated activity on the accuracy of a population code. *Neural Comput.* 11: 91–101.

Albright, T. D. (1992). Form-cue invariant motion processing in primate visual cortex. *Science* 255: 1141–1143.

Britten, K. H., Shadlen, M. N., Newsome, W. T., and Movshon, J. A. (1992). The analysis of visual motion: A comparison of neuronal and psychophysical performance. *J. Neurosci.* 12: 4745–4765.

Carandini, M., Heeger, D. J., and Movshon, J. A. (1997). Linearity and normalization in simple cells of the macaque primary visual cortex. *J. Neurosci.* 17: 8621–8644.

Carandini, M., and Ringach, D. L. (1997). Predictions of a recurrent model of orientation selectivity. *Vis. Res.* 37: 3061–3071.

Deneve, S., Latham, P. E., and Pouget, A. (1999). Reading population codes: A neural implementation of ideal observers. *Nature Neurosci.* 2: 740–745.

Deneve, S., Pouget, A., and Latham, P. (1999). Heeger's normalization, line attractor network and ideal observers. In M. S. Kearns, S. A. Solla, and D. A. Cohn (eds.), *Advances in neural information processing systems,* vol. 11. (pp. 104–110). Cambridge, MA: MIT Press.

Desimone, R., and Duncan, J. (1995). Neural mechanisms of selective visual attention. *Ann. Rev. Neurosci.* 18: 193–222.

Geisler, W. S., and Albrecht, D. G. (1997). Visual cortex neurons in monkeys and cats: Detection, discrimination, and identification. *Vis. Neurosci.* 14: 897–919.

Georgopoulos, A. P., Kalaska, J. F., Caminiti, R., and Massey, J. T. (1982). On the relations between the direction of two-dimensional arm movements and cell discharge in primate motor cortex. *J. Neurosci.* 2: 1527–1537.

Hawken, M. J., and Parker, A. J. (1990). Discrimination and detection mechanisms in the striate cortex of the old-world monkey. In C. Blakemore (ed.), *Vision: Coding and efficiency.* (pp. 103–116). Cambridge: Cambridge University Press.

Heeger, D. J. (1992). Normalization of cell responses in cat striate cortex. *Vis. Neurosci.* 9: 181–197.

Lee, D. K., Itti, L., Koch, C., and Braun, J. (1999). Attention activates winner-take-all competition among visual filters. *Nature Neurosci.* 2: 375–81.

Martinez, J. C., and Treue, S. (1998). Attention does not sharpen direction tuning curves in macaque monkey MT/MST neurons. *Soc. Neurosci. Abstr.* 24: 255–258.

Maunsell, J. H. R., and Van Essen, D. C. (1983). Functional properties of neurons in middle temporal visual area of the macaque monkey. I. Selectivity for stimulus direction, speed, and orientation. *J. Neurophysiol.* 49: 1127–1147.

McAdams, C. J., and Maunsell, J. R. H. (1999). Effects of attention on orientation-tuning functions of single neurons in macaque cortical area V4. *J. Neurosci.* 19: 431–441.

Nelson, M. E. (1994). A mechanism for neuronal gain control by descending pathways. *Neural Comput.* 6: 242–254.

Papoulis, A. (1991). *Probability, random variables, and stochastic process.* New York: McGraw-Hill.

Paradiso, M. A. (1988). A theory of the use of visual orientation information which exploits the columnar structure of striate cortex. *Biol. Cybern.* 58: 35–49.

Pouget, A., Zhang, K., Deneve, S., and Latham, P. E. (1998). Statistically efficient estimation using population coding. *Neural Comput.* 10: 373–401.

Reynolds, J. H., and Desimone, R. (1997). Attention and contrast have similar effect on competitive interactions in macaque area V6. *Neurosci. Abst.* 23: 122–129.

Servan-Schreiber, D., Printz, H., and Cohen, J. D. (1990). A network model of catecholamine effects: Gain, signal-to-noise ratio, and behavior. *Science* 249: 892–895.

Seung, H. S., and Sompolinsky, H. (1993). Simple model for reading neuronal population codes. *Proc. Nat. Acad. Sci. USA* 90: 10749–10753.

Shadlen, M. N., Britten, K. H., Newsome, W. T., and Movshon, T. A. (1996). A computational analysis of the relationship between neuronal and behavioral responses to visual motion. *J. Neurosci.* 16: 1486–1510.

Shadlen, M. N., and Newsome, W. T. (1998). The variable discharge of cortical neurons: Implications for connectivity, computation, and information coding. *J. Neurosci.* 18: 3870–3896.

Skottun, B. C., Bradley, A., Sclar, G., Ohzawa, I., and Freeman, R. D. (1987). The effects of contrast on visual orientation and spatial frequency discrimination: A comparison of single cells and behavior. *J. Neurophysiol.* 57: 773–786.

Somers, D. C., Nelson, S. B., and Sur, M. (1995). An emergent model of orientation selectivity in cat visual cortical simple cells. *J. Neurosci.* 15: 5448–5465.

Spitzer, H., Desimone, R., and Moran, J. (1988). Increased attention enhances both behavioral and neuronal performance. *Science* 240: 338–340.

Tolhust, D. J., Movshon, J. A., and Dean, A. D. (1983). The statistical reliability of signals in single neurons in cat and monkey visual cortex. *Vis. Res.* 23: 775–785.

Troyer, T. W., and Miller, K. D. (1997). Physiological gain leads to high ISI variability in a simple model of a cortical regular spiking cell. *Neural Comput.* 9: 971–983.

van Vreeswijk, C., and Sompolinsky, H. (1996). Chaos in neuronal networks with balanced excitatory and inhibitory activity. *Science* 274: 1724–1726.

Zhang, K., and Sejnowski, T. J. (1999). Neuronal tuning: To sharpen or broaden? *Neural Comput.* 11: 75–84.

# 14 From Foundational Principles to a Hierarchical Selection Circuit for Attention

John K. Tsotsos, Sean M. Culhane, and Florin Cutzu

## 14.1 Introduction

The work described in this chapter spans theoretical considerations, a computer model of cortical circuits applied to real-world scenes, and human psychophysics used to test model predictions. The theoretical work initially addressed the question "Is there a computational justification for attentive selection?" The obvious answer that has been given many times since at least Broadbent—that the brain is not large enough to process all the incoming stimuli—is hardly satisfactory. This answer is not quantitative, and provides no constraints on what processing system might be sufficient. Tsotsos (1989) employed methods from computational complexity theory to formally prove for the first time that purely data-directed visual search in its most general form is an intractable problem in any realization. He claimed that search is ubiquitous in vision, and thus purely data-directed visual processing is also intractable in general. His analyses provided important constraints on visual processing mechanisms and led to a specific (not necessarily unique or optimal) solution for visual perception. The constraints arose because vision was cast as a search problem, and because the combinatorics of search is too large at each stage of analysis. Attentive selection turns out to be a powerful heuristic to limit search and make the overall problem tractable.

Attention is an important mechanism at any level of processing where one finds a many-to-one convergence of neural inputs, and thus potential stimulus interference, a conclusion reached by Tsotsos (1990). This was disputed at first (Desimone, 1990); however, more recent experimental work would appear to be supportive (e.g., Kastner et al., 1998; Vanduffel et al., 2000).

The basic component of the proposed attentional mechanism is a hierarchical neural network that implements a task-dependent, top-down, directed competition among conflicting neural elements, a circuit first described by Tsotsos (1993). Thus the mechanism implements a selective tuning of the visual processing hierarchy. Thus, we name this mechanism the *selective tuning model* of visual attention. In contrast to theories that claim similar conceptual strategies for attention (e.g., Desimone and Duncan, 1995), our model has been fully detailed and simulated on a computer. It provides attentive control to a robotic camera system, and attends both overtly and covertly to task-directed features and objects, using real-world image sequences acquired from video cameras. As such, it is an existence proof that the key elements of the model are realizable and perform as expected.

The exposition will proceed in two parts. The first part provides an overview of the selective tuning model, with particular emphasis on the issue of attentional control. The second part describes a psychophysical study with human observers that tests a basic prediction of the model: that perception is more impaired in the near vicinity than in the far vicinity of an attended stimulus.

## 14.2   The Selective Tuning Model

Complexity analysis leads to the conclusion that attention must tune the visual processing architecture to permit task-directed processing (Tsotsos, 1990). Selective tuning takes two forms: *spatial* selection, realized by inhibiting task-irrelevant connections in the neural network, and *feature* selection, realized by inhibiting the neurons that represent task-irrelevant features. Only a brief summary is presented here because the model is detailed elsewhere (Tsotsos et al., 1995).

The role of attention in the image domain is to localize a subset of the input image and its path through the processing hierarchy in such a way as to minimize any interfering or corrupting signals. The visual processing architecture is a pyramidal network composed of units receiving both feedforward and feedback connections. This general architecture resembles that proposed by Van Essen and colleagues (1992). When a stimulus is first applied to the input layer of the pyramid, it activates in a feedforward manner all of the units within the pyramid to which it is connected. The result is the activation of an inverted subpyramid of units and connections, as shown in figure 14.1. We assume that the degree of unit activa-

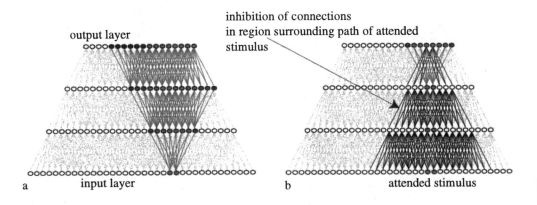

**Figure 14.1**
(*A*) Feedforward activation of the visual processing pyramid and (*B*) its modulation after attentional selection has been applied. Red connections are those affected by the stimulus, gray connections are those which play no role, and black connections are those inhibited by the winner-take-all (WTA) selection process. The top layer is not inhibited by the top-layer WTA, and thus the feedforward divergence of the stimulus to the output layer is seen. If it were inhibited, no other stimulus could reach the output layer, making the system effectively blind to all nonattended stimuli. The model predicts that nonattended stimuli do reach the output layer of the system, but their representation may be incomplete or corrupted by interfering signals (Tsotsos, 1997). The shading of the units' colors reflects the assumption that unit weighting profiles are Gaussian in nature. (See plate 12 for color version.)

tion reflects the goodness of match between the unit and the stimulus it represents. Figure 14.1 shows a visual processing pyramid with four layers, in which each unit is connected to seven units in the layer immediately above, as well as to seven units in the layer immediately below. The input layer (bottom layer) is numbered 1, and the output layer (top layer) is numbered layer 4. Note that feedforward and feedback connections are not shown separately; instead, each reciprocal pair of connections is represented by a single line.

### 14.2.1   Hierarchical Winner-Take-All Processes

Selection relies on a hierarchy of winner-take-all (WTA) processes. WTA is a parallel algorithm for finding the maximum value in a set of variables that was first proposed in this context by Koch and Ullman (1985). It can be steered to favor particular stimulus locations or features, but in the absence of such guidance it operates independently. The processing of a visual input involves three main stages. During the first stage, a stimulus is applied to the input layer and activity propagates along feedforward connections toward the output layer. The response of each unit depends on its particular selectivities, and perhaps also on a top-down bias for task-relevant qualities (see below). During the second stage, a hierarchy of WTA processes is applied in a top-down, coarse-to-fine manner. The first WTA process operates in the top layer and covers the entire visual field at the top layer: it computes the unit with the largest response in the output layer, that is, the *global winner*. In turn, the global winner activates a WTA among its input units in the layer immediately below. This localizes the largest response within the receptive field of the global winner. All of the connections of the visual pyramid that do not contribute to the winner are pruned (i.e., attenuated). This strategy of finding the winner within each receptive field, and then pruning away irrelevant connections, is applied recursively through the pyramid, layer by layer. Thus, the global winner in the output layer is eventually traced back to its perceptual origin in the input layer. The connections that remain (i.e., are not pruned) may be considered the *pass zone* of the attentional beam, and the pruned connections, an *inhibitory zone* around that beam. Although we are not claiming biological accuracy for the WTA process, we are claiming plausibility, because it does not violate biological connectivity or time constraints. During the third stage, the selected stimuli in the input layer repropagate through the network, being processed by the same neurons, but this time without distracting stimuli in each receptive field, as if they had been presented on a blank background. There is no change in identity of the winning neurons in the output layer; the winner initially selected remains the winner, but its value is refined by this process.

### 14.2.2   Examples

The process described above is shown in the examples below. The first example shows the initial and final stages of the processing of a single stimulus item (figure 14.1); the input stimulus spatially spans two input layer units. If the system attends the stimulus in the input layer of figure 14.1A, the configuration of figure 14.1B results. The red lines represent feedforward connections activated by the stimulus; the black lines, connections whose feedforward flow is inhibited (pruned) by the attentional beam; and the gray lines, inactive connections. Red units are activated solely by the red stimulus. The WTA mechanism locates the peaks in the response of the output layer of the pyramid—here, the two remaining red units in figure 14.1B. The attentional beam is then extended from top to bottom, pruning away the connections that might interfere with the selected units. Eventually, the winning units are located in the input layer and isolated within the beam.

The important missing link is the mechanism for localizing the two winners in the output layer. On the assumption that each unit in the pyramid computes some quantity, using a Gaussian-shaped weighting function across its receptive field, the maximum responses of these computations (whatever they may be) will correspond exactly to the two units selected in the output layer (see Tsotsos et al., 1995, for further details, including the mathematical formulation and proofs of its properties). The general question is thus how the mechanism functions if there is more than one stimulus in the input—that is, when there are both target and distractor stimuli in the visual field.

Figure 14.2 shows the sequence of the changes that the visual processing pyramid undergoes in such a situation. Using the same network configuration and showing reciprocal feedforward and feedback connections as a single line, two stimuli are placed in the visual field (input layer, figure 14.2A). They are color-coded red and blue, as are the corresponding connections and units that each stimulus activates. The mauve-colored units and connections are those activated by both stimuli (the relative proportion does not matter here). Much of the pyramid is affected by both stimuli, and as a result, most of the output layer gives a confounded response.

The mauve units respond weakly, due to the conflict that arises when each of those units "sees" two different stimuli within its receptive field. Whatever the optimal tuning properties of a unit may be, nonoptimal input will lead to a reduced response.

Just like a human observer, the model can be provided with a spatial cue to indicate the location of a relevant stimulus. While being presented with a cue, the model determines the location of the most active units in the output layer, and retains this information in the form of a bias in favor of these units. When the subsequent test stimulus appears, this bias remains in place and influences the WTA processes in the next lower layer (figure 14.2B). Finally, the bias propagates backward, layer by layer, each time influencing the WTA processes in question (figures 14.2C, D).

### 14.2.3  Spatial Structure of Attentional Modulation

How does the hierarchical WTA process change the network when more than one stimulus is presented to the input layer? Figure 14.3 summarizes the spatial and temporal structure

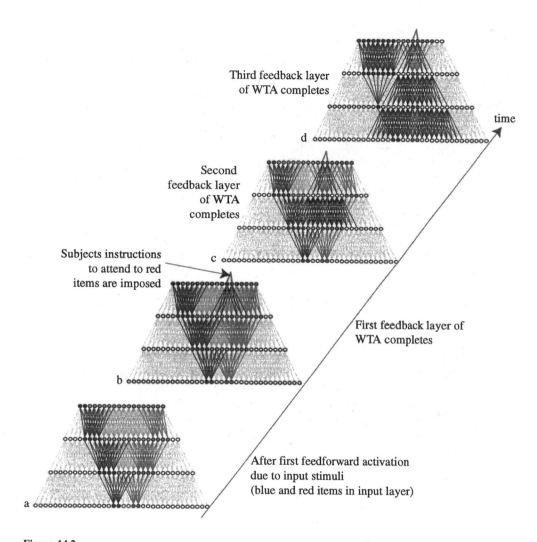

**Figure 14.2**
A four-step sequence showing attentional modulation when there are two stimuli in the input and the system attends to one. (A) The visual processing pyramid at the point where the activation due to separate stimuli in the input layer has just reached the output layer. No attentional effects are yet in evidence. (B) The location selection is applied, and two units in the output layer are identified (location cues can be placed anywhere in the visual field prior to a test stimulus). The first WTA stage then takes place, and the largest responses within the next layer of receptive fields of the selected units are found. The connections not corresponding to those largest response units are inhibited. (C) The results after the second stage of WTA. (D) The results after the third and final stage of WTA. Due to the complexity of the figure, the variations in unit strength due to the Gaussian weighting profile are not shown. (See plate 13 for color version.)

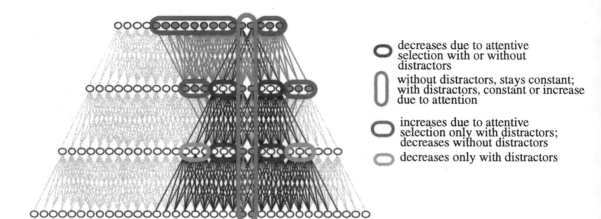

decreases due to attentive
selection with or without
distractors

without distractors, stays constant;
with distractors, constant or increase
due to attention

increases due to attentive
selection only with distractors;
decreases without distractors

decreases only with distractors

**Figure 14.3**
Modulation predictions. Following the changes of a particular unit of the pyramid through the four-step sequence
of figure 14.2 leads to the overall changes depicted in this diagram. Specific portions of each layer undergo
systematic changes as indicated; the changes depend on whether distractors are present or not (and on which
side of the attended stimulus they fall), and their strengths may differ, depending on the distance separating the
attended stimulus and the distractors. The best way to relate this figure to figure 14.2 is to select a specific unit
in the pyramid in figure 14.2A and track its changes over time, as depicted in the sequence from figure 14.2A
through D. (See plate 14 for color version.)

of the attentional changes that are obtained for two stimuli. The details of these changes
depend on whether the stimulus contains unattended distractors in addition to an attended
target, and on the distance between distractors and target. Our model predicts both increases and decreases in unit responses, depending on where a unit is situated relative to
the attended target. Consistent with this prediction, Motter (1993) observed both increases
and decreases in neuronal responses in visual cortical areas V2 and V4, but not in V1,
of monkey when the animal attended to a target stimulus in the presence of distractors.

### 14.2.4   Network Structure and Function

We now describe the WTA circuit employed by our model in more detail. This circuit
involves several different types of computing units arranged in a pyramid (figure 14.4).
*Interpretive units* compute the visual features. *Gating units* compute the WTA result across
the inputs of a particular interpretive unit and then feed the winning input forward to the
interpretive units in the next layer of the pyramid. *Gating control units* control the downward flow of selection through the pyramid and are responsible for the signals that either
activate or suppress the WTA processes. *Bias units* provide top-down, task-related selection via multiplicative attenuation. We term the basic building block of this circuit—one

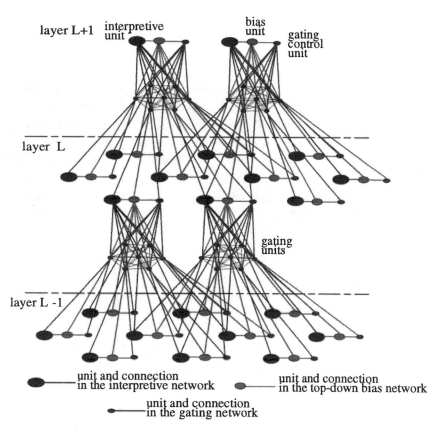

**Figure 14.4**
The circuit that implements the hierarchical selection described in the text is shown; this is a conceptual view and is not intended to correspond to specific neurons and their connectivities. A more detailed explanation of this circuit can be found in Tsotsos et al. (1995). (See plate 15 for color version.)

interpretive unit, the set of gating units on its input, and its associated gating control and bias units—an *assembly*.

The control signal activates or suppresses the WTA process in the next lower layer. This is implemented by turning gating units on or off. Because only connections to one particular target unit are affected, interpretive units may still participate in other computations as needed.

Initially, all gating control signals are zero, leaving all connections open and allowing responses to be computed bottom-up, that is, depending solely on the stimulus (first bottom-up traversal). Next, the control signal becomes unity at the top layer, activating

WTA in this layer and determining the control signals for the next lower layer: winning units pass down a value of unity, activating WTA, whereas all other units pass down a value of zero, suppressing WTA in the next lower layer, and so on (first top-down traversal). As the pruning of connections progresses toward lower and lower layers, first the inputs and then the responses of interpretive units change. Over time, these changes propagate upward toward the top layer (second bottom-up traversal). Once this second bottom-up propagation is complete, active gating units are switched off and become ''refractory,'' so that they cannot be activated again. This inhibition of a previously selected region and pathway is taken from Koch and Ullman (1985), who referred to it as ''inhibition of return.''

Further details about the WTA algorithm and its properties can be found elsewhere (Tsotsos et al., 1995). The algorithm is provably convergent, permits multiple winners, and appears optimal when compared to the provably optimal parallel maximum-finding algorithm of Valiant (1975).

In addition to feedback through gating control units, network activity is modulated by bias units. The bias network has two functions. First, bias units feed *back* task-specific information, such as prior information about the attributes of a task-relevant stimulus. Second, they feed *forward* positional information regarding the winners of the WTA competition. In effect, each layer of WTA computes a higher-order bit of a binary address, and the full address is computed when the first top-down traversal is complete. Thus, the bias network can play an important role in object recognition by conveying the precise position of winning stimulus features. This information allows recognition processes to verify whether the configuration of winning features corresponds to the object to be recognized.

### 14.2.5   A Neural Correlate of the WTA Circuit?

Is there a neural correlate of such a localized WTA network? A strong prediction of such a network is that neurons in each visual area compete with neurons of similar selectivity, and that such a competition takes place separately in each part of visual space and for each attribute or feature. Furthermore, the spatial extent of the competition in one layer corresponds to the receptive field size of neurons in the next higher layer.

Both predictions are consistent with our current knowledge of cortical connectivity. In several species, the long-range intrinsic connections of visual cortex link cortical columns with similar response properties (e.g., orientation, direction, ocular preference; reviewed by Callaway, 1998). In addition, the spatial range of the long-range connectivity in one cortical area roughly corresponds to the receptive field size in the next higher cortical area (e.g., Salin and Bullier, 1995).

In figure 14.4, each unit in the WTA network is shown to be connected to all others. In fact, this connectivity is necessary for a fully parallel implementation of such a network. However, a neural implementation of this network could rely on a lesser degree of connectivity. Figures 14.5A and 14.5B illustrates two possible implementations that differ in their connectivity but are functionally equivalent. The centralized connectivity in figure 14.5B would seem to map more readily onto cortical circuitry. This implementation has been applied to natural scene images, as shown in figure 14.6 (Tsotsos et al., 1995).

### 14.2.6 Is Attentional Control Centralized or Distributed?

Our model makes strong predictions about how attentional control occurs, including the locus of its source, the nature of the decision-making process, and the sites at which these decisions are applied. The original arguments for distributed control and local decision-making are found in Tsotsos (1990) and are rooted in the analysis of the space complexity of the task (number of units, number of connections, number of inputs and outputs for each unit, lengths of connections). However, it is important to consider an alternative strategy. In particular, one may ask whether a centralized attentional decision, taken outside the sensory processing hierarchy, would not also be a feasible strategy. The following paragraphs address this potential alternative explanation.

Consider the set of visual areas where attentive modulation has been observed, and their connections, as shown in figure 14.7.[1] It is evident that attention is applied throughout the processing hierarchy, where it affects individual neurons exactly as predicted by the selective tuning model. Assume that these distributed attentional modulations originate in a central structure, an attentional control center (AC), and are then communicated to the processing hierarchy. To consider this possibility properly, several key questions must be addressed.

**What goals must the AC accomplish?**  At least three goals are important: selection of attended stimuli, suppression of unattended stimuli to remove interference, and coordination of both types of modulations across all levels of the hierarchy.

**What information does the AC require in order to accomplish them?**  To select the most salient items, the AC must necessarily have a global view of the visual field (Milner, 1974). Since task instructions modify the selection of the most salient item, the AC must have access to those instructions. At progressively higher levels of the hierarchy, more and more positional information is discarded, and more and more featural information is accumulated. To recover the discarded spatial information and localize the attended stimulus in visual space, the computations of the processing hierarchy must be reversed. Such a reversal necessitates a local search process over the inputs of each neuron, which must be coordinated across all levels of the hierarchy.

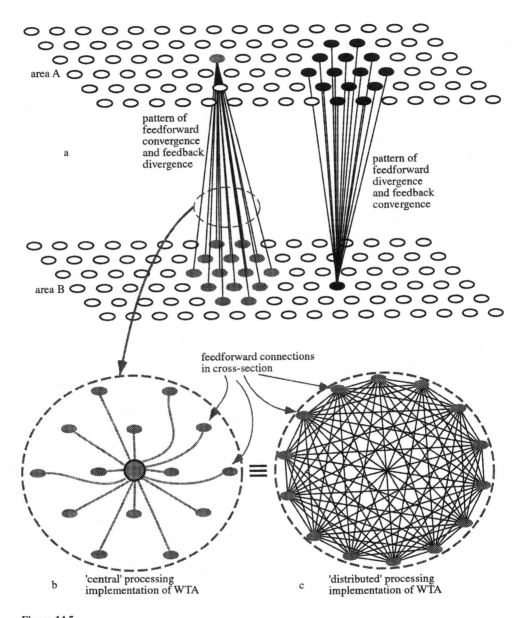

area A

pattern of
feedforward
convergence
and feedback
divergence

a

pattern of
feedforward
divergence
and feedback
convergence

area B

feedforward connections
in cross-section

b   'central' processing
    implementation of WTA

≡

c   'distributed' processing
    implementation of WTA

**Figure 14.5**
WTA circuit proposals. (*A*) Two layers of visual processing are shown, and the feedforward and feedback divergences of connections are highlighted. The patterns of connectivity overlap exactly. The expanded section of the feedforward convergence at the bottom of the figure shows two possible implementations of the WTA circuit. If the WTA is to be implemented in strictly parallel, distributed processing fashion, each unit must be connected to each other as in (*C*). A central processing implementation is functionally equivalent (*B*).

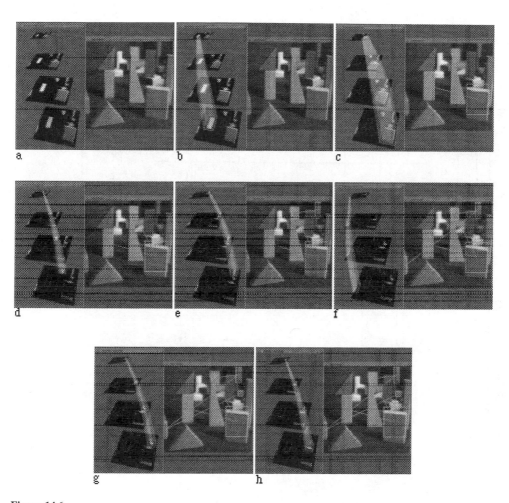

**Figure 14.6**

Example of computer simulation. An image of several colored blocks is the test image. The process operates on a color image; only a gray scale representation is shown here. The algorithm is instructed to search for blue regions, and it attempts to do this by searching for the largest, bluest region first. This test image is shown on the right half of each image; the regions selected are outlined in yellow, with blue lines between them showing the system's scan path. The left side of each image shows a four-level visual processing pyramid. The instruction is applied to the pyramid to tune its feature computations, and the result is that the regions within each layer of the pyramid that remain are those which are blue. The left side of (A) shows the set of blue of objects found. Then the WTA algorithm selects the largest, bluest one first (B), inhibits that region (note it does not appear in (C), and then repeats the process six times. The system does not know about objects, only rectangular regions; thus, although it sometimes appears to select whole blocks, this is due solely to fortuitous camera viewpoints. (See plate 16 for color version.)

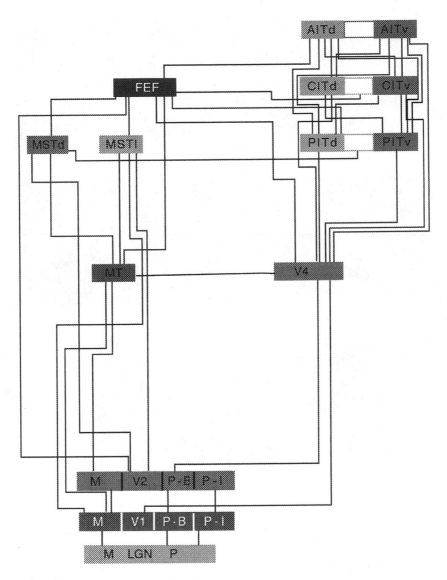

**Figure 14.7**
The network of visual areas of the macaque, where attentional modulation of the kind addressed by the selective tuning model has been observed are shown (V1, Motter, 1993; V2, Motter, 1993; V4, Moran & Desimone, 1985; IT, Chelazzi et al., 1993; MT, Treue & Maunsell, 1996; MST, Treue & Maunsell, 1996; FEF, Schall & Hanes, 1993; LGN, Vanduffel et al., 2000). This diagram is based on the Felleman and Van Essen (1991) diagrams and was created using their software. It is the minimal set of areas to which an attentional control center must connect and provide control signals.

**Where can the required information be found?** A global view is most easily available from neurons in the upper layer of the hierarchy, where receptive fields are largest. On the other hand, precise localization of attended stimuli requires the small receptive fields in the earliest layers of the hierarchy. Thus, the AC requires access to both the highest and the lowest levels of representation. Task instructions seem to have a separate representation, and the AC would require links to any such representation (Corbetta and Shulman, chapter 1 in this volume).

**What connections does the AC need to receive this information?** Since it cannot be determined in advance where salient stimuli appear in the visual field, full connectivity from each neuron in each layer of the processing hierarchy seems necessary.

**What processing must AC perform in order to satisfy its goals?** In order to detect the most salient item in the visual field, it suffices to perform a winner-take-all operation on a representation of saliency (Koch and Ullman, 1985; Tsotsos et al., 1995). At present, it is unknown whether the neural representation of saliency is centralized or distributed, and whether there exists a neural substrate for a winner-take-all operation. However, a centralized saliency representation would appear to require far greater connectivity than is observed in visual cortex. A centralized AC would subsume such a representation and thus would face the same problem.

**How can the AC communicate its decisions to the visual processing hierarchy?** In order to channel information about the attended stimulus through the hierarchy, and to exclude information about unattended stimuli at each level, the AC must have feedback connections to each neuron in each layer of the processing hierarchy.

In the selective tuning model, additional circuitry for attentional control is inserted into the network of interpretive units (red and green parts of figure 14.4). This takes advantage of the locality of information and minimizes both synaptic distance and transmission time for the attentional information flow. Temporal synchronization is accomplished through the gating network (green parts of figure 14.4). Note that the temporal signals are oscillatory, in that they enable attentional feedback only once for each shift of attention. Spatial coordination is accomplished with the help of the top-down selection algorithm.

In the AC model, the same functionality is possible but the resulting architecture is far more expensive. It requires (1) an additional neural area, whose location is unknown at this point; (2) additional long connections to and from each neuron in the hierarchy; (3) an additional delay in moving information to and from the AC; and (4) an enormous convergence of connections in the saliency representation of the AC.

### 14.2.7   Evidence Bearing on the Centralized or Distributed Nature of Attentional Control

Centralized attentional control could, at least potentially, provide synchronized attentional modulation throughout the entire sensory hierarchy. Thus, attentional modulations in V1 and IT neurons would occur simultaneously. A different prediction follows from the distributed attentional control provided by the selective tuning model. In this case, attentional modulations would appear first at higher levels (e.g., IT) and only later at earlier levels (e.g., V1), and the latency would depend on the number of synapses between layers. Unfortunately, evidence on the latency of attentional modulation in different levels of the sensory hierarchy remains unclear. Luck and colleagues (1997) report that neurons in area V4 show attentional modulation about 75 ms after stimulus onset; under the same conditions, area V2 neurons show modulation after 100 ms. Roelfsema and colleagues (1998) observed an attentional latency in area V1 of 200 ms for a curve-tracing and saccade task. These data seem consistent with the selective tuning model of attentional control. In contrast, Chelazzi and colleagues (1993) report attentional modulation in area IT with a latency of about 200 ms, in a situation in which multiple stimuli were presented within a single receptive field. If it can be established that the latency of attentional modulation does not increase from higher to lower visual areas, then this would rule out the localized, distributed control of the selective tuning model. It should be noted there are feedback pathways from AIT to V1 with only one intermediate area, area V4 (figure 14.7), so that the timing differences need not be large.

### 14.3   Psychophysical Investigations

In this section, we psychophysically investigate how visual attention is distributed across visual space. We attempt to measure the *attentional field,* that is, how the degree of attention depends on visual location. This is of course a simplified view, and we are not interested in how attention varies over time or with visual segmentation.

The goal was to map the variation of the attentional field around a target and discriminate between the predictions of the traditional models and of the selective tuning model. Recent psychophysical and neurophysiological studies report evidence for an inhibitory zone surrounding the attended target, in seeming agreement with the model. In the experiments reported on by Bahcall and Kowler (1999), subjects were required to identify two target letters in a circular display of distractor letters. Contrary to the prediction of the traditional models of selective attention, it was observed that recognition performance actually improved with *increasing* spatial separation between the targets.

In a study by Caputo and Guerra (1998) the target, the distractor, and the nontarget elements were arranged in a circular display. Both the target and the distractor stood out from the rest of the display: the target popped out due to its form, and the distractor due to its color. Subjects had to discriminate the length of a longer line segment included in the target. The gist of the results was, once again, that discrimination performance improved with *increasing* distractor–target distance.

Evidence for this lateral inhibition type of effect comes also from neuroscience. Schall and Hanes (1993) recorded from neurons in the frontal eye fields (an area involved in generating intentional eye movements) of rhesus monkeys performing a visual search task. It was found that these neurons initially respond equally to both targets and distractors located in their receptive fields. However, whereas the neuronal response to the target continued until the saccade to the target, the response to the distractor was suppressed, and more so when the target was closer to the receptive field of the neuron.

### 14.3.1 Experiments

The principle of the experimental method was the following: direct the subjects' attention to a *reference* location in the visual field and concomitantly measure their ability to process visual information—the intensity of the attentional field—at different probe locations of equal retinal resolution. By systematically varying the reference–probe distance, one can determine the dependence of the attentional field on distance to the focus of attention.

The experimental requirements were threefold: (1) engaging visual attention—the classical L–T discrimination task was used, and discrimination accuracy was employed as performance measure; (2) directing the attention of the subject to one prespecified reference target location—we resorted to precueing; (3) ensuring equal retinal resolution for all stimuli—we used a circular array display with fixation point in the center.

A typical experimental sequence, shown in figure 14.8, consisted (from bottom to top) of cue image, test image, and mask. The cue, a light gray disk, anticipated the position of the reference target in the following test image. This will be referred to as the peripheral cue condition. It was shown for 180 ms, which is within the time range of effective cueing.

The stimulus set in the test image consisted of six randomly oriented Ls and six randomly oriented Ts, arranged randomly in a ring. The characters were evenly spaced, and were overlaid on light gray disks, as shown in figure 14.8, middle panel. Two of the characters, the reference target and the probe target, were red (bold type in figure 14.8); the rest, the distractors, were black. The orientation of the imaginary line joining the two targets was randomly changed from trial to trial. The radius of the ring was 4° and character size was 0.6° of visual angle.

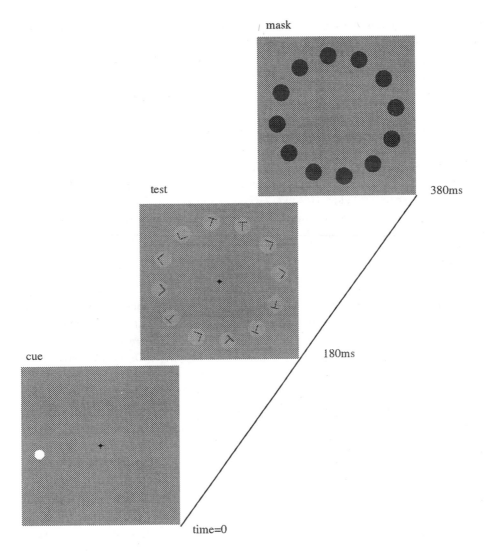

**Figure 14.8**
Peripheral cue condition, experimental trial sequence. (*A*) The cue, a light gray disk, indicated the position of the reference target character in the following test screen. It was shown for 180 msec. (*B*) Test screen, shown for 200 msec. The target characters were red (drawn in this figure with thick lines); the distractors were black. The task is to decide whether the two target characters are same or different. (*C*) Mask, shown until the subject responded.

The task of the subject was to decide whether the two red characters were identical or different, then to press one of two keys on the computer keyboard. After 200 ms the test image was replaced by a mask consisting of red disks positioned at the locations of the disks enclosing the L and T characters in the preceding test image. The role of the mask was to erase the iconic memory of the target letters in the test display. During the mask period the subjects made their response. To ensure that all characters in the ring were perceived at same resolution, the subjects were instructed always to fixate on a cross at the center of the ring.

The main variable of interest in this experiment was intertarget separation, which took on values between 1 (nearest-neighbor targets) and 6 (diametrically opposite targets). Each of the six intertarget separations was tested four times with identical, and four times with different, targets. Thus, each subject performed a total of forty-eight trials.

To demonstrate the effectiveness of the peripheral cue, we also studied a control condition in which the fixation cross was cued by changing its color 180 ms prior to target and distractor onset (central cue condition). Except for the type of cue, the display sequence was identical to the peripheral cue condition. The central cue provided no spatial information about the upcoming target.

### 14.3.2   Results

Eight subjects performed both peripheral and central cue experiments, and their data were pooled. Performance was analyzed in terms of the relative position of targets, specifically, the intertarget separation and the orientation of the imaginary line from reference to probe target. Possible orientations ranged from $-180°$ to $180°$ and were binned into intervals 45° wide. All trials of all subjects with a given intertarget separation and orientation bin were pooled, and the average performance (accuracy) was computed. For each separation, mean and standard deviation of accuracy were computed by averaging over different orientations. For each orientation, mean and standard deviation of accuracy were determined by averaging over different separations.

**Dependence on intertarget separation.**   In the peripheral cue condition, average accuracy was 0.60 in "same" trials and 0.66 in "different" trials (figure 14.9B). In the central cue condition, average accuracy was slightly lower, with values of 0.50 in same trials and 0.55 in different trials (figure 14.9A). The error rate plots also show that in the peripheral cue condition, accuracy increases with the intertarget separation (ANOVA: $F = 4.5$, $p < 0.01$). This is consistent with the results of Bahcall and Kowler (1999) but directly contradicts the predictions of a spotlight model. In the central cue condition, accuracy does not depend significantly on intertarget separation. Because peripheral and central cue conditions were identical except for the cue, the difference in performance represents a genuine attention effect.

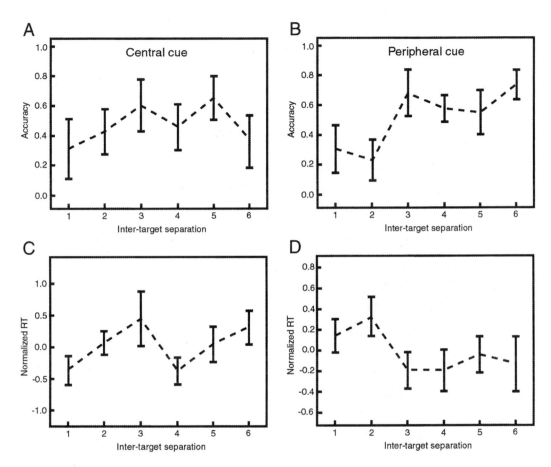

**Figure 14.9**
Dependence of accuracy on intertarget separation. Abscissa: distance between the two targets. Ordinate: mean accuracy; standard deviations correspond to different orientation values. (*B*) Peripheral cue condition; there is a significant improvement in accuracy beyond an intertarget separation of 2 for this set of targets and cues. (*A*) Central cue (control) condition; subjects are cued to the fixation point. There are no significant performance differences with changes in separation. Response time vs. intertarget separation. (*C*) The control condition. There is no significant difference of response time as a function of separation when the subjects are cued to the fixation point. (*D*) The peripheral cue condition. Subjects spend more time on smaller intertarget separations and still are not as accurate as for large separations.

In addition to the effect on accuracy, intertarget separation affects response times (figures 14.9C, D). In the peripheral cue conditions, response times increase as accuracy decreases, demonstrating that there is a true loss of performance, rather than merely an altered speed–accuracy trade-off.

**Dependence on intertarget orientation.** We analyzed the effect of intertarget orientation because we considered this to be a potential confound for the effect of intertarget separation. Also, in preliminary experiments we found that performance peaked near zero orientation (i.e., same elevation). Reassuringly, the present data showed no significant effect of intertarget orientation under either the peripheral or the central cue condition.

### 14.3.3 Discussion

These results can be interpreted as follows. A peripheral cue directs attention to the reference target, and the inhibitory surround of the attention field impedes the discrimination of nearby probe targets, but not of probe targets at greater distances. In contrast to the experiments of Bahcall and Kowler (1999) and Caputo and Guerra (1998), the focus of attention in each trial is known. Future experiments will test the effect of cue size on the attentional field, and will try to provide a more accurate measure of the size of the inhibitory surround with finer spacing of probe locations.

### 14.4 Conclusions

There are at least two strategies for modeling biological information processing. The most common approach is to develop a mathematical framework (in its simplest form, fitting curves to sets of data) that can account for experimental data (the data-fitting approach). Such models may provide some predictive power for experiments of the same type. The second strategy is to develop a model from first principles of information processing, without direct incorporation of any particular data sets (the first-principles approach). If the model is defined appropriately, it is possible to have the same explanatory power as the data-fitting approach, and there are also at least two other major benefits. For vision, the data-fitting approach does not directly lead to an algorithm that can take images as input and produce the measurements being modeled, whereas the first-principles approach does. Thus, in a very real sense, data-fitting solves only a part of the problem of understanding the nature of information processing that leads to the data. Second, the first-principles approach has much broader predictive power because it makes no early commitment to a particular experimental paradigm, a necessary ingredient of the data-fitting approach.

The selective tuning model was derived in a first-principles fashion. The major contributor to those principles derives from a series of formal analyses performed within the theory of computational complexity, the most appropriate theoretical foundation to address the question Why is attention necessary for perception? The model displays performance compatible with experimental observations, and does so in a self-contained manner. That is, input to the model is a set of real, digitized images and not preprocessed data. The predictive power of the model seems broad.

• An early prediction (Tsotsos, 1990) was that attention seems necessary at any level of processing where a many-to-one mapping of neurons is found. Further, attention occurs in all the areas in concert. The prediction was made at a time when good evidence for attentional modulation was known for area V4 only (Moran and Desimone, 1985). Since then, attentional modulation has been found in many other areas, both earlier and later in the visual processing stream, and it occurs in these areas simultaneously (Kastner et al., 1998). Vanduffel and colleagues (2000) have shown that attentional modulation appears as early as the LGN. The prediction that attention modulates all cortical, and perhaps even subcortical, levels of processing has been borne out by recent work from several groups (e.g., Brefczynski and DeYoe, 1999; Gandhi et al., 1999; Vauduffel et al., 2000).

• The notions of competition between stimuli and of attentional modulation of this competition were also early components of the model (Tsotsos, 1990); these, too, have gained substantial support over the years (Desimone and Duncan, 1995; Kastner et al., 1998; Reynolds et al., 1999).

• The model predicts an inhibitory surround that impairs perception around the focus of attention (Tsotsos, 1990). This, too, has recently gained support (Caputo and Guerra, 1998; Bahcall and Kowler, 1999; Vanduffel et al., 2000).

• The model further implies that preattentive and attentive visual processing occur in the same neural substrate, which contrasts with the traditional view that these are wholly independent mechanisms. This point of view has been gaining ground recently (Joseph et al., 1997; Yeshurun and Carrasco, 1999; Braun et al., chapter 11 in this volume).

• A final prediction is that attentional guidance and control are integrated into the visual processing hierarchy, rather than being centralized in some external brain structure. This implies that the latency of attentional modulations *decreases* from lower to higher visual areas, and constitutes one of the strongest predictions of the model.

Additional predictions of the selective tuning model are the spatial and temporal modulations of visual cortical responses around the focus of attention (figure 14.3), and the existence of a WTA circuit connecting cortical columns of similar tuning (figure 14.5). The selective tuning model offers a principled solution to the fundamental problems of visual complexity, a detailed perceptual account of both the guidance and the consequences of visual attention, and a neurally plausible implementation as an integral part of the visual cortical hierarchy. Thus, the model "works" at three distinct levels—computational, perceptual, and neural—and offers a more concrete account, and far more specific predictions, than previous models limited to one of these levels. We are working to extend the model in several directions, and are particularly interested in seeing how its architecture might map onto the actual neural circuitry of visual cortex.

## Note

1. We thank Dan Felleman for sharing the software used to create the original figures for Felleman and Van Essen (1991).

## References

Bahcall, D., and Kowler, E. (1999). Attentional interference at small spatial separations. *Vis. Res.* 39: 71–86.

Brefczynski, J. A., and DeYoe, E. A. (1999). A physiological correlate of the "spotlight" of visual attention. *Nat. Neurosci.* 2: 370–374.

Britten, K. (1996). Attention is everywhere. *Nature* 382: 497–498.

Callaway, E. (1998). Local circuits in primary visual cortex of the macaque monkey. *Ann. Rev. Neurosci.* 21: 47–74.

Caputo, G., and Guerra, S. (1998). Attentional selection by distractor suppression, *Vis. Res.* 38: 669–689.

Chelazzi, L., Miller, E. K., Duncan, J., and Desimone, R. (1993). A neural basis for visual search in inferior temporal cortex. *Nature* 363: 345–347.

Crick, F. (1984). Function of the thalamic reticular complex: The Searchlight Hypothesis. *Proc. Nat. Acad. Sci. USA* 81: 4586–4590.

Desimone, R. (1990). Complexity at the neuronal level. *Behav. Brain Sci.* 13: 446.

Desimone, R., and Duncan, J. (1995). Neural mechanisms of selective attention. *Ann. Rev. Neurosci.* 18: 193–222.

Felleman, D., and Van Essen, D. (1991). Distributed hierarchical processing in the primate visual cortex. *Cereb. Cortex* 1: 1–47.

Gandhi, S. P., Heeger, D. J., and Boynton, G. M. (1999). Spatial attention affects brain activity in human primary visual cortex. *Proc. Natl. Acad. Sci. USA* 96: 3314–3319.

He, S., Cavanagh, P., and Intriligator, J. (1996). Attentional resolution and the locus of visual awareness. *Nature* 83: 334–337.

Joseph, J. S., Chun, M. M., and Nakayama, K. (1997). Attentional requirements in a "preattentive" feature search task. *Nature* 387: 805–807.

Kastner, S., De Weerd, P., Desimone, R., and Ungerleider, L. G. (1998). Mechanisms of directed attention in the human extrastriate cortex as revealed by functional MRI. *Science* 282: 108–111.

Koch, C., and Ullman, S. (1985). Shifts in selective visual attention: Towards the underlying neural circuitry. *Hum. Neurobiol.* 4: 219–227.

Luck, S. J., Chelazzi, L., Hillyard, S. A., and Desimone, R. (1997). Neural mechanisms of spatial selective attention in areas V1, V2, and V4 of macaque visual cortex. *J. Neurophysiol.* 77: 24–42.

Maunsell, J., and Ferrera, V. (1995). Attentional mechanisms in visual cortex. In M. Gazzaniga (ed.), *The cognitive neurosciences* (pp. 451–461). Cambridge, MA: MIT Press.

Milner, P. (1974). A model for visual shape recognition. *Psychol. Rev.* 81: 521–535.

Moran, J., and Desimone, R. (1985). Selective attention gates visual processing in the extrastriate cortex. *Science* 229: 782–784.

Motter, B. C. (1993). Focal attention produces spatially selective processing in visual cortical areas V1, V2, and V4 in the presence of competing stimuli. *J. Neurophysiol.* 70: 909–919.

Olshausen, B. A., Anderson, C. H., and Van Essen, D. C. (1993). A neurobiological model of visual attention and invariant pattern recognition based on dynamic routing of information. *J. Neurosci.* 13: 4700–4719.

Reynolds, J. H., Chelazzi, L., and Desimone, R. (1999). Competitive mechanisms subserve attention in macaque areas V2 and V4. *J. Neurosci.* 19(5): 1736–1753.

Roelfsema, P. R., Lamme, V. A., and Spekreijse, H. (1998). Object-based attention in the primary visual cortex of the macaque monkey. *Nature* 395: 376–381.

Salin, P.-A., and Bullier, J. (1995). Corticocortical connections in the visual system: Structure and function. *Physiol. Rev.* 75(1): 107–154.

Schall, J., and Hanes, D. (1993). Neural basis of saccade target selection in frontal eye field during visual search. *Nature* 366: 467–469.

Treue, S., and Maunsell, J. H. R. (1996). Attentional modulation of visual motion processing in cortical areas MT and MST. *Nature* 382: 539–541.

Tsotsos, J. K. (1989). The complexity of perceptual search tasks. *Proc. Int. Joint Conf. Artif. Intell.*, Detroit, August, pp. 1571–1577.

Tsotsos, J. K. (1990). A complexity level analysis of vision. *Behav. Brain Sci.* 13(3): 423–455.

Tsotsos, J. K. (1993). An inhibitory beam for attentional selection. In Harris and Jenkin (eds.), *Spatial vision in humans and robots* (pp. 313–331). Cambridge, UK: Cambridge University Press.

Tsotsos, J. K. (1997). Limited capacity is a sufficient reason for attentive behavior. *Cog. Conscious.* 6: 429–436.

Tsotsos, J. K., Culhane, S. M., Wai, W. Y., Lai, Y., Davis, N., and Nuflo, F. (1995). Modeling visual attention via selective tuning, *Art. Intell.* 78: 507–545.

Valiant, L. (1975). Parallelism in comparison problems. *SIAM J. Comput.* 4(3): 348–355.

Vanduffel, W., Tootell, R., and Orban, G. (2000). Attention-dependent suppression of metabolic activity in the early stages of the macaque visual system. *Cereb. Cortex* 10: 109–126.

Van Essen, D., Anderson, C., and Felleman, D. (1992). Information processing in the primate visual system: An integrated systems perspective. *Science* 255: 419–422.

Yeshurun, Y., and Carrasco, M. (1999). Spatial attention improves performance in spatial resolution tasks. *Vis. Res.* 39: 293–306.

# Contributors

**Narcisse P. Bichot**
Laboratory of Neuropsychology
National Institute of Mental Health
Bethesda, Maryland

**Erik Blaser**
Department of Cognitive Science
Rutgers University
New Brunswick, New Jersey

**Geoffrey M. Boynton**
The Salk Institute for Biological Studies
Systems Neurobiology Laboratories
La Jolla, California

**Jochen Braun**
Institute of Neuroscience
and School of Computing
University of Plymouth
Plymouth, Devon, UK

**Maurizio Corbetta**
Departments of Neurology, Radiology,
Anatomy, and Neurobiology
Washington University School
of Medicine
St. Louis, Missouri

**Sean M. Culhane**
Department of Computer Science
University of Toronto
Toronto, Canada

**Florin Cutzu**
Centre for Vision Research
York University
Toronto, Canada

**Sophie Deneve**
Department of Brain and Cognitive
Sciences
University of Rochester
Rochester, New York

**Robert Desimone**
Laboratory of Neuropsychology
National Institute of Mental Health
Bethesda, Maryland

**John Duncan**
MRC Cognition and Brain Sciences Unit
Cambridge, UK

**Sunil P. Gandhi**
Department of Psychology
Stanford University
Stanford, California

**Charles D. Gilbert**
The Rockefeller University
New York, New York

**David J. Heeger**
Department of Psychology
Stanford University
Stanford, California

**James W. Holsapple**
Veterans Affairs Medical Center
and Department of Neurosurgery
State University of New York—
Health Science Center
Syracuse, New York

**Alexander C. Huk**
Department of Psychology
Stanford University
Stanford, California

**Minami Ito**
The Rockefeller University
New York, New York

**Laurent Itti**
Department of Computer Science
University of Southern California
Los Angeles, California

**Christof Koch**
California Institute of Technology
Computation and Neural Systems
Pasadena, California

**Peter E. Latham**
Department of Neurobiology
University of California
at Los Angeles
Los Angeles, California

**Nilli Lavie**
Department of Psychology
University College London
London, UK

**D. Kathleen Lee**
California Institute of Technology
Computation and Neural Systems
Pasadena, California

**Zhong-Lin Lu**
Department of Psychology
and Program in Neural, Informational,
and Behavioral Sciences
University of Southern California
Los Angeles, California

**John H. R. Maunsell**
Howard Hughes Medical Institute
Division of Neuroscience
Baylor College of Medicine
Houston, Texas

**Carrie J. McAdams**
Division of Neuroscience
Baylor College of Medicine
Houston, Texas

**Brad C. Motter**
Veterans Affairs Medical Center
and Department of Neurosurgery
State University of New York—
Health Science Center
Syracuse, New York

**Alexandre Pouget**
Department of Brain and Cognitive
Sciences
University of Rochester
Rochester, New York

**Adam Reeves**
Department of Psychology
Northeastern University
Boston, Massachusetts

**John H. Reynolds**
The Salk Institute for Biological Studies
Systems Neurobiology Laboratories
La Jolla, California

**Jeffrey D. Schall**
Vanderbilt Vision Research Center
Department of Psychology

Vanderbilt University
Nashville, Tennessee

**Christian Scheier**
California Institute of Technology
Computation and Neural Systems
Pasadena, California

**Shinsuke Shimojo**
California Institute of Technology
Computation and Neural Systems
Pasadena, California

**Gordon L. Shulman**
Departments of Neurology, Radiology,
Anatomy, and Neurobiology
Washington University School of Medicine
St. Louis, Missouri

**George Sperling**
Departments of Cognitive Sciences,
and of Neurobiology and Behavior
University of California, Irvine
Irvine, California

**Kirk G. Thompson**
Laboratory for Sensorimotor Research
National Eye Institute
Bethesda, Maryland

**John K. Tsotsos**
Centre for Vision Research
York University
Toronto, Canada

**Katsumi Watanabe**
California Institute of Technology
Computation and Neural Systems
Pasadena, California

**Erich Weichselgartner**
ZPID Institute for Psychology
Trier University
Trier, Germany

**Gerald Westheimer**
The Rockefeller University
New York, New York

# Index